ON

SLIGHT AILMENTS:

THEIR

NATURE AND TREATMENT.

☞ Based on Recent Medical Literature.

GOULD'S MEDICAL DICTIONARIES.

BY GEORGE M. GOULD, A.M., M.D.,

Ophthalmic Surgeon to the Philadelphia Hospital, Editor of "The Medical News."

THE STANDARD MEDICAL REFERENCE BOOKS.

THE ILLUSTRATED DICTIONARY OF MEDICINE, BIOLOGY, AND ALLIED SCIENCES. Being an Exhaustive Lexicon of Medicine and those Sciences Collateral to it: Biology (Zoölogy and Botany), Chemistry, Dentistry, Pharmacology, Microscopy, etc. Including Pronunciation, Accentuation, Derivation, and Definition of all Words. With many Useful Tables and numerous Fine Illustrations. Large, Square 8vo, 1633 pages. Full Sheep, or Half Morocco, *net*, $10.00; Half Russia, Thumb Index, *net*, $12.00.

THE STUDENT'S DICTIONARY. Including all the Words and Phrases generally used in Medicine, with their proper Pronunciation and Definitions. With Tables of the Bacilli, Micrococci, Leucomains, Ptomains, etc., of the Arteries, Muscles, Nerves, Ganglia, and Plexuses; Mineral Springs of the U. S.; Vital Statistics, etc. Small Octavo, 520 pages. Half Dark Leather, $3 25; Half Morocco, Thumb Index, $4.25.

THE POCKET PRONOUNCING MEDICAL LEXICON. (12,000 Medical Words Pronounced and Defined.) Containing all the Words, their Definition and Pronunciation, that the Student generally comes in contact with; also elaborate Tables and a Dose List in English and Metric System, etc. 317 pages. Full Limp Leather, Gilt Edges, $1.00; Thumb Index, $1.25.

These books may be ordered through any bookseller, or upon receipt of price the publishers will deliver free to the purchaser's address. *Full descriptive circulars and sample pages sent free upon application.*

P. BLAKISTON, SON & CO., Publishers, Philad'a.

35,000 COPIES HAVE BEEN SOLD.

ON

SLIGHT AILMENTS:

THEIR

NATURE AND TREATMENT.

BY

LIONEL S. BEALE, M.B., F.R.S.,

FELLOW OF THE ROYAL COLLEGE OF PHYSICIANS; PROFESSOR OF THE PRINCIPLES AND PRACTICE OF
MEDICINE IN KING'S COLLEGE, LONDON, AND PHYSICIAN TO KING'S COLLEGE HOSPITAL;
LATELY PROFESSOR OF PATHOLOGICAL ANATOMY, AND FORMERLY PROFESSOR OF
PHYSIOLOGY AND OF GENERAL AND MORBID ANATOMY IN KING'S COLLEGE.

SECOND EDITION,

ENLARGED AND ILLUSTRATED.

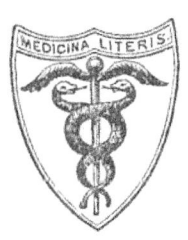

PHILADELPHIA:

P. BLAKISTON, SON & CO.,

No. 1012 WALNUT STREET.

1895.

PUBLISHERS' NOTICE.—This new revised edition of Dr. Beale's "Slight Ailments" is published simultaneously with the London Edition, by special arrangement between Dr. Beale and P. Blakiston, Son and Co. It is, therefore, the only authorized edition, and contains all the Additions, Illustrations, and a complete Index, as in the London Edition.

TABLE OF CONTENTS.

Introductory.

Slight ailments and civilization; Interest in the patient; Attention and kindness; Tact and treatment; Quackery and tact; Humbug; Vulgarity; Decillionths of grains; Credulity and imposition; Imposture and nonsense; Principles of conduct; Studying slight ailments; Self-supporting dispensaries; Remedies in slight ailments; Knowledge derived from microscopical observation; Intermolecular circulation.. 17–41

Of the Tongue in Health and in Slight Ailments.

Characters in health; The dorsum of the tongue; Fungiform and filiform papillæ and their covering; Epithelial cells; Fungi and low organisms in the mouth; Bacteria; Tongue in various derangements; Importance of secretion; Dry and moist states of the tongue; Exciting the flow of saliva; White moist furred tongue; Bright red tongue; Dry brown tongue; Hæmorrhage; Cracks and fissures; Changes in the mucous membrane of mouth and fauces; Inhalers, bronchitis kettle; Of the use of spray; Metallic and other tastes in the mouth; Aphthæ, thrush, sores, and ulcers in the mouth; Treatment of aphthæ; Offensive breath; Use of purgatives; Use of mercury... 41–75

Appetite—Nausea—Thirst—Hunger.

Impaired appetite; Loss of appetite; Voracious appetite, bulimia; Nausea; Treatment of nausea; Objections to alcohol; Thirst............................. 75–84

Indigestion: Its Nature and Treatment.

Indigestion, dyspepsia; Nerve-fibres of intestinal canal; Nerve-ganglia and plexuses; Gastrodynia; Heartburn, pyrosis, or waterbrash; Flatulence, wind in the stomach; Treatment of ordinary forms of indigestion; Of condiments; Influence of cold; Indigestion from failing glands, as in old age; Of pepsine and its uses Method of preparing pepsine.. 84–111

Of Constipation.

Importance of regular action of bowels; Impaction of fæcal matter in large intestine; Influence of the reabsorption of fluid in causing constipation; Hæmorrhoids or piles.. 111–122

Treatment of Constipation.

Of the action of enemata; Hygienic and dietetic treatment of constipation; Exercise, cold-bath, rubbing, moist applications, etc.; Diet; Of taking fluid; Smoking tobacco; Of purgatives in constipation; Drastic and hydragogue purgatives; Saline purgatives; Friedrichshall and other waters...................... 123–144

2   xiii

Diarrhœa.

Ordinary diarrhœa; Nature and causes of diarrhœa; Treatment of diar-
rhœa... 144–152

Intestinal Worms.

Threadworms; Large round worm; Remedies to be used.................. 152–154

Vertigo—Giddiness.

Vertigo, swimming in the head; Causes; Aural vertigo, treatment, etc... 154–157

Biliousness—Sick Headache.

Biliousness; Derangement of the liver; Treatment of biliousness; Action of
east wind; Jaundice; Yellow atrophy; Sick headache; Treatment of sick headache; Treatment of sick headache during the attack; Starving; Treatment of
sick headache in the intervals between the attacks; Of the management of sick
headache when the patient continues at work; Drowsiness; Wakefulness and
restlessness........ 157–186

Neuralgia—Rheumatism.

Nervousness; Neuralgia; Treatment of neuralgia; Rheumatic pains; Treatment of rheumatism; Free sweating; Diet in rheumatism; Warm clothing. 187–202

On the Feverish and Inflammatory State.

Of catching cold; Preliminary changes and attendant phenomena; Rise in the
body-heat in all fevers and inflammations; Is there increased oxidation in fever
and inflammation? Method of ascertaining the temperature of the body; Fever,
rigors, hot stage, sweating stage; Of free secretion leading to recovery; Principles of treatment of a cold; Management of affections beginning like a cold. 202–219

Of the Actual Changes in Fever and Inflammation.

Phenomena of fever and inflammation; Of a flea-bite; Alterations of calibre
of small arteries; Influence of nerves in determining the degree of contraction;
Of the ganglia governing the calibre of small arteries; Nerves to capillary vessels; Demonstrating the nerves distributed to capillaries; Mechanism by which
the capillary circulation of man and animals is regulated; General vascular disturbance resulting from local injury; The formation of pus in and near the capillaries in inflammation and fever; The passage of blood and living particles
through the walls of capillary vessels, Diapedesis; Hæmorrhage; Spontaneous
movement; Vital phenomena. 219–248

Common Forms of Slight Inflammation.

Formation of mucus, mucus corpuscle; Bioplasm of mucus; Dryness of the
mucous membrane; impaired sensibility; counter-action; counter-irritation;
Cracks and fissures about the lips; Principles of treatment; Conjunctiva, inflammation of; Treatment of inflamed eyes; Sore throat; treatment of sore throat;
Gargles; Running from the ears; Inflammation of stomach and intestinal canal;
Chilblains; Treatment; Boils; Carbuncle; Changes preparatory to the occurrence of disease; Concluding remarks... 248–276

Index 277

CORRIGENDIUM.

On page 202, between the second and third paragraphs, the follow ing heading has been inadvertently omitted:

ON THE FEVERISH AND INFLAMMATORY STATE.

SLIGHT AILMENTS:

NATURE AND TREATMENT.

INTRODUCTORY.

EACH one of us has, no doubt, suffered at times from slight derange ments of the health—derangements which are not dependent upon or likely to determine structural change in any tissue or organ in the body —due to temporary disturbance, to an alteration in the functional activity of tissues and organs, which may be soon succeeded by a return to the healthy state. In many instances the derangement depends upon the altered rate at which normal phenomena are performed. Perhaps, in consequence of changes in the blood itself or in the tissues outside the vessels, the blood flows too slowly or too quickly through the capillaries. These tubes often become unduly distended or relaxed. Disturbed action in the adjacent nerve-fibres is thereby occasioned, and pain or discomfort is in consequence experienced.

Among civilized nations a perfectly healthy individual seems to be the exception rather than the rule. I do not remember having seen more than two or three men in the course of my life who had never experienced any form of illness, and did not know what it was to feel out of sorts. It is indeed very rarely one meets with any one who has reached the age of thirty who will not admit that at various times he has suffered from many different, though slight, derangements of health. We are indeed often told by persons, whose prospects of longevity are nevertheless good, that they have scarcely passed a week without the occurrence of a very decided departure from the healthy state. The most healthy among us occasionally feel unwell and are less up to work than is usual. Some complain of feeling fatigued, others tell you they are uncomfortable, or complain of being irritable and annoyed at slight troubles, which would not ruffle them in the least if they were in ordinary health. How few of those who take a very active part in the work of the world know what it is to enjoy uninterrupted health ! Most have to work on in spite of lassitude, or headache, or muscular or nerve pains, or indigestion, or some other discomfort which continually troubles them. How many of us experience a confused feeling, an indisposition to mental exertion, a distinct sense of fatigue after what we cannot but regard as very moderate mental application ! Many people take dismal so-called constitutional walks, not because they enjoy the exercise or from necessity, but because they have heard that this sort of penal servitude —walking for walking's sake—is necessary to keep themselves in a condition which some call health. Many a man thus imposes upon himself the regular performance of the most dreary form of task-work, and forces himself to go through his monotonous labors when his inclination would lead him to take rest and probably to go to sleep. In many instances the inclination would have the support of the reason.

Some, again, who are considered to be in perfect health, scarcely know what it is to sleep soundly and rise refreshed, with spirits buoyant, energetic, with a desire for work. Men and women there are, and in every class of society, poor as well as rich, hardworking as well as idle, who scarcely ever eat without discomfort, and suffer still more if they do not take their usual meal. Few, indeed, of those who live in cities pass through life without being troubled with various derangements connected with the action of the stomach and intestinal canal.

You will, of course, desire to know whether all these disturbances are necessary consequences of our civilization—of our somewhat artificial mode of living—or whether by altering our habits we could acquire and maintain a state of perfect health. Unquestionably not a few suffer because they are ignorant of the proper way of managing themselves in order that they may work most advantageously, or because they give way to habits of self-indulgence as regards the quantity and character of their food and drink. Many probably, from inherited weakness of various organs, would suffer more or less under any circumstances, and it is our duty to study the many ordinary slight ailments, in order that we may be able to mitigate the sufferings of our patients, if we cannot make them strong and vigorous. In this direction there is much to be done, and I cannot help thinking that of late years, in our zeal for pathological discovery, we have devoted less attention to functional disturbance than for the interests of the community might reasonably be looked for from us, and for the interests of true medicine might be expected.

What is the meaning of these slight, but perhaps very frequent, disturbances or derangements of the changes which take place in an organism whose tissues are in a perfectly normal state ? When any departure from the healthy state occurs, it is obvious that the processes by which the equilibrium of physiological action is preserved are temporarily deranged and out of order. An unusual or exceptional change—increased or diminished ordinary action—results. In many instances some time must elapse before the exceptional gives place to the ordinary activity, and by slight excess of action in one or other direction the balance is restored.

A little too much food, or food of a bad kind, or badly cooked, or food eaten at the wrong time, or too quickly—a glass of bad wine, bad milk, or bad water, to say nothing of a dry east wind, or a cold damp atmosphere, has occasioned such disturbance in the normal changes in the body, as to cause even the strongest and exceptionally healthy to feel for a time far from well. Every generation has thus suffered, and we have not yet discovered exactly how a healthy person should proceed so as to keep every organ and every tissue in his body in a perfectly healthy state under the necessarily varying conditions to which it is exposed, so that each may continue to act for the longest possible time, and all gradually fail together in old age, until at last action ceases in natural and inevitable death.

As it is our particular work in life to reduce disease and suffering to the utmost extent that is possible, it is undoubtedly our duty to carefully study and investigate, as far as we are able to do so, the nature of such slight aches, pains, discomforts, and derangements from which nearly all suffer. Not a few people magnify their slight ailments, but, on the other hand, some persons are no doubt inclined to under-estimate the importance of, or to ignore altogether, aches, pains, and disturbances, the early recognition of which might be of great advantage, by enabling the doctor to interfere at once, and perhaps prevent serious illness, or even save that particular life.

You will certainly be very frequently called upon to prescribe for slight ailments, and you will often be asked how this and that bodily derangement or discomfort may be avoided, upon what it depends, and whether it is not indicative of some change more serious than mere temporary disturbance of ordinary action. You will be expected to fully explain how many a slight ache or pain is caused, and you will often be asked to lay down rules of health, by the practice of which it may be avoided in the future. Very disappointed will the sufferer feel if you make light of his suffering, and dismiss him with the suggestion that, being only functional derangement, it is of no consequence. A little study and intelligent observation among sick people will teach you not to be too off-hand in giving advice, and will suffice to impress upon you the fact that very grave symptoms and the most excruciating pain may result from temporary derangements of no real consequence, and that, on the other hand, the most terrible morbid changes in important organs may exist for years, and run their course without the patient being cognizant of any unusual symptoms, or conscious that anything in his organism had been going wrong.

I propose, then, that these lectures should be devoted to the consideration of the nature and treatment of slight ailments. Could we examine the tissues ever so minutely, it is doubtful whether we should discover the slightest departure from the healthy state. No structural change whatever is induced, and even in cases in which there is decided departure from the normal physiological action, and where considerable pain and distress may be experienced, the accumulation in the blood of some product that should be quickly eliminated,—a slightly altered state of the fluid that transudes through the capillary walls and bathes the tissue elements,—is probably all that would be found, and would indeed be quite sufficient to account for the symptoms.

In the course of our inquiry questions of the greatest interest will present themselves, and although the present state of our knowledge does not enable us to give a full and satisfactory explanation of all the phenomena, say, of an *Ordinary Cold* or a *Sick Headache*, I feel sure that a more full consideration of the slight disturbance of physiological actions which are continually occurring even in the healthiest among us, will assist us in understanding those more complex changes which occur in actual disease.

The plan I propose to adopt will not only enable me to bring under your notice thus early in my course some of the simplest and most common derangements you will be called upon to correct, but I shall be able to direct your attention to practical matters of great importance with regard to the action of remedies and methods of prescribing and administering many ordinary medicines—matters of greater importance than ever in these days, when so few among you enjoy the advantages formerly gained by apprenticeship, and become acquainted with the art and mystery of preparing drugs and compounding medicines and dispensing pills and potions.

I shall make use of very few learned terms, and when obliged to employ hard words shall give their exact meaning and derivation, and I shall try to describe the derangements I have to consider in the simplest manner possible. In case any of you should think I am too outspoken as regards the confessions I shall have to make of ignorance concerning the real nature of some of the simplest and most common of the slight ailments, I would only remark that, as there is so much real knowledge in medicine, and as the labors of our predecessors have established so many great truths and principles, we may surely freely admit that there are many things which we do not know, without fear of losing the confidence of the public. In my opinion, it is the very worst thing for the interest of true medicine when any of her followers act in such a way as to lead those who are completely ignorant of our work to suppose that we have acquired in some mysterious way knowledge that we cannot communicate to others, or that we have means of investigating disease which cannot be pursued or understood by ordinary mortals. We have no remedies of a secret nature, no occult arts of preparing or combining them so as to increase their virtues. All that we know can be learned by any one who chooses to spend the time and take the trouble requisite for mastering our art and the branches of science upon which it is based.

There is no doubt still manifest a slight tendency here and there to credit some of us with the possession of mysterious power to control disease, but there is no excuse for this. Whenever naturally self-reliant enthusiasts act as if they were really the fortunate and favored possessors of a power of detecting and controlling morbid processes that was not to be acquired by other men, the advance of medical truth will be retarded. In every age self-confidence has commanded faith and devotion, and with the aid of these the evolution of the extraordinary and marvellous from the ordinary and intelligible is not difficult. I should feel very sorry if in after days I should discover that any of my pupils have deviated from the right path, as some who have studied medicine had done, and had tried to make people believe they possessed powers and influences over disease which they did not possess. So terrible a falling away from the high standard raised by our predecessors and handed down to us would be a sad disgrace, and is most painful to contemplate.

Of the patients who come under our care, many will be the subjects of but slight ailments, with the general nature of which any well-educated and experienced practitioner would no doubt be well acquainted. But if you go into practice fresh from the wards and the pathological department, and at once undertake the treatment of sick people,—if you pass from the investigations of important structural changes to the practical consideration of functional disturbance, and especially if you look too exclusively from a purely scientific stand-point, you will meet with many things that will puzzle you. The patients you treat will not be satisfied, and you will be disappointed and annoyed, because they are not contented with the advice you give. Perhaps you will feel in consequence out of heart or thoroughly disgusted with practical professional work.

It has been said that the physician should be a consolation to the patient, but many a physician fresh from the study of severe forms of disease would, I fear, afford poor comfort to a dyspeptic, or to a person suffering, say, from functional nervous disturbance, and would hardly know what to say to a patient in whose body he could discover no actual

disease of tissues or organs.   The patient might describe many unpleasant and even alarming sensations and symptoms, which to him were of
course of grave consequence, and all the comfort that he could get from
such a medical adviser might be that, as there was no organic disease, he
might go away and bear his complaints as best he could.   Medical
advisers of purely anatomical and pathological habits of mind are certainly apt to disappoint or even offend unscientific patients, and, without
deserving it, gain for themselves the unenviable reputation of being
thoughtless and unkind—regardless of others' suffering, and, if not
objectionable, very far from agreeable ministers of relief.   People do
strongly object to follow the advice of such advisers, however correct it
may be ; and perhaps the least unfriendly among the patients of such a
doctor would, out of kindness and in the most quiet and confidential
way, recommend him as soon as possible to change his vocation.

You ought, therefore, to learn how to investigate the nature of
slight ailments and how to relieve them, and, if the conditions which
give rise to them are beyond our means of control, how to reduce the
severity of the patient's sufferings.   If the patient's malady is, unfortunately, ever so intractable or incurable, he will be much more grateful
to you for your attention, and for doing what you can to relieve him,
than he would be if you favored him with the most learned and
elaborate disquisition concerning his case, even if it was accompanied
with the demonstration that his illness was profoundly interesting and
afforded an exceptionally perfect illustration of very remarkable pathological phenomena.   You will generally find that if a man has pain in
his stomach, especially if accompanied with excruciating spasm, he will
not be satisfied with the assurance that he will be better when the wind
is dispersed.   However interested we may be in studying the natural
history of disease, the patient desires our assistance to disperse wind
that torments him, and wants remedies which will relieve his sufferings
as soon as possible.   I think you will agree in the opinion that such a
patient is not more unreasonable than most doctors themselves would
be under similar circumstances.   If you know your work, you can be of
use both in getting rid of the flatus and in relieving the pain.   If from
ignorance of the use of simple remedies you tell the patient that
nothing can be done, the chances are that he will go to some intelligent
person, professional or non-professional, who may, perhaps, give him a
dose of Bicarbonate of potash or some Sal volatile.   He is at once
relieved, gets well in the course of a few hours, and loudly praises the
adviser of the successful treatment.   On the other hand, anything but
praise in such a case would fall to your share.   I fear that the patient
would give you a very bad character, and he might possibly speak of you
as a most ignorant person and incompetent practitioner.   Though, perhaps, not acquainted with the great value of such simple, commonplace

things as Bicarbonate of potash and Sal volatile, and some other simple medicines which are very efficacious in curing various unpleasant aches and pains, you might nevertheless be well informed as regards the management of serious cases, and, in fact, a well-informed and good practitioner. Those of you who are going to take part in country practice ought to be especially careful to try to do all you can to please as well as to help your patients. There may be no other medical adviser within many miles, and it is most unfortunate if any of the people in your neighborhood should be prejudiced against you. You must, indeed, think over people's individual peculiarities, be ready to pardon their susceptibilities, and try your utmost not to offend them. The most painful differences have been occasioned from want of care on this head ; and many a coolness between patient and practitioner, which has lasted for years, and has caused much suffering and misery, might have been altogether avoided, if the practitioner had exhibited a little amiability and exercised ordinary caution and self-control early in his acquaintanceship. Not a few differences with patients may sometimes be traced to the practitioner's ignorance of common things he ought to know, or to an attempt upon his part to introduce new customs in dealing with his patients with which they are not familiar.

You will find some useful hints to guide you in country practice and much information on conducting different branches of practice in a very useful little book to those about to enter upon the practical duties of professional life, lately written by Dr. Diver, entitled *"The Young Doctor's Future ; or, What shall be my Practice?"*

But, further, the study of the slight ailments is of no small importance to medical men, for it is of the greatest consequence that we ourselves should be in good health. Attendants of the sick should themselves be well, and each one of us should recognize the importance of keeping himself in a healthy state, that he may be cheerful and hopeful in the presence of the sick. It never does for the doctor, while listening to the sorrows of his patients, to be continually reminded of his own discomforts, and constantly thinking, if he does not actually say, that he is far worse than his patient, and more worthy of attention, sympathy, and commiseration. The sufferer suffers less if he has healthy, cheerful people about him. Dwelling on the fact of pain, and talking about it, seems to increase it. Many patients suffering from temporary derangements are in a low, despondent state. Such a frame of mind is more commonly due to temporary deranged action of the stomach and liver than to any other circumstance. Though you may be equally or even more dyspeptic and may feel very wretched, you must be careful not to add to the general depression by discoursing about your own ailments, but must encourage and cheer the patient, and speak hopefully. All

this is not very easy to do if we are not well.   The doctor who is suffering aches and twinges is to be pitied, for he must not allow himself to
complain.   He must not make wry faces while he is inquiring into his
patient's case.   An ailing or hypochondriacal doctor will be of little
use, will get into discredit with patients, and will be disappointed with
himself; and it will probably happen that some, it may be, ill-informed,
but more worldly-minded medical authority in his neighborhood will
get the patients who ought to be in his more deserving hands.   This,
I fear, is not unfrequently the secret of many a failure in practice.

Those of you who, like many excellent men who have preceded you,
feel inclined to condemn the delicate attention, the excessive care, the
extreme solicitude for minute perturbations of sensation or emotion of
the invalid, characteristic of some very successful and favorite doctors,
should pause, and try to look a little from the patient's point of view.
Even a philosopher who feels ill, though he may be sure that there is
not much the matter with him, may nevertheless desire some skilled
and experienced medical adviser who will appreciate his aches and
pains, who will consider his complaint, and listen patiently to the story
of his woes, who will take a cheerful view of his case, and express himself accordingly, instead of suggesting possibilities of pathological
degeneration in the gloomiest phraseology.   You may be able to relieve
many a sufferer by suggesting some very simple remedy.   A dose of
bicarbonate of potash or lime-water after meals may be all that is
requisite to restore him to health.   Little may be needed, but still that
little assistance is required.

Many of the apparently slight disturbances or ailments may be due
to some grave pathological change, which would be entirely passed over
by one who had had little experience in medical observation, but would
be full of significance to the well-informed practitioner.   On the other
hand, we often find that apparently serious illness is really due to temporary and functional derangement only.   Do not, therefore, be too
hasty in giving an opinion concerning the import of uncertain and in-
definite symptoms.   You should remember that the most perfect
machines sometimes go wrong without a flaw being discoverable just
before the occurrence, it may be, of a complete breakdown.   No
wonder that the tissues and organs and the marvellously minute and
delicate structures of a living being may fail in a hundred ways without
giving any notice even to their owner.   The most careful scrutiny and
minute examination may fail to demonstrate any fault or flaw; nay,
even after the body had ceased to work, after its death, the changes
resulting in its destruction may elude the most careful investigation.
We know that, for example, hydrocyanic acid, by its action on the
nervous system, will kill a living organism in a few seconds, but as to
the exact changes which the acid works in the nerve structures and

their living particles, we know nothing. The same is true of many other modes of death. The flaws existing in tissues in disease are not always to be demonstrated, though possibly many at least may be demonstrable, if we only knew exactly how to render them evident and distinct.

Practitioners who will not endeavor to help their patients who are suffering from slight ailments had better not attempt to practise medicine at all, because they will almost certainly fail, seeing that a large percentage of our patients, fortunately for themselves, do not suffer from grave pathological changes. Nevertheless they require intelligent medical assistance. There is not one amongst us who gives his attention to those patients only who are suffering from very serious forms of disease. You must therefore understand the nature of slight derangements, and you must know how to relieve them. You must not treat the complaining patient with contempt, and tell him there is nothing of any consequence the matter, and that he may go about his business. If we behave in this manner the public will lose confidence in us, and great numbers of people will seek and accept advice from mere pretenders, and from wiseacres who profess to discover the most wonderful and exceptional phenomena in very ordinary cases, or who, while thus trying to gain the ear of the patient, make the most of every opportunity of casting a slur on those who have honestly studied and practised their profession. Knowing little or nothing of morbid changes, and of the sciences upon which the investigation and treatment of disease rests, many of these professing healers are, in a way, extremely clever, and not a few have the advantage of a marvellous development of that peculiar mental endowment called "tact"—a most desirable possession for every one who has to treat and take care of sick people, if, in addition, he is honest and good. I would have you take note, however, that this word "tact" has a very comprehensive and elastic meaning, and is in these days equally applied to an honest desire on the part of any one to avoid wounding the feelings of a sensitive person, or needlessly vexing such an one when it is necessary to communicate unpleasant things, and to the successful exercise of glaring imposture and pitiless humbug. One now and then gets, in a sense, an instructive, though a very painful and profitless lesson, as to the means by which the good opinion of people unlearned in medical and other matters may be gained by a practitioner who is sadly deficient in knowledge and in experience, and who is perfectly conscious of his defects, but knows well how to make up for them. A master of tact, and determined to avail himself of the advantage he thus possesses in the struggle for existence, he convinces, he persuades, and, in short, flourishes where many a good man would fail, and, perhaps, where many such have already failed. Nevertheless, do not let me lead you to conclude that

3

tact is another name for humbug, any more than that kindness and politeness imply insincerity; but it is only too true that some makers of fortunes have been indebted for their success to cunning, cuteness, and tact, rather than to hard work, goodness, or intellectual power ; and he who thinks very highly of tact, and acts upon his opinion, must be very careful lest he slide too far down the incline, which may lead him on from the display of tact to the habitual exercise of humbug, and at last to giving way to utter heartlessness and selfishness of the lowest order.

Unless the highly competent and intelligent practitioner exercise due care as regards what he says and what he leaves unsaid, he may entirely fail to gain the confidence of his patient.   Many a good, honest, and intelligent man unconsciously helps to drive the patient into bad hands. Grave pathological changes may be overlooked, and trifling aches and pains magnified by the patient into indications of serious and dangerous disease—from want of care and attention as regards the manner in which the practitioner expresses himself concerning aches and pains.

But there are persons who would be easily influenced by what the quack says, who would go away from the honest, well-informed medical practitioner, with the idea that he knew nothing whatever about his business, and was quite ignorant of the nature of the changes taking place in the organism, and of the method by which these changes might be modified when they were not properly performed.   This is unfortunate, but there is no help for it.   Every upright practitioner has been placed in this most unhappy position more than once in his life. Should you find yourselves so situated, the best thing is to say very little, and be as patient as possible, leaving matters to be set right by time.   While doing our utmost to preserve and extend the high repute always enjoyed by the medical profession, we must be careful not to play into the hands of pretenders, and this we shall certainly do if we needlessly offend fanciful and crotchety patients, for by thus acting we practically dismiss them to be preyed upon by quacks.

There are few matters of greater interest or consequence to us than the consideration of the manner by which we may succeed in gaining the confidence of our patients, without making promises which cannot be fulfilled, and, indeed, without saying anything of which an upright, intelligent, and high-minded gentleman of kindness and consideration could in the least degree feel ashamed.   Some men have the natural gift of inspiring confidence at once, just as others have unfortunately to contend with natural defects resulting in exciting in the minds of others anything but confidence.   Still you must bear in mind that he who is to afford real help to people as a medical adviser, must be trusted and believed in by his patients.   It is, therefore, our duty to study and train ourselves so that we may inspire confidence in those who place themselves under our care.   In this endeavor we are, so to say, often heavily weighted. To gain the esteem, especially of people unlearned in matters medical, it may, indeed, be necessary to promise more in the way of cure than truthfully a man of sound judgment would be able to do. We are often placed at a disadvantage, and a vulgar, ignorant pretender, brimful of assurance and conceit, will sometimes succeed in gaining the confidence even of an intelligent patient, when men of a higher order of mind have hopelessly failed. In not a few instances the patient pays most dearly for the mistake he has made, but it may be long before he finds out that he has made a mistake at all, and still longer before he confesses he has done so when he does find it out. It is the conceit rather than the ignorance of the dupe which renders him an easy victim of the quack.

On Quackery and Medical Humbug.—To those of us who have passed thirty years or more working and thinking amongst sick people, and studying with the aid of accurate scientific instruments the nature of the actual phenomena occurring in the tissue elements, and in the fluids of the body in departures from the healthy state, it seems as extraordinary as it is disappointing, that men of undoubted intelligence and well acquainted with the ways of the world, should sometimes select for their medical adviser, not only an ignoramus, but a medical pretender—an impudent fellow, who acts up to the conviction that if he only talks nonsense with sufficient audacity he will prevail, because even among highly educated people, it is very exceptional to meet with one who is sufficiently acquainted with anatomy, physiology, and chemistry to detect the true character of his insolent balderdash. But such complaint is not new. Galen ("Meth. Med.," l. i.) remarks in the time of the Roman Empire, "What gives vogue to a physician is not science, but skill in flattery. To him who is the best sycophant, everything becomes easy. To him every door is open. In a short time he becomes rich and powerful." "The asses of Thessalus had parcelled out the art of healing into the most minute subdivisions of practice. Rome swarmed with special curers. Some, for instance, confined their practice to the treatment of the uvula, or the eyelashes, or certain kinds of cutaneous eruptions. Some restricted their attention to the treatment of aged men, others to that of the strong and robust. Some would cure only with herbs, others by means of gymnastic exercises."

One would, however, have thought that certain people of intelligence and culture would have preferred as their medical attendant one whose position alone rendered it evident that he could not be a quack or an ignoramus, and at least take the very little trouble required to discover among the four or five hundred public medical officers, whose work and repute are known, or at least among the two or three thousand medical practitioners whose training and character are recognized, one adviser who would not only treat them with judgment and intelligence, but satisfy and please them in other ways.   Instead of taking the little trouble required, how often is the recommendation of some old woman, who declares she has been cured of the most serious and extraordinary maladies after the most distinguished members of the profession had completely failed, taken and acted upon without further inquiry.   It is quite extraordinary what large practices may be made in a short time by the puffing of influential people, not one of whom has perhaps taken the trouble to ascertain whether the practitioner so extolled is really deserving or not of the high praise and recommendation he has had the good luck to enjoy.

Sometimes it would appear that some extraordinary vulgarity of manner on the part of the fortunate doctor had been set down as indicating originality of mind or unusual genius.   The art of looking wise and saying nothing seems to be the secret of success in not a few instances.   Sometimes success in small talk, a bustling manner indicative of overwhelming business; while, occasionally, peculiarity or perfection of dress appears to have won the respect and confidence of patients, and secured to the elegant doctor a considerable practice.   You will not, however, feel astonished at all this if you consider how very ignorant of all subjects bearing in any way upon physiology and medicine are the generality even of so-called well-informed people. Not a few of the intellectual classes, the leaders of thought, great classics and mathematicians, lawyers, public speakers and writers, do not take the slightest interest in any department of natural knowledge, and are so incapable of entering into scientific modes of thought and work, that they can be deceived and cheated by the most commonplace pretender.   The efficacy of the thousandth, or millionth, or decillionth of a grain of charcoal is deemed by them a question open to inquiry and to be determined by experiment.   The utter suppression of experiments upon the lower animals seems to them but reasonable, magnanimous, and right.   The ignorance and prejudice fostered by the teaching and advice of persons wholly ignorant of science and by nature strongly opposed to all attempts to inquire into the nature of things, constitute the chief obstacles to sanitary improvement, and encourage the maintenance of conditions adverse to health and the perpetuation of diseases still annually destroying thousands, but which ought long ago to have become unknown in England.

It is easy for those who make light of the facts of medical and sanitary science, and who pretend to believe in the virtue of minute globules, to retort by accusing us of attempting to constitute ourselves into a sort of trades-union, which condemns all who do not fall in with its views. The writers in our public journals, however, ought to be able to see through such false charges and commonplace cries, and expose them. But to condemn as a trades-union a body of men engaged in the furtherance of the greatest of all blessings, the health of the community, is most unjust. Our profession encourages and rewards individual merit, and allows and sanctions individual success,—permits the freest competition between its members, limits neither the hours of work nor the freedom of thought,—encourages all to aspire to equal, and, if it may be, to excel the greatest of those whose lives and works are recorded in its annals,—endeavors to protect the unlearned and uninstructed from imposition and wrong, and refuses to sanction on the part of its members any secret method of healing, however useful it may be, or the use of any medicine the ingredients, composition, and method of producing which are not published to the world for the advantage of all. There is not the faintest justification for urging a complaint of the kind against the medical profession. Anything like what is called trades-unionism amongst us, if possible, is one of the most improbable of improbable eventualities.

We only insist that the real knowledge which has been handed down to us, and which is still being added to by the work of thousands of practitioners in all parts of the world, shall not be considered in any way comparable with or related to any so-called medical systems which are based upon the assumption that any effects result from the exhibition of quantities of various medicines supposed to amount to a millionth of a grain or less. We maintain that the dicta upon these and other medical matters received as true by a section of the public are opposed to facts of anatomy, physiology, and chemistry, to observation and experiments, by which, on the other hand, the principles upon which medicine is based are continually being tested and verified or modified.

To ascertain whether such a quantity as the decillionth of a grain acts in any way is impossible, any attempt to do so would be foolish, since no one can be sure that one-decillionth of a grain of anything in the world can be obtained. Such supposed fractional part is beyond the limits of physiological, chemical, or other method of investigation. It is invisible, intangible, undemonstrable, and as a medicine exists only in imagination, and can be proved by assertion only. In fact, it is not even possible to imagine particles of a degree of minuteness considerably less extreme than these. But it is useless to attempt to reason on such absurdities. I am ready to admit that there are persons who believe that the decillionth of a grain of opium will produce an effect upon man's organism, just as there are people who hold that the earth is flat, that living things are machines, that spontaneous generation occurs, that vaccination is detrimental, and a number of things which may have been conclusively proved or disproved, as the case may be, or concerning which there can be no evidence one way or the other, or which are altogether beyond the reach of thought.

In this country we are proud of what is called liberty of opinion, and

3 *

we cannot prevent our friends and neighbors from holding and propagating beliefs, views, and doctrines which from the stand-point of fact and reason may be inadmissible. Many of the questions upon which there is wide difference are really open to discussion, and where there is doubt all ought to keep their minds open to conviction if evidence should be adduced, but many assertions which are commonly and frequently advanced are not reasonable,—not open to discussion. The assertion, for example, that the decillionth of a grain of opium produces an effect on the human organism is one of these. Many years ago I saw in a hospital in the south of Europe a poor woman who was dying of cholera—was indeed obviously within an hour or two of death. The attending physician examined her and prescribed " Opium." I asked him what quantity of the drug he had ordered the patient to take, and after some calculation he said, " The decillionth of a grain." Now, I shall no doubt be considered by some who prescribe millionths and decillionths a very prejudiced person, but I decline to discuss with a man who believes, or professes to believe, either that he was actually giving this quantity of opium, or that such an imaginary amount of that drug would, if it could be introduced into the body, produce any effect whatever upon the organism

It would not be reasonable to expect that the public generally should be sufficiently informed concerning medical and scientific questions to enable them to form a judgment as to the relative merits of different systems of medical treatment, any more than we can expect them to investigate such questions as spiritualism or to determine the nature of, and right method of dealing with, certain forms of contagious disease. All thoughtful and reasonable professional men have, however, strong cause of complaint when they find that persons of intelligence holding positions of authority—law-makers, ministers, and distinguished political chiefs—so express themselves as to lead the public to suppose that it is as reasonable to place confidence in a man who prescribes the millionth of a grain of charcoal or the decillionth of a grain of opium as in one who orders ten or twenty grains of the first or a tenth of a grain of the last.*

I doubt whether anything in modern times is upon the whole more disgraceful to an enlightened community than the spread of a disease so certainly preventible as Small-Pox. Only think of the absurdity of having to provide, at enormous expense, accommodation for thousands of people suffering from and spreading this loathsome disease when every case might have been prevented by vaccination. And we go on year

---

* It is remarkable how very few persons seem to realize the tremendous difference between such fractional parts as hundredths, and thousandths, and millionths, billionths, and decillionths.

after year allowing people to pay fines for the privilege of enjoying the right to catch Small-Pox and to communicate it to others.

Intelligence as regards one department of knowledge is often associated with extraordinary ignorance and credulity concerning others; nay, the same individual sometimes manifests the extreme of scepticism as regards certain things, while in others he is unsurpassed for his credulity. You will find some persons sceptical concerning demonstrable and demonstrated facts, and faithful and believing in respect of fictions of the imagination and dicta of the most nonsensical character. The most profound knowledge of logic, mathematics, law, classics, or metaphysics will not protect a man from imposition and quackery as regards the nature and management of the ailments of his body, and there are not a few persons distinguished for great intellectual power who have been duped by quacks, while they altogether mistrusted the true statements of honest, straightforward medical practitioners. There is nothing more extraordinary than the trust often reposed in what is false, and the doubt, disbelief, and suspicion indicated concerning that which is true.

In the matter of medical advice, and not uncommonly in high quarters, humbug sometimes rules supreme. Character, experience, unremitting work often go for nothing. In England and in America there is nothing more wonderful than the great success obtained by persons utterly ignorant of their calling. There still lurks much belief in mysterious and inexplicable actions as regards medicines and in the wonder-working powers of some who prescribe them. This it is, possibly, which enables the self-praising, vulgar empiric to exert a favorable impression upon those who are at best but very ill-informed concerning matters of health and disease. It is curious how some even of our very simplest prescriptions get handed about from one to another in consequence of some wonder-working power they are supposed to possess, which would, I fear, vanish in a moment if only they were translated into English. Still we may hope that the time is not far distant when we may order Carbonate of soda, Hydrochloric acid, and such like simple medicines, which often afford the greatest relief, without enveloping them in a cloak of mystery. People would often be much astonished if they knew what cheap and common drugs they sometimes bought at extravagant prices in various highly-puffed patent medicines of secret composition, not a few of which simple remedies we are prescribing every day.

It is hardly reasonable to expect that we should be able to persuade people, especially those who are well off, to live like reasonable creatures; but those who are completely ignorant of medical knowledge, and who come to us for advice and assistance, go a little too far when they suggest or dictate to us the kind of advice we are to give, the medicines we are to order, and the methods of treatment which we are to adopt, we having been studying during many years the nature and causes of disease, while they are utterly ignorant of the whole matter. And yet this is no imaginary picture; there are people who know nothing of science, and who have never seen anything of sick people, who nevertheless talk as if they were thoroughly experienced in the science and practice of medicine. Such persons sometimes condemn us because we decline to "consult" with men who practise according to conjectural principles based neither on experiment, observation, nor experience. Certain rich, influential, and fashionable persons having patronized and embraced some absurd medical conceits, profess to be grievously offended with some practitioner, who perhaps has been studying and teaching medicine for half a lifetime, because he declines to adopt measures which the patient himself desires out of mere caprice should be carried out.

It has been my lot to study, on more than one occasion, the well-turned phrases and persuasive sentences by which a popular prescriber of decillionths, brimful of tact, managed to bring conviction to the minds of people of intelligence, and at the same time to impress them with his profound knowledge and intelligence, though all the time he was writing nonsense, and probably knew that he was doing so. But, as is well known, cleverly stated nonsense often hits the mark, and will continue to do so for many a long year. Men high among the most intelligent and most learned, nay, men who have been looked up to as men of the world, have often been humbugged in matters medical, and even profound lawyers have failed to distinguish medical nonsense from medical sense, and mere sham science from real scientific knowledge. Those who are always gauging the value of evidence, and devoting themselves to the extraction of truth, seem to be specially susceptible to medical and scientific imposition. But there is hardly a department of human endeavor in these days in which you will not find audacious humbugs influencing opinion, and gaining for a time notoriety and renown at the hands of their dupes.

But if we raise our voice ever so gently against nonsense and imposture, some of the writers belonging to the organs of so-called public opinion hold up to reprobation what they denominate the proverbial jealousy, the intolerance, the illiberality, and the narrow-mindedness of the doctors. The comments in the supposed interests of the public and the strictures passed upon us are sometimes most comical, but you will find sometimes, I fear, that your work is rendered very difficult in consequence. If you attend, through a very long and serious illness, a patient, who, from the badness of the times, is unable to afford you any remuneration for your services, and you hear that as soon as he was able to get about he placed himself under the care of a distinguished quack, who found it necessary to see him every day, and received a handsome fee each time, you are to consider your-selves fortunate in belonging to a liberal profession, and though you receive nothing for your work, you are not to feel jealous of the quack who is well paid perhaps for doing nothing, perhaps for the mistakes he has made. If, after having ridden over hundreds of miles of ground of the roughest country in the roughest weather to attend the sick poor around you, finding not only medicine for all, but food and medical comforts for not a few, you one day discover that the only people within ten miles of you enjoying an income of more than a hundred a-year have, out of the purest kindness, invited a celebrated homœopath to visit them, and he, also out of kindness, has seen and prescribed for a number of your patients at half the fee he usually receives, and has been paid more money by your poor patients in a week than you will receive in a year, you are to feel thankful that you live in a free country, where opportunity is afforded to all. If, after having served the offices of House Surgeon, House Physician, and many minor appointments in a public Hospital, and qualified with honors, the wealthiest of your neighbors gives it out that you are very kind to the poor, and that the servants are well satisfied with you, while he and the members of his family, when there is anything the matter, send over to —— for a dis-tinguished eclectic doctor of philosophy who graduated abroad, and is supposed to have had great experience, but whose early history and training are involved in obscurity, patiently submit. If he neither knows the test for albumen, nor its import when present in the urine ; if he discards as useless physical examination of the chest ; and disapproves of the stethoscope, microscope, and other "medical toys," because by prolonged inquiries into the mysteries of the magnetization of the solids and fluids of the body he, as he says, has detected molecular anti-gyrations of a most important character in the component particles of the brain and nerves,—and if by the administration of gyrating "similars" in the shape of small globules, largely composed of sugar of milk, this celebrity professes to be able to combat pathological phenomena before they could establish disease, do not be indignant.   You may be expected to preserve an attitude of deferential awe or respect whenever the distinguished and eminently successful authority is spoken of. You may not discover his name on the medical register, and you may find that as soon as any patient is indiscreet enough to become very seriously ill, some "ordinary" medical practitioner, perhaps your-self, is requested just to attend as "a matter of form." You may possess incontrovertible evidence that the distinguished person is utterly ignorant of the very elements of medicine, but you must not be sur-prised to find out, notwithstanding, that his important services have been judged to be worth more than five times as much as the county pays for your own conferred upon hundreds of poor people, and extending

C

over a much longer period of time. We may, no doubt, derive some
consolation from the reflection that we belong to a truly liberal profession,
and do not practise merely for the purpose of receiving pay. You may,
perhaps, think it hard that unqualified and only partly legally qualified
charlatans are not prevented by law from humbugging innocent people,
as is the case in some countries which have not reached the high degree
of civilization which we enjoy, but rather you should feel thankful that
the Government does not pass laws which might conduce to the further
impoverishment and degradation of legally qualified medical men who
attend the poor of the district in which they live. No doubt many
highly influential law-making persons agree with eclectics, animal mag-
netizers, hydro-, homœo-, and other "paths," in the opinion that it is
degrading for a genius, a conjurer, or a certain cure to submit to the
ordeal of examinations on elementary anatomy, physiology, and medicine conducted by unpractical theorizers, and presided over by the
narrow-minded supporters of "medical trades-unions"!

After all, it must be conceded that the most popular of quacks
seldom enjoys more than a short-lived reputation. He has to make
hay while the sun shines, for he may soon have to give place to a greater
quack than himself, and pass into obscurity. On the other hand,
although we may in every way receive far less than our due, we belong
to a body rightly proud of its history and confident as to its future.
Resting on science, medicine must progress as knowledge advances.
As information spreads, respect for real work will increase. The regard
for the medical practitioner will be higher in the future than it has been
in the past, and by and by the numbers of those who appreciate our work
and put trust in us will include as many as the most enthusiastic among
us could desire.

We are, as I have remarked, sometimes placed in a position of great
difficulty, and much perplexed as to the course we ought to take.
Occasionally, regard for the honor of the profession would seem to
require a course of action which might not coincide with the interest of
the patient or be in accordance with that consideration and kindness
which, under all circumstances, should be extended to the sick and
suffering.

If we carefully bear in mind that the credit and honor of us all are
of higher consequence than individual success, or personal loss, or
even injustice—if we explain that we have nothing to keep secret, no
mysteries to protect or preserve—that on the contrary we desire that
the knowledge we possess should spread, and that all possible means of
relief and all methods of preventing disease should be widely diffused ;
that we court inquiry into the principles upon which our methods of
investigation and treatment are based, and desire that our reasonings
thereupon should be examined and criticised, we shall seldom, I think,

experience difficulty in deciding how we ought to act in almost any case that may arise. We must, in short, endeavor to act for the advantage and honor of the profession without in the smallest degree, or in any way sacrificing the interests of the sick person, and without wounding the feelings of the patient or his friends. In these, and in all other difficulties we encounter, we shall act upon the maxim *Fac recte nil time.*

Of Studying Slight Ailments in the Dispensary Department of the Hospital. — Great principles as regards the treatment of disease may, without doubt, be learned and taught, and the influence of important remedies illustrated in the case of slight ailments as well as in grave disorders. The circumstance that little attention, comparatively speaking, has been paid to this part of medicine in modern systematic works, makes me particularly desirous to bring it under your notice.

You may learn a good deal about man's slight derangements if you study in the dispensary department of the hospital, or in public dispensaries, and I strongly advise you to take advantage of the opportunities that may offer. Do not be deterred from spending time in this department, although you may hear disparaging observations concerning out-patient medical work, both from professional and non-professional people. It is now the fashion to condemn the system upon which the dispensary department of most of our hospitals has long been successfully conducted. To those unacquainted with the facts, there seems much that is plausible in the objections raised, but it will be found that the desire, on the part of some enthusiasts in charity organization, to improve the out-patient department of hospitals is supplemented by a much stronger desire to do everything to encourage the so-called self-supporting dispensary system, based on the hypothesis that working-men and others are degraded if they receive relief from their sufferings without paying something. The "facts" and the value of the arguments advanced may be judged by the oft-repeated assertion that a fourth of the population of London receives gratuitous medical treatment.

There is a class of philanthropists whose dictum it is that every one ought to pay for medical advice, and that if he cannot pay enough to remunerate a practitioner he should combine with others placed in a similar position, and so form a club to which a salaried medical officer is appointed. The "self-supporting" system is, however, in many instances, not a reality, while any one who knows much of the working classes, knows that the demand for medical help and medical comforts usually comes at a time when little or no money is being earned. Thousands of pounds are to be collected for starting these "self-supporting" dispensaries, which, therefore, are "self-supporting" only in name. Charitable persons are to give in order that certain members of the population may be doctored at half the usual cost, or less than that. I have seen a great deal of the poor and of out-patient hospital practice, and as I have not met with the so-called evils of the system, I cannot advocate the proposed remedies.   Many of the energetic legislators in connection with medical charity seem to think that no one who suffers from a pain in his stomach should be relieved until he has either paid for help, or has proved that he is a really necessitous and impecunious person.   I believe that if some of the new suggestions were carried out, the profession would not only receive less, but would have to give more advice for nothing than they do now.

Up to this time the Dispensary departments of our hospitals have been of the greatest service to the poor, and of great advantage to those who are studying medicine.   It is there we learn to interpret the curious descriptions given by people in so many different ways of the aches and pains they experience—there we learn to recognize the difference between apparent and actual suffering—there we are taught to quickly discern different forms of disease, and to acquire that ready method of investigation which is so valuable in after life.   Moreover, some of the hardest workers among us prefer to give their services out-and-out rather than receive the pittance which seems to be considered by some reformers as payment for services rendered,—and pitied and possibly despised as poor doctors whose services are valued at a very small sum *per annum*, and to be obtained by right by those who promise to pay a few pence per week.

Although complaints may be made of the rate at which people are gratuitously seen and dismissed, the out-patient hospital physician, in fact, seldom misses an important case of actual disease, while of his real use to the poor there can be no question whatever.   Slight ailments are prescribed for and relieved, while serious cases of disease are detected and at once transferred to the wards, without those inquisitorial investigations which seem to form a very important factor in model sick-poor relief and centralization and general organization.   It is doubtful if, by any system that can be inaugurated, a poor patient will be more quickly relieved and cared for than by the one which has been gradually built up by members of our profession, and is now in useful operation in hundreds of institutions.   To teach providence to all classes is very laudable, but there is no good reason why this desirable lesson should be taught by lowering the status of the medical practitioner.   We must never forget that our work is to relieve suffering as promptly and as efficiently as possible, and it is on all grounds better that we should sometimes give our services altogether than accept what is called remuneration of a very inadequate character.

The Treatment of Slight Ailments conducted on the same Principles as that of Serious Diseases.—There is, lastly, this very cogent reason which impels me to direct your attention thus early in my course to the consideration of slight ailments. It will be found that many of the principles upon which the treatment of trivial derangements is conducted obtain in the management of graver maladies. This is a matter of the highest practical importance, and in not a few instances you will find that attention to the relief of slight ailments will afford you great assistance in determining the proper course to pursue in the treatment of very serious forms of acute disease. For example, I shall be able to show you that the treatment of a grave disorder like acute rheumatism is based upon facts and reasoning which apply equally to slight affections of a rheumatic nature. Fevers and inflammations of the very slightest character afford lessons of the greatest value concerning the management of every disease of that class.

By observing carefully the action of remedies in slight ailments, we may gain knowledge which will be of the greatest use to us, and especially in the treatment of slight derangements of our own health may we hope to gain very definite information concerning the precise action of some of the most important of the medicines we employ. I am sure that any one who has experienced the change in his sensations which occurs after taking a few doses of ammonia in the course of an ordinary cold, or has noticed the pleasant alteration which occurs during an attack of quinsy as soon as diuretic and sudorific remedies have commenced to act, or is practically acquainted with the relief afforded in sick headache by a grain or two of gray powder or calomel, will be quite convinced of the usefulness of medicine, will not altogether despise the views and practice of forty years ago, or feel reduced to advocate the administration of colored water to his suffering contemporaries, or will propose to leave a number of cases of different forms of disease without any medical treatment whatever, in order that he may observe what has been naïvely termed the "natural history of disease," the patient, of course, not wishing to complicate the interesting inquiry by desiring the relief of his suffering and quick convalescence.

There are many valuable points connected with prescribing, which are of the utmost importance, and which are to be learned from the practitioner who is well acquainted with the management of slight ailments. I have often heard the remark that our predecessors knew more about the treatment of disease than we of this generation do. There is some truth in this; and I am sure that many old practitioners now living are more successful in relieving the aches and pains of their patients than some of the young ones, who may, nevertheless, have a far more intimate knowledge of the diagnosis of obscure forms of disease and of the minute pathological changes which have damaged tissues and organs. Those of you who have worked under country practitioners enjoy a great advantage in this respect, and will be aware of many things connected with the art of prescribing for symptoms, of

4

which, even men who have highly distinguished themselves in our medical classes and medical examinations, may be in total ignorance. Nor do I see how this very desirable practical information can be gained in any better way. I may try to convey to you some of the wrinkles I have learned from my own masters, but shall only very imperfectly succeed. To offer remarks on the details of treatment when prescribing for the sick person in the country surgery is advantageous, but to give in lectures or at the bedside at the hospital detailed information as to the combination of remedies in pills and mixtures, and a number of things of considerable importance practically, would be tedious, and would take so long a time, that I could not expect a class to listen to such matters with attention. I shall, therefore, only venture to trouble you now and then with details as regards prescribing, but it will be well for you to take note of prescriptions, which I have frequently found of great value in the management of cases of deranged health.

Importance of Knowledge derived from Microscopical Investigation. —In all healthy changes, in all derangements, in all forms of disease, thousands of very minute particles, each of complex arrangement and composition, are implicated. It is by the united action of multitudes of these that the broad phenomena evident to us as healthy actions, derangements, morbid changes are occasioned. Do not, therefore, cast a slur on the consideration of minute details, do not neglect the facts arrived at by microscopical investigation. Rather, on the other hand, try to acquire the power of seeing in imagination the very particles which are involved, and of contemplating the phenomena proceeding in connection with them.

Bear in mind that around and in the interstices between the molecules of matter composing each elementary part of a living organism changes are constantly taking place. Remember that of the matter of the elementary part the bioplasm only lives and is the seat of *vital action*. The formed material which results from the death of particles of the bioplasm is the seat of physical and chemical changes only.

These elementary parts are so small that a thousand thousand of them might not occupy more than a cubic inch. Each of them during life is the seat of incessant change. Towards the bioplasm of each, streams of fluid, holding various substances in solution, continually tend, and, having reached it, part with certain constituents, there to be made into living matter, while the fluid, deprived of these, again traverses the formed material, and is taken up by the blood or is otherwise disposed of. Thus the formed material or tissue of every organ of the body is being constantly bathed by fresh portions of fluid, bringing and taking away, dissolved in it, things required for use or things which must be got rid of. This continual movement of fluid characterizes everything living from the lowest to the highest. In every form of plant and animal it is present and essential. When the flow is impeded derangement results, and degeneration and decay may commence ; when it stops, death takes place, and the portion of tissue thus losing the preservative influence exerted by the never-ceasing currents of fresh portions of fluid through its most minute interstices, undergoes chemical decomposition, just as a portion of tissue taken from a dead animal would do if kept artificially at a temperature of 100°. The deleterious gases and other poisonous substances formed, if there is no vent by which they can escape altogether, may pass into the blood and contaminate or actually poison every drop of the nutrient fluid, or may, by transudation into adjacent tissue, destroy it by causing the death of its living matter. In this way a large portion of tissue may soon be involved, and the death of the individual must shortly follow.

There is, in fact, a constant circulation — a constant interchange of gases and certain solid matters dissolved in fluid, some of which are appropriated as nutrient material, while others are removed as products of decay. This never-ceasing circulation goes on around and amongst the smallest particles of tissues and organs. Slow-moving tiny streamlets bathe the very molecules of the cells or elementary parts, and thus minister not only to the growth and increase of the bioplasm, but by aid of these currents alone can the formed material of the different tissues be preserved in a healthy and active state.

What may be correctly termed an *active inter-molecular circulation* is one essential condition of a healthy state of tissues, and it will be well for us to occupy a few minutes' time in its consideration.

In plants the inter-molecular circulation is equally essential, and the constant removal of fluid consequent upon evaporation from the surface of the leaves is one of the most important of the operations concerned in establishing and maintaining a very free circulation of fluid around and in and out of every living cell of the plant. Even in the lowest, simplest, and most minute of living forms inter-molecular circulation begins with existence and never ceases until death takes place. It is one of the phenomena constant in and characteristic of every form of life, but it is peculiar to living things. There is nothing like it in any non-living matter.

The importance of the continual flow of fresh particles of fluid through all the formed material or tissue of every part of the organism cannot be exaggerated. The rate of flow changes from time to time, and though it may sometimes take place very slowly, the movement never stops as long as life lasts, without derangement, damage, or destruction of the portion of tissue involved. You must try to picture to yourselves these never-ceasing movements of fluid simultaneously proceeding in every elementary part of every tissue of the organism, though it may be less than the thousandth of an inch in diameter. It is obvious that the activity of

these movements will in some measure depend upon the quantity of
fluid taken up by the blood.   If the nutrient fluid is habitually deficient
in water, more especially if it be surcharged with only slightly soluble
materials, there will be slow molecular circulation and a tendency to the
deposition of some of these slightly soluble matters in tissues where the
circulation is slowest.   It is in this way that urates are deposited in
fibrous tissues where ordinarily the circulation is slow, in cases of gout.
Substances may be introduced from time to time into the blood which
have the property of exerting a solvent action on these slightly soluble
compounds.   In this way their deposition may be prevented, or, if deposited, their resolution and reintroduction into the blood, and at last their
excretion from the body, may be effected.   The knowledge of the phenomena proceeding in the interstices of tissues enables us to understand precisely how many of our remedies act.   The careful consideration of such
minute changes may enable us to suggest methods of treatment in
various cases of great importance and value.   We may act upon the
formed material itself, rendering it more soft or more firm, help or interfere with the deposition of insoluble matters in its substance, influence
the growth of bioplasm, assist the removal of products of its death, and
bring about many changes of the greatest consequence in treatment.
Many of the diseases we have to diagnose and treat are due to a disturbed state of this inter-molecular circulation, and not a few of the
most serious morbid changes result from diminished activity of the flow.
Thus many matters which ought to be washed away accumulate in the
interstices of the tissues and impede their action.

When we can restore this molecular circulation to its normal state
derangements of various kinds are at once relieved, and in treating many
forms of established disease our principal object is to increase the activity
of the inter-molecular currents in the interstices of the tissues involved.
This object may be fulfilled in several ways.   In many cases free perspiration and indraughts of water will effect it ; sometimes the administration of frequently repeated doses of alkali promotes increased activity
of the inter-molecular circulation, and assists the solution of imperfectly soluble matters which have been deposited, or are in course of
deposition.

Looking from the point of view I have indicated, it will be well to
consider, for example, what is the precise action of quinine when it cures
in a few hours certain forms of obstinate lumbar pain.   What happens
when local thickening of the subcutaneous areolar tissue and inflammation of the sebaceous glands, that may have lasted for months, subsides
in a fortnight or less under the influence of biniodide or other preparation of mercury.

In cases in which too much nutrient material has been day by day
introduced into the blood for considerable periods of time, slow circula-

tion or stagnation of some of the molecular currents in various tissues and organs of the body will occur. Partial starvation, or at any rate a very moderate diet for several weeks, will again promote the flow. Free perspiration will have the same effect. The inhibition daily of several tumblers of water will, by favoring the transudation of fluid from the blood, also benefit the patient by washing out the tissues in their interstices, and interfering with the deposition of imperfectly soluble matters. Water containing alkalies or salts of vegetable acids, particularly the citrates and tartrates, will, by exciting free action of the skin and kidneys, also help to re-establish currents in the several tissues and organs in which the molecular circulation has become unduly slow or has even ceased.

Further, when we consider the close proximity of the nerve-fibres distributed to the capillaries to the very thin walls of these tubes, we shall not feel surprised that nerve changes are among the prominent and constant phenomena of disturbed molecular circulation. Any change occurring in the composition of the blood, leading to a diminished tendency on the part of the fluid constituents to permeate the vascular walls, must produce an effect upon the nerve-fibres just outside the capillary vessels. If the capillary vessels are over-distended or insufficiently filled with blood, these nerve-fibres are disturbed and will transmit impressions to the nerve-centre, which may react upon the nerves distributed to the muscular fibres of the small arteries, resulting in dilatation or contraction, and may cause a more general and more widely distributed nervous disturbance. But this part of the question will be more conveniently discussed when we have to consider the vascular phenomena of Inflammation and Fever.

OF THE TONGUE IN HEALTH AND IN SLIGHT AILMENTS.

I shall in the first place speak of the characters of the tongue. Few things it used to be supposed were of greater consequence than the recognition of the varied character which the dorsal surface of the tongue assumes in various cases of actual disease, and of slight derangements of health.

That the importance of the characters of the tongue as an indication of internal disease has been exaggerated by some physicians is undoubtedly true, but that it is altogether useless as an indication is certainly an incorrect inference. Any one who is at the pains to notice the alterations in his own tongue under varying conditions of health will convince himself that there is something to be gained by noting the changes of the tongue in disease. If you are to form a correct estimate of the value of the changes in the characters of the tongue, you must be well acquainted with the appearance of the surface of the healthy organ and with the exact nature of the structures which exist upon its dorsal

4 *

surface. Now, I dare say that few among you have had the curiosity to examine the back of the tongue, and see what is to be discovered there by microscopical examination.

If you scrape off a small piece of the soft matter from the surface of the dorsum of the tongue, place it on a glass slide, and, after adding a drop of water, cover it with a piece of thin glass, and examine it under a quarter of an inch object-glass, you will find, though the tongue be in a perfectly healthy state, a great many objects of interest, of which I shall have to speak presently.

I dare say that many who tell patients to put out their tongues sometimes do it as a matter of routine. I have known a rather absent doctor tell the patient to put out his tongue several times in the course of a few minutes' medical conversation. Patients are sometimes a little prosy, and if there is not much the matter with them, you may not attend as diligently as you ought to do. You lose the thread of the discourse, and while your wits are wandering you may cry out quite unconsciously, almost as if your command was the result of some reflex and habitual action, "Put out your tongue," although the organ has been already more than once displayed for your examination.

General Characters of the Surface.—The character of the tongue undoubtedly is very much influenced by the state of the stomach. The mucous membrane which lines every part of the alimentary canal is, as you know, continuous with that which lines the mouth and covers the tongue. Whenever there is a little gastric disturbance the tongue usually participates in the change. The relation between the two phenomena is, however, a complex one, and not very easily explained. Of the fact, in very many cases, there is no doubt, as many may easily prove by observations upon themselves.

The appearance of the tongue, as I shall explain more in detail further on, is also in some measure affected by the state of the circulation, by the character of the blood itself, as well as by the rate at which the epithelium ($\epsilon\pi\iota$, upon, and $\tau\iota\theta\eta\mu\iota$, to place) on its surface grows, arrives at maturity, and decays and falls off. Sometimes the epithelial cells remain intimately adherent to the tissue beneath upon which they are placed, and from which they seem to grow. The epithelium, or rather a layer of it, is frequently very easily detached, but sometimes it adheres very firmly. If the epithelium on the dorsum of the tongue is very thick and adherent, the tongue looks pale, and perhaps *white*. On the other hand, if the epithelial layer is very thin the tongue is *red*.

If you look at the under surface and sides of the tongue in the looking-glass, you will observe that these parts have a deep red appearance. The epithelium upon the sides, and the deep aspect of the tongue, consists of a layer so thin that the color of the blood is seen through the epithelial tissue. The degree of redness varies according to the

distention of the vessels; and depends upon changes in vascular distention like those which determine the redness or pallor of the skin. In
blushing, the small vessels of the skin of the cheeks are suddenly
distended in consequence of an inrush of blood permitted by the sudden
yielding and dilatation of the little arteries continuous with them, and
the same phenomenon under certain circumstances occurs in the vessels
of the tongue.

The Dorsum of the Tongue.—On the dorsal surface of the tongue
generally, the epithelium (ἐπι, upon, and τιθημι, to place) is arranged to
form a layer of considerable thickness, so that in many places the red
color of the blood is not seen. In health the general color of the
dorsal surface inclines to pale red, but in certain forms of disease it
becomes of a bright red color, almost like raw beef, and it is in consequence sometimes spoken of as " beefy." This seemingly raw condition depends partly upon the desquamation and falling off of a good
deal of epithelium, so that the layer covering the subjacent structures
is much reduced in thickness, and partly upon the capillaries being distended with blood. You can see the deep red color of the blood
through the epithelial layer, and the tongue looks raw. The mucous
membrane of the stomach and of other parts of the intestinal canal
participates in this change. There is desquamation of the epithelium
and undue turgescence of the vessels beneath.

**On the Fungiform and Filiform Papillæ, and of their Epithelial
Covering.**—In health there are to be seen here and there over the
dorsal surface little spots, which are of a bright red color. Upon
more careful examination, it will be found that the red spots are really
small papillæ with a constricted neck, in shape resembling that of a
mushroom, and known as the *Fungiform* (fungus) *Papillæ.* The
epithelium investment of the fungiform papillæ is extremely thin, and
the blood-vessels and terminal nerve networks lie just beneath. The
papillæ in question always appear red, and can therefore be easily
detected here and there amongst the filiform or conical papillæ which
are more uniformly spread over the dorsal surface of the tongue.

The epithelium covering the surface of the filiform papillæ is so
thick that we cannot suppose sapid substances could quickly pass
through it, or between the edges of the overlapping cells, and come in
contact with the nerves beneath. These filiform (*filum*, a thread, and
forma, likeness) papillæ have probably nothing to do with the sense of
taste, but are important organs of touch, much concerned, it may be, in
the process of placing the food in the proper position for mastication
and deglutition. It is the fungiform papillæ and the soft red mucous
membrane at the sides and back of the tongue, and that of the palate
and fauces, which are concerned in taste.

As regards the color of the tongue, it may be remarked, generally,

that if the epithelial layer on the organ is thin, the tongue will be red ;
if very thick, it will be white ; if rather dry, of a dull brown or dark
brown color ; and if there is an abundant accumulation of soft and
moist epithelium upon its surface, of a very opaque dirty white.

Epithelial Hair-like Processes of the Filiform Papillæ.—In the central part of the dorsum of the tongue the epithelial sheaths of the filiform
papillæ are very long, and indeed form elongated thread-like filaments,
closely resembling hairs in structure. You may snip off a few of these
hair-like bodies from your own tongue, or scrape portions of them from
the central part of the back of the surface with a knife. The specimen
is then to be placed in a watch-glass in a little weak glycerine. After the
processes have soaked for a time they may be placed on the glass slide,
covered in the usual way with thin glass, and examined under the microscope, first under an inch power, and then under a quarter of an inch
object-glass. You will find these long hair-like processes are composed
of layers of scaly epithelium imbricated and superimposed one upon the
other. The longest of the epithelial filaments project from the dorsal
surface of the tongue, perhaps, for more than the twentieth part of an
inch. Small particles of food often become entangled amongst these
epithelial extensions of the filiform papillæ. If you scrape the central
part of the back of the tongue a short time after you have taken a
meal, and examine the matter as just described, you will almost invariably find a number of oil globules, and very frequently starch
globules, portions of muscular fibres, and other things, according to the
nature of the last food taken.

Of the Epithelial Cells.—The layer on all the papillæ of the tongue
varies in thickness from time to time. The several epithelial cells composing the layer necessarily differ in age. The oldest of these cells are
those which are outermost, or situated at the greatest distance from the
surface on which they grow, and the youngest are those which are
nearest the vessels. Passing outwards we meet with cells gradually
advancing in age. The oldest are constantly decaying and falling off.
These mix with the food, and, no doubt, during every meal we swallow
them in thousands. But the old epithelial cells upon the tongue and
mucous membrane of the mouth undergo other changes, with the
general nature of which it is important that you should be acquainted
The changes in the epithelium should therefore be carefully studied as
opportunities of making the examination occur.

**Of Fungi and Low Organisms in and amongst the Epithelium of
the Tongue and Mouth.**—If, then, you look at the old epithelial cells
detached from the mucous membrane of the mouth, from the inside of
the cheek or the tongue, under high magnifying powers (from three to
twelve hundred diameters), you will find that the cells contain a number
of very minute spherical or oval particles, while multitudes of very

delicate filaments are often seen amongst them. ("Microscope in Medicine," pl. XXXVIII., fig. 1, p. 272.) Now these minute spherical and oval particles, situated in the formed material of the cell, and most numerous at its outer, that is, in its oldest part, are very low and simple organisms in an early phase of development. They have been called *micrococci* (μιχρος, little, and χοχχος, a grain), and have received other names. In this state they have not reached their full development. They are the living germs of organisms which exhibit different characters in their fully developed state. Each is capable of producing millions of descendants in a few hours. Some of them, probably, under certain circumstances, become elongated, and evolve bacteria of various forms; others may form the long thread which used to be called *Leptothrix buccalis.* ("Microscope in Medicine," pl. LXXXI., p. 492.) Some, perhaps, may be the germs of *Oidium albicans* and other fungi. It is, probable, indeed, that many different species of fungi may be developed from the spherical or oval germ-particles, existing in connection with the older epithelial cells on the surface of the mucous membrane of the mouth. The germ-particles themselves, although they closely resemble one another in appearance, may have been derived from different species of organism. The various species of germs grow and multiply under different circumstances. The growth and multiplication of such minute organisms has much to do with the appearance which the tongue presents in the same person at different times, as well as its character in different forms of derangement and disease.

It has been stated by more than one observer that *Sarcina ventriculi* is often present in the fur of the tongue, but I have never found it in this situation, though I have examined the fur in very many cases during the past thirty years. In cases in which sarcinæ were found in the stomach, I did not find them on the tongue or in other situations. I am afraid that many mistakes have been made with regard to the identification of *Sarcina ventriculi.*

Old epithelial cells, like other old and formed tissue or other dead organic animal or vegetable matter, are very soon invaded by the germs of low vegetable organisms, always very numerous in their vicinity, which grow at their expense and live upon their substance. Not only on the surface of the cells, but in their substance, the fungus germs are found, and frequently project from them, forming little collections, which may be detached from time to time.

Amongst the hair-like epithelial processes projecting from the free extremities of the filiform papillæ, are often found masses which have a granular appearance under low magnifying powers. When examined under objectives magnifying more than three hundred diameters, these masses will be found to consist of millions of spherical and oval fungi or micrococci, grouped together, each little mass of bioplasm being surrounded by, and separated from, its neighbors by clear structureless material, which probably has been formed by it.

Amongst the epithelial cells in every part of the mouth you will often find some very long extremely delicate filaments, which, if examined under high powers, will be found to exhibit a number of transverse markings. These grow and freely multiply in the fluids of the mouth at the usual temperature of that cavity. Many are found between the teeth, and in the tartar you will meet with numbers of vegetable organisms. Indeed, it is probable that the deposition of the tartar is intimately connected with changes occasioned by the living vegetable organisms in question, which belong to the genus *Leptothrix*. ("Microscope in Medicine," pl. LXXXI., fig. 3, p. 92.) Many of the filaments, long and short, exhibit peculiar movements, some vibrating to and fro, others taking a spiral course.

In many cases you will find whole forests of vegetable organisms consisting of many different species, and of the same species at different periods of growth, upon the dorsal surface of the tongue. These increase in number in cases of derangement of the digestive organs, and in many forms of disease.

The growth and multiplication of these low organisms at the very entrance of our bodies, and so placed that they must pass in immense numbers into the stomach whenever we swallow anything, is a fact of great significance in connection with certain conclusions respecting the action of these low organisms upon the solids and fluids of man's body. Of late years, the idea that such organisms constitute the active particles concerned in the propagation of contagious disease,—are, in fact, the actual *materies morbi*,—has been increasingly popular. The first question you will ask will probably be this :—Do these germ-particles perform any distinct office or function in connection with the solution of food or digestion, or do they merely live and grow upon the old epithelial cells and the *débris* of the food which must needs undergo change in such a situation, and at the temperature of the inside of the mouth? We find such bodies in animals as well as man, and though they are found in greatest number in certain derangements, multitudes are constantly present in the most healthy individuals. They have no doubt grown and multiplied under similar conditions and without varying in character for thousands of years.

Wherever organic matter is undergoing change and disintegration in an organism, or outside it, at the temperature of man's body, or some degrees lower or higher than this, and in some cases at a much lower temperature, such organisms exist in countless multitudes, and grow and multiply at the expense of the disintegrating organic matter. In the autumn there is not a leaf in which you will not find millions of low vegetable organisms in various stages of development and growth. As the organic matter of the dying leaf or plant undergoes change, and the decomposition of its more unstable compounds commences, the circumstances specially favorable for the growth and multiplication of many of the microscopic fungi are established. Fungus germs exist in the air at every part of the earth's surface at all times. Though by no means constantly present in precisely the same amount, some are always to be detected in appreciable numbers, if the air is properly examined. Many coming into contact with the moist surface of the leaf about to decay, find there a surface favorable for their development. The spores germinate, and from the surface of the tissues of the plant the growth easily makes its way into the substance.

But is it not remarkable that any one should believe, on the one hand, that the decay of the leaves is due to the fungi, or, on the other, that the decay is the cause of their development, growth, and multiplication? All that can be proved by facts and observation is, that as the leaf grows old, substances are formed which are easily appropriated by the fungi. The germs of fungi are present and are ready to develop just at the time when the appropriate pabulum is formed. The fungus does not spring from the leaf, neither is the leaf caused to grow old by the fungus, and its deterioration begins before the growth of the fungus commences. The fungus is in no sense either the cause or the consequence of the decay. And in the case of the higher animals and man, at least in many instances in which low organisms are associated with morbid processes, these last are neither the cause of disease nor are they produced by it. Fungus germs and micrococci of various kinds, being present, will grow and multiply whenever the surrounding conditions become favorable for the multiplication of each particular kind. If these conditions remain for a considerable time unfavorable, the germs, if present, remain quiescent, and may at last die, though probably most of such germs retain their vitality in a quiescent state for many years, and some perhaps for centuries.

Nor are microscopic fungi found only at this period of the year (autumn) in connection with dead and decaying vegetable tissue. In the vegetables and fruit we eat are countless multitudes of living growing organisms. Look, for instance, at the cells of a piece of lettuce or of the leaf of the watercress, nay, even those in the leaf and stem of the young and rapidly growing mustard and cress. There you will find, if you examine thin sections or the separated cells under a magnifying power of three hundred diameters or more, millions of little bodies, each of which is capable of giving rise to countless multitudes in a very short time. If you carefully study the revolving living matter of the cell of the leaf of the Vallisneria, you will have no difficulty in discerning some of these very low organisms in close proximity to the living matter of the plant itself. So very near, indeed, is the lowest living particle to the highest during its life, that no wonder the material of the latter falls a prey to it at last. The instant matter ceases to live it is invaded and appropriated by the ever-growing bacterium—the most constant, the most unchanging and universal of all kinds of living things—and of all the survivor; but whether this be of all things the most fit to survive, you may decide if you can.

As it is with regard to deteriorating vegetable tissues, so it is with regard to decaying animal tissue. Whether the body be in a state of health or disease, wherever tissue is about to undergo active disintegrating chemical change, wherever decomposition is taking place, or is approaching, the conditions may be favorable for the growth and multiplication of certain low organisms, the germs of which are present. Long before any changes akin to deterioration and decay are ordinarily supposed to commence, even from the very earliest period of construction and growth, fungus germs are ever present, ready to grow and multiply should the death and disintegration of a living particle occur. No wonder, then, that we find so many low organisms growing in connection with the old decaying epithelium of the mouth and of the tongue, of the œsophagus, and other parts. Under certain circumstances, the fungi grow and multiply to a vast extent lower down the alimentary canal, as I shall presently explain. We cannot suppose that such organisms do any harm; for patients suffering from maladies in which the alimentary canal seems to be almost filled with bacteria recover, without damage to any textures having been occasioned.

I have not studied the epithelium from the mouth of a savage who has never been in contact with civilized man, but, without having actually looked, I think I may feel pretty confident that low vegetable organisms would be found growing in the cells just as they grow in those of our own mucous membrane, and the species are probably precisely the same.

In lower animals, organisms of the same general character abound. If you examine the tongue of the dog or of the cat, of the sheep or of the ox, you will find that the same sort of changes are constantly going on. Everywhere the old epithelial cells are being invaded by low vegetable organisms, which grow and multiply as they do in the epithelial cells of man himself. Multitudes, of course, pass down into the stomach, and, under ordinary circumstances, many are probably destroyed during digestion by the action of the gastric juice and bile, and other fluids, which are poured into the alimentary canal. Those that are not destroyed certainly do no harm. In the healthy state they either do not grow and multiply at all during digestion and assimilation, or only to a very slight extent.

In the case of the lower animals, the introduction of fungi into the stomach goes on constantly and upon an enormous scale. Every mouthful of water consumed by sheep, oxen, and other animals, teems with myriads of low vegetable and animal organisms in various stages of existence ; and in the food they take, fungi in various stages are present, as well as the sporules of many different species. These low organisms are, therefore, always passing into the bodies of the animals in countless multitudes. But although millions of living fungi are always entering the alimentary canal of man and animals without doing harm, and probably without growing and multiplying there to any great extent, there are circumstances under which a different state of things is observed. If the stomach is out of order, if the bile and other secretions are deranged, or from some temporary or permanent impediment to their escape are not poured into the alimentary canal in proper quantity, phenomena totally unlike those characteristic of the healthy state are induced. Many an infant has suffered from the extraordinary development of bacteria in its alimentary canal, and some children die from the state of things thereby induced. But the bacteria cannot correctly be regarded as the cause of the departure from the normal state. That is to be sought in the secretions and in the action of the glands prior to the multiplication of the organisms.

I have seen every part of the cavity of the stomach, and the small and large intestine of an infant filled with curdled milk which had not undergone the slightest digestion, and every particle of which, when under the microscope, seemed to be almost composed of bacteria, so abundant were these bodies. Sometimes, however, bacteria grow and multiply in the milk of the mother before it has escaped from the breast, and the changes effected in the milk by the growth and multiplication of the organisms, it need scarcely be said, render it quite unfit for the sustenance of the infant ; and such milk, were it taken, would, except perhaps in the very strongest children, give rise to serious derangement of the digestive organs. In such a case the maternal secretion must have been out of order at the time of its secretion, or the bacteria would not have grown and multiplied in it. It is certain that in such secretions and in the glands that produce them, bacteria-germs are always present, but do not increase and multiply until long after the secretion has been discharged from the gland.

In face of such facts, it is difficult to accept the doctrine that bacteria, fungi, and such like low organisms are morbific, or disease-producing agents, or are of themselves productive of harm to the organism into which they pass. It is astonishing that, notwithstanding, these facts, which can be verified by any one—facts with which many of us have been familiar for the last thirty years and more—should at this time be unknown to, or somehow escape the cognizance of, some who have been recently studying the life-history of these very organisms..

5   D

The knowledge of such broad general facts renders it difficult, I think, to accept off-hand the doctrine that such organisms are somehow intimately connected with the origin and communication of many of the most serious diseases of man and animals. Of late years, however, the theory that such organisms, which are invariably present in all decaying healthy normal structure, or closely allied organisms, or their pathologically modified descendants, constitute the actual poison of most of the contagious diseases which invade us, has spread far and wide, and has been accepted by many as a general principle.

There is, probably, not a part of the body of any one of us of a quarter of an inch in diameter where bacteria-germs are not present. Certainly every time we eat, myriads are carried into our alimentary canal ; and every time we breathe, except in the very purest atmosphere, multitudes pass into the air-passages. So small are these bacterial germs, that they would pass without the slightest difficulty through basement membrane and through the interstices of any of the tissues of the organism ; and yet the public is taught that there is some intimate connection between bacteria, and dust, and morbid phenomena. Erroneous notions are spread far and wide by sensation lectures, under such a title as " Dust and Disease." The dust which causes disease is of a most exceptional kind. It has been said that the air of the Swiss mountains is devoid of bacteria. But is the health and vigor of the inhabitants of the Alps to be compared with that of the workers on the Paddington Dust Heaps? As a fact, ordinary bacteria are harmless enough ; they exist in us without disturbing us in any way, but they only grow and multiply in great numbers when circumstances become favorable. I can give you positive proof that bacteria germs exist not only upon the surface of the skin and mucous membranes, but in the internal organs, in the interstices of healthy tissues, and in the blood itself. Some years ago I examined the layers of a fibrinous clot which had been slowly formed from the blood in the interoir of a large aneurism of the aorta of a man who died of the disease. The body was examined six or eight hours after death. The aneurism had existed for many years ; and probably some of the layers of fibrin which had been deposited were almost as old as the aneurism itself. Now I found that in all parts of the firm, laminated, leather-like material, which served to greatly increase the thickness of the wall of the aneurismal sac, there were indications of disintegrating changes having taken place. Upon carefully examining minute pieces of the fibrin under high powers, multitudes of bacteria and their germs were discovered without difficulty. But the older layers in the outer part were here and there softened, and portions of the fibrinous matter seemed eroded, many small masses of soft and broken-down material being present. All these teemed with bacteria, moving, growing, and multiplying.

Now these bacteria, like the fibrin in which they were growing and multiplying, were very close to the blood and within the vascular system ; internal to the various tissues constituting the wall of the vessel, which was dilated to form the aneurismal sac. The bacteria must have been growing and multiplying in the lifetime of the patient, and probably for many months before his death occurred. They could not have got into the position in which they were discovered from the outside, for it is hardly conceivable that such an organism as a bacterium could have found out, while outside the body, that within the vascular system there was material suitable for its growth and multiplication. Neither is it possible the bacteria could have made their way from without to the situation in which they were found, nor could they have effected, in the course of a few hours, the extensive erosions and softening discovered. Such theories could not be sustained with any show of reason. The only conclusion, therefore, which is in accordance with the facts of the case and with common sense, is that which I have before adverted to : viz., that bacteria-germs exist at all times in all parts of the body, even in the blood itself during the healthy state.

I conclude that as long as the normal state of things exists, the living bacteria-germs in all parts of the organism do not grow and multiply, but that when any change occurs of the character of that which results in chemical decomposition, these bacteria-germs multiply. This multiplication proceeds, although we are alive, just as it takes place in dead animal and vegetable matter. And it will occur in every part of every one of us a very few hours after death.

So that you see if bacteria-germs constitute the actual, material, living particles by which contagious disease is propagated, they must be peculiar bacteria, totally different from the ordinary bacteria-germs which exist, and have existed everywhere. The ordinary bacteria may certainly grow and multiply enormously on the mucous membranes of the body, in follicles of the mucous surfaces, and in viscera,—intestinal canal, bladder, and passages therefrom, nay, even amongst the elements of healthy growing tissue, without causing any disease at all. Bacteria-germs, low fungi, and low algæ exist in connection with the tissues and fluids of every human organism, and, as you may convince yourselves at any time, millions of these are unquestionably present during every moment of existence in health on the surface of the dorsum of the tongue. Multitudes, as I have said, pass down the alimentary canal every time we swallow food or fluid. Such ordinary bacteria and their germs do us no harm whatever. But please do not infer from what I have said that putrid fluids loaded with bacteria are innocuous or to be recommended. Organic matter in a state of putrefactive decomposition when introduced into the alimentary canal gives rise to pathological phenomena irrespective of the bacteria it may contain.

Some have attempted to surmount the difficulty of accounting for the origin of such a multitude of bacterial species or varieties, each having the power or property of causing a definite disease, by the conjecture that ordinary bacteria, like higher organisms, are themselves the subjects of pathological evolutional changes. It is surmised that the ordinary bacterium living under altered conditions, might give origin to a pathological bacterium, and these might further change, and thus give rise to new disease-producing organisms. In this way, conjecture is added to conjecture, and the evolution of one hypothesis leads to the evolution of another. New forms of being are assumed, and pathological prodigies are added to the multitudinous new creations of the evolutional imagination. As a fact, we find that pathological phenomena become less distinct as we descend in the scale of created beings, and it is doubtful if in the lower simpler forms of life any phenomena occur to which the term pathological or morbid is strictly applicable. That an Actinia or a Hydra may suffer from pathological change is certain, but organisms much lower and simpler than these, are probably incapable of undergoing change which could be properly regarded as morbid or pathological.

The suggestion of bacteria taking upon themselves a sort of pathological transformation, and developing by degradational evolution a bacterium of vileness and virulence potent to produce, it may be, new and fatal forms of disease, strikes me as a wonderful conjecture, even in these days of rampant scientific fancy, and as gratuitous as it is unnecessary. The broad facts of nature are entirely opposed to it. So far from any observations yet made being in its support, there is potent evidence against such an hypothesis. Conditions which in high and complex organisms would result in pathological phenomena, in these low forms merely determine an alteration in the rate of growth and multiplication. The change in such an organism as the yeast plant, which seems to correspond to the formation of pus in man and the higher animals, is but more rapid multiplication, by the division and subdivision of the living matter (bioplasm), of the minute and simple organism. The bacterium would appear to be much lower and simpler as regards the varied conditions under which it lives and grows than the yeast plant. Indeed, the bacterium is one of the most constant and unchangeable of all forms of life, and if altered forms spring from it, they soon revert to the primitive universal constant form.

Still, it might be said, that it is possible that great change in surrounding conditions might cause the development of bacteria with new disease-causing powers, from pre-existing harmless or disease-producing varieties or species. There are, however, serious objections to adopting such an hypothesis, among which, by no means the least, is the necessity of accepting several minor hypotheses involved in the acceptance of the major. It is most difficult to see how and why the supposed new forms should begin. Indeed, looking broadly, one most striking fact in connection with bacteria is, that countless millions of similar forms resulting from endless repetition have been produced without change in power through past ages. We must be very careful as regards the acceptance of so-called evidence of change in property and power of organisms of this low class. It is, I readily admit, not unreasonable to suppose that changes within certain definite limits may occur, but in some cases what seem to be new forms, are probably but temporary modifications, the descendants of which soon resume the old type. Divergence and reversion in a limited and very moderate degree, and possibly in forms of life much higher than the bacterium, may occur, and be frequently repeated, without ever leading to or resulting in any lasting change of type.

Time will probably show that many of the pretentious statements which have been made concerning the fungus germ hypothesis of contagious disease, are groundless.

It has been clearly shown, that as the bioplasm of man's body acquires increased power of growth, it also acquires increased power of resisting the destructive influence of external conditions. The movements of the morbid bioplasm of the pus-corpuscle will continue long after those of the healthy bioplasm of the white blood-corpuscle have ceased. It is certain, that other forms of morbid bioplasm originating in man's body exhibit far greater resisting power than that manifested by pus. These and many more cogent and striking facts are wholly ignored by writers of the bacterial school, and by those whose general views are founded on highly partial considerations, and whose judgment seems to have been warped from the first by the assertions and extraordinary delineations of speculative observers like Hallier. In spite of all that has been urged in favor of a bacterium hypothesis, it must at this time be admitted that in no case has the specific bacterium of any definite disease been identified. The ordinary bacterium is certainly the least varying of all living forms. The organism that grew and multiplied in the dead bodies of the Pharaohs is probably identical with that which is associated with the decomposition of the organic matter of the human body in our own time. Nor is there any reason to suppose that, should the world last as long, any alteration will take place in the characters, mode of growth, and disintegrating activity of the bacterium some thousands of years hence.

It seems to have been forgotten that the chemical substances in many putrefying organic matters act as poisons to the living matter of the tissues and organs of the body. These substances passing to the bioplasm quickly destroy it, and the material around each living mass, no longer being traversed by fresh particles of fluid as in health, passes into decomposition; and so the process goes on, until a considerable pro-

5 *

portion of tissue is destroyed, and passes into a state of putrefaction. In many such cases the blood itself is poisoned, and it may be at an early period of the change. But for all this, an exceptional state of things is in the first instance necessary. The phenomena, which in the higher organisms ordinarily interfere with the growth and multiplication of the ever-present bacteria, must have given place to very exceptional changes, and these, not the bacteria, must be regarded as the true cause of the disease.

It has been objected that the *materies morbi* of contagious diseases cannot consist of the modified living matter of the body itself, because the healthy living matter rapidly undergoes change when removed from the seat of its growth, and very soon dies. But he who accepts this apparent objection must at the same time ignore most important facts, and must forget that, for example, healthy ciliated cells retain their vitality for many days after the death of the body ; the bioplasm at the base of the hair, and that in the deep layers of the cuticle, also resists the destructive influences which quickly kill the living matter of many other parts of the healthy body. But, worse than all, the important fact I have urged in favor of my view remains unanswered, and is, indeed, wholly ignored by those who accept hypotheses concerning very difficult questions, which have the great advantage of being well talked of, but little thought about.

In concluding my remarks on this very important and highly interesting question, I venture to ask you to bear in mind that the bacterium and its germs are intimately associated with every kind of animal and plant, in its healthy and morbid state and during every period of existence, from its earliest embryonic condition to the time of death at the most advanced age. Whether it is some special bacterium which directly causes the results consequent upon the introduction of a specific poison into the organism, or whether the active particle, the *contagium* or *materies morbi*, is of a totally different nature, altogether independent of bacteria and allied organisms, must be regarded as still an open question. Some statements, it must be admitted, have been recently made in favor of the hypothesis that there are bacteria and bacteria—that the real contagious bacterium is an organism altogether apart from the harmless bodies so intimately associated with the tissues and fluids of every one of us ; but, as I have endeavored to show, the arguments hitherto advanced are by no means convincing. Further, as I have endeavored to explain, it has been conjectured that the horrible death-carrying bacteria of various orders have been somehow derived from the harmless form by pathological transformations, or developed in the course of evolutional struggles proceeding through the ages, or that they are the product of a constantly altering environment. But, it need scarcely be said, many new facts must be discovered, and much must be learned concerning special bacterial phenomena before the problem can be solved. I have alluded to these views here in order that the most important points may be before you, and I hope, in considering them, you will keep prominently before your mind's eye this one universal, ever-existing, unchangeable organism, which, possibly the first formed of all life, has outstood every change, and is probably destined to outlast every other living form, which is domiciled in every organism on the face of the earth, is found in almost every kind of food and drink, flourishes in the human mouth, and the germs of which are to be found in every part of man's body, and which is conjectured to be closely related to the living forms which cause various contagious diseases, and to have given origin to them.

The Tongue in various Derangements.

I shall now proceed to consider a little more in detail the changes which occur in the tongue, which are of special interest to us, and the peculiar characters assumed by the organ in different states of health. The subject has received great attention from the very earliest ages, and not only from medical practitioners. It is in all respects worthy of your most attentive consideration. Not a few persons, ignorant of medicine, have been in the constant habit of studying the state of the tongue. To many it is a matter of grave anxiety through life, and men have been known to use the looking-glass every day for half a century or more for the purpose of observing the daily changes which occur. Especially does the tongue excite the greatest attention and interest among the members of that large section of civilized man which knows not what it is to feel perfectly well—to be free from discomfort of every kind, and not to ail anything.

It has been already stated that changes in the tongue are frequently associated with somewhat similar changes occurring in other parts of the very extensive system of mucous membrane concerned in the preparation, digestion, and absorption of food. We have now to consider how such extensive changes are probably occasioned. One part of the mucous tract may participate in the phenomena occurring, it may be, at a considerable distance. This participation is doubtless due to the circumstance that the nerve-centres presiding over the several actions occurring in different parts of the mucous membrane of the alimentary canal are connected together by commissural fibres. The actions of the numerous minute nerve-centres are also harmonized and co-ordinated by intercommunicating cords.

The extensive gastro-intestinal tract of mucous membrane is indeed supplied with one system of nerves, the great characteristic of which is extensive distribution and intimate intercommunication, so that when one portion is deranged the action of others is often disturbed. In certain forms of disease a local affection of very limited extent often provokes an altered and pathological action of twenty or thirty feet of intestine or more, and may affect the character of the secretions from gastric and intestinal glands at a great distance from the seat of actual lesion.

Very slight changes as regards diet will lead to reduction of the secreting action of the stomach glands. The mucous membrane often becomes less moist than it should be, and the secretion from every part is reduced, though it would be incorrect to say that the membrane became dry. The mucous membrane of the mouth and the glands connected therewith may participate in any altered action going on in the stomach. In practice we invariably find that in fevers, and indeed in any slight attack of feverishness, when the temperature of the body has risen only two or three degrees, in short, in the common pathological change which everybody has experienced when he has taken cold, there is imperfect action and deranged secretion in the stomach. For several hours, it may be for two or three days, there is in most cases defective formation of the substances which form the all-essential constituents of saliva, the gastric juice, and other secretions poured into the intestinal canal. One consequence is that the ordinary desire for eating is not present, and if the person eat well in spite of his disinclination to do so, further derangement, perhaps severe pain and indigestion, may add to his troubles, if he has not the good fortune to escape by free vomiting or by the occurrence of diarrhœa, or both. Under such circumstances it is, therefore, the best plan to starve, or, if the person is weak and feeble, he might take milk, beef-tea, or strong soup in very small quantities, at short intervals of time (an hour or two hours) until healthy action returns.

It is probable that under the circumstances I am considering, the various materials out of which the mucus which is secreted on the surface of the mucous membranes and by the glands connected with them, are not separated from the blood, or are present in an altered state. In fevers, and even in slightly feverish conditions, I believe that those complex compounds from which the cells of the salivary glands form saliva, and those out of which the gland cells of other parts of the alimentary canal develop the marvellous and peculiar substances which play so important a part in digestion and ultimately in nutrition, are not drawn from the blood through the walls of the vessels. This deranged action of an extensive system of glandular organs necessarily affects the composition of the blood (which also suffers in other ways), and thus the action of every tissue and organ in the body may for a time become more or less deranged.

When we come to consider the nature of the changes occurring in feverishness, we shall see that in all fevers, and in every febrile condition, digestion, and the action of the alimentary canal are invariably disturbed, and often to an alarming extent. Every intelligent mother knows that in infants and in young children the febrile state often commences with derangement of the stomach, and may be occasioned by improper food, as, for example, hard, unripe apples. In this way important alterations in the blood and general derangement of the system result from pathological phenomena, which start from disturbance in the action of, it may be, only a small portion of the mucous membrane of the alimentary canal.

It is very important that the organs whose action is disturbed should be permitted to rest for awhile. You will find after a time there will be good evidence of returning action, and possibly of undue action. A greater amount of action than occurs in health may be noticed, but this is soon followed by reduced activity, and at length the proper degree of action. By degrees the normal state of health is re-established, without any permanent lesion or structural change of any kind having been induced. In such derangements, if by any means we can cause the return of secreting action, if we can get these various glands to act freely, the abnormal condition will be relieved, and the normal or healthy state restored, sooner than if matters are left to right themselves. In this way the patient would gain an important advantage. I think I shall be able to convince you that we can be of use, not only by effecting the expulsion of the irritating matters from the stomach or bowels, but also by diminishing the febrile condition set up in these cases, and in others in which febrile development is more obscure and difficult to trace. It will be well for me, before further discussing this part of the matter, to draw your attention to one or two other points of general interest in connection with the febrile state.

In an ordinary cold the mouth is often more or less dry or clammy. The throat, as you know, feels dry and rough, and the appetite becomes impaired. Little gastric juice is formed under these circumstances, and probably the quantity of intestinal fluid that ought to be secreted is much less than usual. You will also notice, if you pay careful attention to the matter, that the kidneys do not secrete in the normal degree, while the bowels are often constipated. You will find, when you are suffering in this manner, that if you take a warm bath or a hot air or vapor bath, by which the free action of the skin will be excited, the unpleasant sensations cease, and at least for a time you feel very much better. You may even experience complete relief. If you take a few doses of *Nitrate of Potash*, or *Bicarbonate of Potash*, or *Liquor Ammoniæ Acetatis*, or some other saline which acts on the skin and kidneys, you will be greatly relieved.

This relief is, I think, consequent upon the removal of certain substances from the blood which had been accumulating in that fluid to its

detriment, and which as they circulated caused derangement of action
in many tissues and organs in the body. I shall have frequently to
direct your attention to the general and often widespread changes which
result from deranged actions confined to very limited areas of tissue or
organ, and shall show that, at least in a number of cases, this may be
explained by the alterations induced, directly or indirectly, in the character and composition of the blood. Hardly any of the ordinary
physiological changes of the body can be deranged without some
alteration taking place in the character of the blood. The action of
the digestive organs will be disturbed at once, and of this we shall soon
have indications in the loss of appetite and various unpleasant sensations in the stomach, as well as by the altered state of the tongue.

Of Dry and Moist States of the Tongue.—One of the commonest
changes observed in the tongue is undue dryness,—a condition which
may depend upon a variety of circumstances. The moisture of the
parts within the mouth varies greatly, and even, in most persons, the
mouth is not equally moist at all periods of the day and night. The
activity of the process of secretion varies much at different times; the
quantity of fluid in the interstices of a thick tissue like the skin or the
dorsal surface of the tongue is by no means always the same, and varies
with every change in the tension of the walls of the capillaries, the
pressure of the circulation, the activity of the lymphatics, and a number
of other circumstances. Lastly, it is obvious that the varying rate of
evaporation from the mouth and nasal passages will alone cause alterations in the tongue as regards its moisture.

The dryness of the dorsal surface of the tongue, a change which is
not uncommon in many forms of disease, cannot be attributed only to
changes taking place upon the surface of the mucous membrane, for the
secretion of fluid by the glands beneath might entirely compensate, or
more than compensate, for the loss of fluid by evaporation. In many
cases the dryness seems to be due to alterations which take place
beneath the mucous membrane affecting the nutrition of the deep cells
of the cuticular coverings of the papillæ, and in part to the change in the
composition of the blood itself and an altered state of the blood distribution, as determined by dilatation of the little arteries, consequent
upon relaxation of the circular muscular fibres, occasioned by change in
some part, peripheral or central, of the nerve apparatus which governs their
calibre. In ordinary health the moist condition of the tongue is due partly
to the transudation of fluid through the walls of the vessels towards the
epithelial and other tissues, and partly to the presence of fluids secreted
in varying quantities and poured into the cavity of the mouth, particularly the saliva. · The surface of the tongue and inside of the mouth
are thus kept moist. The moisture of the tongue and interior of the
mouth will, however, be very much favored if the air we breathe is

moist, while in the opposite state of things the tongue will become more or less dry from evaporation. Obviously a greater amount of fluid will be required to maintain the mouth in a moist state in dry than in damp weather. The quantity of vapor communicated to the expired air which traverses the cavity of the mouth is liable to variations according to changes which occur in the lungs and air passages. The blood, as it traverses the capillaries of the lungs at different times, contains very different quantities of fluid, and therefore during some periods much more vapor will be given off from the blood to the air about to be expired than at other periods. Not only so, but the rate of exhalation of watery vapor from the blood is influenced by a number of complex conditions which are continually undergoing change, but which I must not attempt to consider here. Every time we expire through the open mouth, the air laden with moisture is driven over the mucous membrane of the mouth and tongue. However dry the *inspired* air may be, it becomes nearly saturated with moisture as it leaves the air-cells of the lungs. This damp air playing over surfaces it traverses assists in keeping them moist.

The mouth and tongue, however, may readily become dry, and a very unpleasant state of things will be experienced. Those who have acquired the bad habit of sleeping with the mouth wide open frequently suffer from the derangement in question. We should close the mouth before falling asleep, and during sleep we should breathe freely through the nose. In cold weather it is important that the cold air which is inhaled should pass over the surface of the mucous membrane of the nasal passages, in order that it may be warmed before it reaches the windpipe and lungs. The air which receives a supply of moisture is better adapted for the further complex chemical changes effected by respiration, which changes, as many of you are no doubt aware, are most actively carried on during the period of sleep. Always advise your patients to get into the habit of keeping the mouth closed and breathing through the nose, not only during sleep, but generally, for, especially in cold weather, it is important upon many grounds that the inflowing air should take this circuitous route rather than the more direct one by the mouth.

As soon as the mucous membrane of the mouth or adjacent passages gets dry, a desire for fluid will be experienced. The person longs for a little water, and when he gets it he moves it about in all parts of the mouth, so as to thoroughly moisten the mucous membrane; but this operation requires to be very frequently repeated, as the surface when moistened with water gets dry much sooner than when bathed with the natural fluids of the mouth. In many cases you will find glycerine and water, in the proportion of one part to five or six, more effective than pure water. A little lemon-juice may be added to make the mixture more palatable, and sometimes you will find that linseed tea with glycerine will be better than water.

If the mouth becomes very dry, articulation will be difficult or impossible. No one can speak properly if his mouth and tongue lose their ordinary moist condition, and you may have noticed that many orators who are accustomed to address audiences for a considerable period of time are obliged to sip water every now and then. In perfect health the quantity of saliva that flows into the mouth varies remarkably at different times, and the proportion is diminished in any little derangement of the system. The mouth feels more or less dry and uncomfortable until the free secretion of the salivary fluid is resumed. Some speakers are seen to take a few drops of fluid every four or five minutes, and I much fear that in some of these cases the dry state of the mucous membrane has resulted from the introduction during a long period of time of too much alcohol into the system, a practice which soon causes most important changes in the blood, and eventually leads to impairment of the action of the most important of the secreting glands.

Of Exciting the Flow of Saliva.—In many cases in which the secretion of saliva is deficient, the increased action of the salivary glands may be excited in a very simple manner. Anything which promotes the flow of saliva, and induces the glands of the mouth to secrete more freely, will, to some extent, relieve a dry state of the mouth and tongue. Commonly, the mere irritation, stimulation, or excitation of the sensitive nerve-fibres spread out beneath the epithelium of the mucous membrane of the mouth, brought about by the contact of some pungent or acid material, is sufficient to cause a very free salivary secretion. A small piece of lemon just placed in the mouth will often give rise to a very free flow of saliva; and there are various pungent materials which are introduced into the mouth for the very purpose. The mere moving about in the mouth of some solid body, such as a smooth pebble, will, through reflex action, promote the secretion of the saliva. The pebble acts upon the nerves, and an increased flow of saliva follows. This is owing not only to the expulsion of the secretion already formed, but to increased secretion of salivary fluid by the gland-cells.

Sialogogues.—We have many remedies which belong to the class of Sialogogues (σιαλον, saliva, and αγω, I expel). *Horse-radish,—Mezereum, —Ginger,—Pyrethrum*, the root of *Anacyclus Pyrethrum*, the old *Pelletory of Spain*, are examples of well-known sialogogues. But there is one better known to most of you, though its use as a sialogogue is in these days almost entirely limited to some of the nautical people—I mean *tobacco*, which if used at all should be smoked, not chewed, and smoked only in moderation, and in the open air.

Certain salts also excite the secretion of the salivary glands. *Chlorate of Potash (Dose,* twenty grains in water) and *Nitrate of Potash (Dose,* five to twenty grains dissolved in a wineglassful of water) are among the best. Sucking *fused nitre* (nitre balls) is an old and very favorite treatment for many slight ailments.

You may now get *Nitrate of Potash,* generally known as *Nitre, Chlorate of Potash, Bicarbonate of Potash and Soda,* and a number of other useful saline remedies, compressed into small lozenges or pilules containing five grains each. One or two may be allowed to slowly dissolve in the mouth three or four times a day, half an hour or more after a meal, and you will find they will cause a very free flow of saliva. When the mouth becomes very dry at night, it is a good plan for the sufferer to sip now and then a little cold *Linseed tea* (one tablespoonful of *Linseed* infused with a pint of boiling water; when cold the seeds may be strained off and a little sugar added). Or the viscid fluid may be flavored with lemon juice, and sweetened with glycerine in cases in which it is not desirable to give sugar. Or, a mixture of the latter with water,—one of glycerine to five or six of water may be used.

But the most important and most potent of all our medicines used for increasing the action of the salivary, and most if not all other glands in the body, is Mercury. You will find when you have to prescribe for a dry, uncomfortable state of the mouth, that if you give only half a grain of calomel, or even considerably less than this, within five or six hours a free secretion of the saliva into the mouth will occur, and the mucous membrane of the mouth, fauces, and neighboring parts will become moist and more comfortable. All the little labial and buccal glands will secrete more freely. Instead of *Calomel,* you may give one or two grains of *blue pill* or *gray powder.* The last (*Hydrargyrum cum Cretâ*) is the mildest, and perhaps the best, of all the mercurial preparations we use. In children's ailments it is one of the most efficient remedies handed down to us. In the days of my apprenticeship, we used to keep equal parts of powdered *Rhubarb* and *Hydrargyrum cum Cretâ* already mixed, and gave from one to six grains of the mixture to children, according to age. I continue to use this most useful prescription. The only objection is its nastiness, even in jam; but for older children and adults the powder may be made into pills with a little *Extract of Henbane.*

White Moist Furred Tongue.—In some conditions the tongue presents a very peculiar appearance, being very white in consequence of the accumulation of a quantity of soft moist epithelium on its surface, with mucus and secretions from some small glands, with multitudes of bacteria, fungi, and the *débris* of food. This state of tongue is seen in its most remarkable degree of manifestation in acute rheumatism.

6

Unfortunately, we have many opportunities of studying the tongue in this serious malady in the wards of our hospital, which often contains several well-marked cases of the disease.

I do not know anything you can do in the hospital tolerably early in your student days, that will be of more real use to you afterwards, than making observations upon the characters of the tongue in different forms of disease. I strongly advise you, with the permission of the house physician, to go into the wards when he makes his visits, and institute a careful examination of the tongue in several well-marked cases of disease. Describe what you see, and repeat the observations on each case every day or every other day. It is better not to undertake more than two or three cases at one time. Make microscopic examinations of the fur every now and then, and keep careful records and drawings of the results. From time to time you will notice how frequently improvement in the state of the patient coincides with, or is just preceded by, satisfactory changes in the state of the tongue. Of course you will meet with exceptions, and you will easily find cases which might be adduced in favor of the opinion that the appearances of the tongue are so variable and so uncertain that nothing of importance clinically is to be gained by taking note of the state of the organ. To rely exclusively on changes in the tongue would undoubtedly be unwise and misleading, but I think not more so than it would be to observe exclusively other individual signs and symptoms of disease. We do gain important information from the tongue, and I strongly advise you to study the changes which occur in its appearances.

Pale Tongue, Anæmia (α, priv., αἷμα, blood, literally bloodlessness). In anæmia the blood is poor and defective in red blood-corpuscles. In *anæmic* persons, and in those suffering from various forms of disturbed digestion, the tongue is flabby, the vessels being imperfectly filled with blood, and the blood itself poor in red corpuscles. The dorsum of the tongue appears pallid, and a quantity of moist epithelium adheres to its surface. The tongue itself is sometimes visibly larger, swollen or sodden, œdematous (οἴδημα, from οἰδέω, to swell), as well as soft and flabby. The edges are much indented and marked with impressions of the teeth. This state of tongue improves under the influence of quinine and other tonics, and other remedies which improve the digestive power of the stomach.

In Slight Chronic Rheumatism (Rheuma, ῥέω, to flow) the tongue is frequently white, covered with what we call a thick, blankety fur. The white furred tongue is more moist than is the organ in the normal healthy state; its epithelium is abundant and sodden, and everywhere invaded by fungi. Numerous low organisms are actually growing and multiplying very rapidly in the moist, soft, imperfectly-formed epithelium which continues to be developed and to accumulate while the rheumatic state lasts. Various organic matters also collect, and decomposition may take place in the spongy mass, which is formed in such great abundance. The various fluids of the mouth also contribute to increase the thickness of the white fur so characteristic of the disease.

In many temporary derangements of the stomach and bowels we also find this moist furred condition of the tongue, and it may last for a few days at a time. The tongue of inveterate smokers is generally white and dirty. Some persons constantly have a foul tongue, although they are nevertheless in good health. A constantly dirty tongue, like some other departures from the normal state, is not incompatible with considerable vigor, good working power, and longevity.

Bright Red Tongue.—In striking contrast with the white blankety tongue is the red tongue, which is met with in certain forms of fever, the surface being smooth, of a bright red color, sometimes appearing raw, and not unfrequently being dry and glazed. The red tongue is often seen in scarlet-fever. In the early stage of the disease the tongue is often furred, and the red fungiform papillæ are seen to project through the adherent epithelium, and appear as bright red spots. But in a few days the superficial layers of epithelium of the tongue and of the lining membrane of the mouth and fauces are detached, desquamate (*de*, from, *squama*, a scale), and then the whole surface of the tongue is red. The fungiform papillæ are swollen and the vessels much distended, the surface more or less uneven, and we have the appearance somewhat resembling that of a strawberry—hence, *the strawberry tongue.*

The smoothness and redness of the tongue last for some time, for the old cells of epithelium having been completely detached, some time must elapse before the new cells have sufficiently accumulated to prevent the red color of the blood being so distinctly seen in the vessels beneath. The raw, beefy character of the tongue is also observed towards the close of many exhausting diseases, as phthisis (φθίνω, to corrupt), and some forms of pyæmia. Aphthous sores also form sometimes in conjunction with this state of the tongue, and must be treated as described in page 66.

The Dry Brown Tongue.—Strictly speaking, the dry brown tongue is hardly ever seen in slight ailments, and I shall only say a few words about it here for convenience' sake. Do not forget that a state of tongue somewhat resembling it may result from sucking liquorice, black currants, or black cherries; and other dark fruits may produce temporary staining of the tongue. These give to it a very peculiar appearance which you ought to be able to recognize at once, and it is well also to bear in mind that the juices of some fruits, or other fluids having the property of staining the tongue or skin, are sometimes applied, in order to puzzle us.

In typhus and typhoid fever, and many other low conditions, the tongue may become brown or more or less black, owing to changes occurring in the epithelium, which, with mucus and secretions from various glands, has accumulated upon its surface and has got dry. If the feverish condition reaches any considerable degree of intensity, as I have already told you, the moist surfaces about the mouth soon become very dry and cease to secrete. They are no longer bathed with healthy moisture, the mucus is no longer formed, and the secretion of the salivary and other glands is diminished to such an extent as to render the process of deglutition (the swallowing of the food) extremely difficult. This is one of the reasons why we give patients suffering from fever, milk and beef-tea, and put them on slop diet. All the nutrient matter required should be introduced in actual solution, or in a very moist state, as in the form of pap ; or you may have finely divided solid matter suspended in beef-tea, soup, or milk, and thus much nutritious matter may be given in cases where it is absolutely required to support life. In milk, as you are probably aware, some nutrient materials are dissolved, while fatty matter exists as very minute globules suspended in the fluid, and therefore in a state in which it is very easily absorbed into the blood.

In many cases great relief will be afforded if the nurse will occasionally paint, as it were, the dry mucous membrane of the tongue and mouth with a little weak *glycerine and water* (one part to nine or ten of water) with a camel-hair brush. This is very necessary in some severe forms of fever in which the tongue and mouth get very dry and painful. After the tongue has been dry for several days, it is not unusual for deep fissures to form upon its surface, and these fissures sometimes go quite through the mucous membrane, and even reach the vessels and nerve-fibres in its substance. Escape of blood (hæmorrhage) frequently occurs, and the blood accumulates and helps to form the dry brown matter which adheres to the tongue. Sometimes much of the hæmoglobin of the blood is disintegrated while the blood circulates, and may make its way through the capillaries without rupture ; but more generally the blood escapes from the capillaries in the usual manner, in consequence of their over-distention and the formation of longitudinal rents or fissures in their walls. Unless sensation is previously numbed by the presence of morbid substances in the blood, the occurrence of the fissures is associated with much pain, discomfort, and distress.

The blood from the vessels and the viscid mucus which collects upon the tongue and lips, together form dark brown or black flaky masses (*sordes*, from the Latin, *sordes*, dirt, filth), which accumulate about the mouth and often firmly adhere to the surface of the teeth. These may sometimes be pulled off, but generally leave a raw and sore surface beneath.

The dry brown tongue passes by gradations into the black tongue, characteristic of some of the very worst forms of fevers which occurred in former days, and which are even now occasionally met with in the East. As the severity of the feverish state passes off, the tongue begins to clean, usually first at the edges. This "cleaning" results from the growth of new epithelium on the deep surface, and the detachment of the old cells with mucus, fungus growths, particles of food, and probably a little blood, which have been accumulating and have adhered to the surface during the illness. As convalescence approaches, all this is cast off. To prevent this altered and partly decomposed organic matter, *débris*, etc., being swallowed, the mouth should be frequently rinsed out with *Condy's fluid* and water (one teaspoonful to a tumbler of water), or a very weak *Solution of Sulphurous acid* (one part of the *Sulphurous acid, Acidum Sulphurosum* of the Pharmacopœia, to five or six parts of water), or of *Hyposulphite of Soda* (five grains to an ounce of water).

Hæmorrhage.—Just now I used the word hæmorrhage, and as this was, I think, the first time I have had to employ the term, it is desirable that I should explain its meaning, and tell you exactly what happens when *hæmorrhage* takes place. The word is derived from two Greek words, αἷμα, "blood," and ῥηγνύμι, "to break forth." Hæmorrhage means, therefore, a breaking forth of blood. In former days we used to be told that there was such a thing as the passage of blood corpuscles through closed membrane, through the walls of vessels, in some mysterious manner, without any rupture or solution of continuity in their walls. This was called *hæmorrhage by exhalation*, and in my student days the opinion was still entertained that red blood corpuscles might traverse a capillary wall by "exhalation." At an earlier period, the capillaries used to be spoken of as exhalant vessels, and their function was regarded by some as opposed to that of the absorbents.

Under certain circumstances blood corpuscles may pass through the thin walls of capillary vessels without the vessels being destroyed or permanently damaged. In all cases, however, an opening, it may be temporary only, in the vascular wall does exist. The capillary is not actually torn across, but when it becomes much distended by the accumulation of blood within it, the thin vascular walls are stretched and rendered very thin. Longitudinal rents or fissures result, through which the blood corpuscles, a few at a time, easily escape. When the pressure is relieved, the elastic wall of the vessel will contract, and the fissures close up, the capillary transmitting the blood as freely as it did before.

The term *Hæmorrhage*, then, is strictly correct, and always means the breaking forth of blood from a vessel, large or small.

Chronic Cracks and Fissures of the Tongue.—This state of tongue

is very common in persons who have long suffered from weak digestion.
The tongue is generally rather pale, quite moist, and from time to time
becomes covered with white fur, which is often distributed in patches.
The cracks are usually rather deep, very irregular in arrangement, and
differ much in number in different cases.   For the most part they are
permanent, but occasionally new ones form and the older ones increase
in depth.   The papillæ at the edges of the fissures occasionally become
sore.   Aphthous patches of irregular shapes may appear and increase in
size, extending often to the bottom of the fissures, and sometimes the
tongue becomes so sore that eating solid food is a painful process.   The
cracks may go on separating until a raw surface is exposed at the bottom.
This is often exquisitely painful ; and if any alcohol, pepper, or salt
substance is taken, the almost bare nerve fibres exposed in the fissures
are instantly affected.   Not unfrequently in such cases the pain and discomfort are so great that the patient is deterred from eating, and in consequence the general health suffers.   A moderate degree of the condition of tongue referred to is extremely common.   It does not usually
interfere with longevity or predispose to any more serious derangements.
Those who suffer in this way are obliged to be very careful in diet and
ought to live very moderately.   If they exceed in any way, digestion
becomes deranged, the tongue gets foul and very sore, and some days
must pass before the usual state of health returns.   In such cases the
bowels are sluggish, but you will generally find that mild purgatives only
in small doses can be borne.   Three or four grains of *compound rhubarb
pill*, two or three nights running, with perhaps a little *effervescing
citrate of ammonia*, soda or potash, or some such simple saline, three or
four times daily, will be of use, and expedite the return of the normal
state.   Carbolic acid lotion (one part to one hundred of water) is also
a good application, especially if the fissures are associated with the
presence of aphthous spots, with vegetable growths on the surface, but
the lotion is not a pleasant one to use.   See also page 71.

There is, however, another form of cracked tongue common enough
and very chronic, which is not to be cured in this simple manner.
There are cracks and fissures here and there, but in some situations the
surface is too smooth.   The appearance is such as to lead one to think
that, in the course of very slow pathological changes many of the
papillæ have undergone change, and have at last wasted and dis-
appeared, just as the villi of the small intestines do in certain forms of
disease.

The state of tongue which I am considering may last for years,
getting better and worse many times.   It is usually relieved, and in not
a few cases cured, by *Iodide of Potassium*.   The remedy must be taken
for two or three or more weeks at a time, then stopped for a short
period, and resumed again.   You may begin with two grains, and

gradually increase the dose to five or six grains three times daily, and it is a point to give it dissolved in as much as half a pint of water.

Some cases improve rapidly on *Iodide of Mercury.* You may order from the thirty-second to the sixteenth of a grain of the *Perchloride of Mercury,* that is, from thirty to sixty drops of the *Liquor Hydrargyri Perchloridi,* with five grains of *Iodide of Potassium,* and a little *Syrup of Ginger,* and perhaps twenty minims of *Battley's Liquor Cinchonæ,* in four ounces of water, an hour after food, twice or three times a day, for two or three weeks at a time. These cases, and especially if they are cured by the medicine I have recommended, are generally considered to result from syphilis, but I feel confident that all are not of this nature. It is a grave mistake to suppose that everything cured by mercury and iodide of potassium, or some other iodide, *must* be syphilitic in its nature and origin. These remedies are most useful in the treatment of many conditions which have nothing whatever to do with syphilis. Some who read these words will, however, assert that I am mistaken, and that in cases in which the patient had never had an attack of syphilis, the poison must have been introduced into the organism in some obscure and unknown manner, or that it got into the organism through its predecessors, one or more generations back. This is a mere dictum. It cannot be disproved, but it rests on no sound foundation of fact or observation, and I attach little importance to such assertions when they rest on authority only.

Changes in the Mucous Membrane of the Mouth and Fauces.— Associated with the changes taking place in the epithelial surface of the back of the tongue, we have in many cases, also, corresponding changes in the mucous membrane of the mouth, the palate, the fauces, and the throat. The mucous membrane of all these parts is continuous, and no wonder the different sections are sometimes affected in the same manner. The action, also, not uncommonly extends downward through the narrow chink of the *Glottis* (γλῶττα, the tongue) into the *Larynx* (Λάρυγξ, the larynx) and wind-pipe, or *trachea* (τραχύς, rough). The voice may become hoarse in consequence of the mucous membrane being swollen, dry, and otherwise altered. Not unfrequently this dryness extends to the *posterior nares,* and affects the mucous membrane at the back of the nose, giving rise to a very painful sensation, a slight degree of which most have experienced when an ordinary cold is about to come on.

If you look in the looking-glass at the back part of the widely opened mouth, when a cold is coming on, you may see the mucous membrane of a darker red than usual, and here and there it may appear glazed and dry. Not only so, but if you try a simple experiment you will discover that an important change has taken place in the sensitiveness of the

surface of the delicate mucous membrane of the soft palate.   In health
the slightest touch will excite movements of deglutition by reflex action,
but when the membrane is dry and sore, there is no such sudden
response, and contraction of the pharyngeal muscles (φάρυγξ, the throat)
follows very slowly, or does not occur at all.   You may touch the palate
firmly without any effort to swallow being excited.   This benumbed
state of the highly sensitive surface generally is only temporary, and
consequent upon the changes which have occurred just beneath the
epithelium, where extremely delicate afferent nerve fibrils are distributed
in immense numbers, but the condition may occur frequently, and some
persons are hardly ever free from some slight derangement of the
mucous membrane of the soft palate, fauces, and upper part of the
Pharynx (φάρυγξ, the throat).   In the treatment of this state of
things, inhalation of steam simple, or with a little ammonia or camphor,
is often of use.   Simple forms of apparatus are now made for the purpose.

Inhalers are now largely sold.   Many are made of china, and are so
arranged, that various volatile substances may be very easily inhaled
with the steam of warm water.   The latter alone often affords great
relief in irritable states of the mucous membrane of the throat and air
passages.

Bronchitis Kettle.—The air of the sick-room may be rendered moist
by arranging an ordinary kettle in such a manner that the steam comes
direct from the kettle-mouth into the room, instead of going up the
chimney.   The spout of the kettle may be lengthened by adding a foot
or more of tin tube, or the special bronchitis kettle made for the purpose may be used.

In derangements of the kind, the application of astringent substances
to the palate and fauces often affords relief.   You may apply with a
large camel-hair brush a little of the Glycerine of Tannic Acid, the Glycerinum Acidi Tannici, or a solution of Nitrate of Silver (five to ten grains
to the ounce of distilled water), three or four times daily.   A few
minutes after application the mouth should be gargled out with cold
water or salt and water (one teaspoonful or more to half a pint); but
the best plan of treating such affections, especially if they are chronic,
is the direct application of the astringent or other solution, in the form
of spray, as I will now describe.

Of the Use of Spray.—Of late years very many remedies have been
applied to parts about the mouth in the form of spray, and great advantage has resulted.   The practice was first employed in the treatment of
diseases of the larynx, and many very ingenious instruments have been
invented for the purpose of obtaining a cloud of watery vapor in a very
minute state of division.   Spray producers have of late been very much

simplified in structure, as well as rendered much more perfect. There are two principal forms of apparatus. One in which the "spray" consists of high pressure steam, a stream of water with the required substances dissolved in it, being minutely divided into spray by the steam as it issues from a tube communicating with a reservoir. The steam is obtained by boiling water in a strong copper boiler specially made for the purpose and heated by a spirit-lamp. In the other, the requisite degree of pressure required for sufficiently comminuting the liquid to be converted into spray is obtained by a little india-rubber ball bellows. Both forms may now be obtained of the surgical instrument makers for a few shillings, and are well adapted for use in the treatment of affections of the mucous membrane of the mouth, throat, nose, and larynx. The solution containing the material to be projected against the mucous membrane may be much stronger if the steam spray producer be used than if the air instrument be selected, because, in the first case, the solution converted into spray is diluted in strength by the steam which is used. Some of the best spray producers are those used by Professor Lister in surgical operations.

In cases of dryness of the mouth, tongue, and throat, water alone may be used in the form of spray, or water with the addition of one-tenth part of pure glycerine. *Alum* spray solution is a powerful astringent. Ten grains of *Alum* to the ounce of water is a good proportion. The same quantity of *Tannic Acid* may also be tried. The spray solution of *Carbolic Acid* may contain two grains to the ounce of water. Of *Chloride of Sodium*, that is common salt, from two to twenty grains or more to the ounce of water. *Chlorate of Potash* five to fifteen grains to the ounce. *Nitrate of Potash* solution may be used of the same strength. The spray solution of *Nitrate of Silver* should contain a grain to the ounce of distilled water.

You must be careful to filter the spray solution before you use it, and you must prevent dust from getting into it, as the fine tube of the spray producer is very easily obstructed by any small solid particle, and is cleaned with difficulty. I find it a good plan to cover the end of the tube which dips into the solution with a piece of muslin, which may be tied round it. In this way any solid particles which may be suspended in the fluid will be entirely prevented from entering the spray-tube at all. The spray instruments, the tubes of which are made of vulcanite, and which are worked by the hand, answer very well for ordinary purposes when five minutes' application two or three times a day is sufficient, but for more prolonged use a good steam apparatus is the best. Simple spray producers worked by the hand can be readily obtained. I think, as time goes on, we shall find that the spray method is well adapted for the treatment of certain forms of skin disease, and many other cases in which it is not used at present.   There is no difficulty whatever in the use of the spray producer, and the patient can be easily taught to use the apparatus himself.   For some time past I have had a large spray producer of the form used by Professor Lister in constant use.   It answers perfectly for many purposes, and I often employ it for disinfecting persons, clothes, or rooms.   When attending any case of contagious disease, I can expose every part of my clothes, as well as my hair and hands, to the action of a twenty or thirty per cent. solution of carbolic acid.   So quickly can the steam be generated that the whole process does not take more than ten minutes or a quarter of an hour.

Metallic and other Tastes in the Mouth.—Patients not unfrequently complain of very peculiar tastes in the mouth, described as metallic, salt, acid, sweet, bitter, and even fæcal (Fæx, dregs.)   The odorous matter of some putrid smells is unquestionably sometimes absorbed into the blood from the inspired air, and afterwards exhaled, the smell and taste of the breath remaining for many hours after the individual has left the neighborhood of the odoriferous matter.   In various derangements of the stomach the most peculiar tastes are experienced, and by patients are compared to the flavor of rancid butter, valerian, vinegar, and many other things.   Generally speaking, the symptoms complained of may be relieved by exciting the excreting organs.

Purgatives, especially small doses of *Calomel* or *Gray Powder* (one to three grains) repeated every third or fourth night for a fortnight or longer, usually afford relief.   *Exercise, free perspiration* in a warm bath, *Diuretics* and *Sudorifics* are also useful.

Thrush, Aphthæ,—Sores and Ulcers in the Mouth.—Sores of the mucous membrane of the mouth are exceedingly common.   These superficial sores are spoken of as *Aphthæ*, from the Greek ἅπτω, I inflame.   The derivation is not a very good one, for, although no doubt the aphthous spots are associated with inflammation, they are not caused by this process.   The meaning of this, like those of many other scientific terms, has changed as our knowledge has advanced.   Aphthæ are little superficial ulcer-like depressions, sometimes with infiltration and consequent thickening of the tissues around, which form upon the surface of the mucous membrane.   Sometimes the epithelium only seems to be affected, but more often the sore extends deeper, and damages the structure of the mucous membrane itself.   Aphthæ are extremely common in weak, ill-nourished infants, but are not unfrequently met with at all ages.   In advanced age the disease occurs, especially in those who have suffered from prolonged exhausting maladies.   In various forms of chronic phthisis, and in some forms of pyæmia, they are present, and may cause great discomfort to the patient.   It is difficult to explain precisely the changes which initiate the formation of aphthous sores, as, for example, those which are so frequently formed on the side of the tongue, just where the organ comes in contact with some tooth which is undergoing decay. The formation of a little painful ulcer is the result. Such ulcers very often affect the mucous membrane lining the lower lip, just where the orifice of a labial gland is situated. Upon examination, we find upon the aphthous spot a quantity of soft, moist material, which consists largely of epithelial *débris*, imbedded in and everywhere invaded by fungi, especially a form of *Oidium albicans*, in various stages of development.

Now it has been supposed that the fungi are the cause of the aphthæ. The spores of the fungi, it is said, grow and multiply on the surface of the mucous membrane, and thereby cause inflammation and ulceration of the surface. Secretion takes place and the epithelium becomes soft and spongy, and thus the growth and spread of the fungus is favored. The constituents of all organic secretions at the temperature of the body very soon undergo decomposition, and the germs being already present, fungi would soon develop, and would grow there and multiply. So that, instead of the fungi *causing* the disease, it is more probable that morbid actions on the surface of the mucous membrane give rise to changes favoring the development and the growth of the vegetable organism, and that in these prior changes the true origin of the disease is to be sought for. Fungi and their spores are, as I have said, invariably present, and their mere presence cannot possibly explain the development of the obstinate little ulcers which are now and then found in persons who are in good health, though they trouble such only for a very short time. I say in good health, but have little doubt that I use the term incorrectly, and though I cannot tell you the precise particulars in which the normal condition is departed from, the fact of the development of aphthæ is, I consider, proof that the person affected is not in perfect health. The affection is not purely local, and it is most probable that the occurrence of the spots in the mouth is preceded by, and intimately connected with, an altered state of the blood. These little aphthous ulcers are sometimes very difficult to get rid of, and of course a great number of *infallible* remedies have been discovered. Some of the most useful applications I will now refer to.

Treatment of Aphthæ.—Honey and borax, the *Mel Boracis* of the Pharmacopœia, is a well-known remedy for aphthæ, and is equally efficacious in children, adults, and old people. Chlorate of potash also seems to exert some influence. In the case of adults the best remedies are those which are known to chemically change the fluids upon the surface of the spots which favor the development of fungi, and upon which they live. *Tincture of Perchloride of Iron*, or the *Liquor Ferri Perchloridi* of the British Pharmacopœia, is a very potent local remedy.

It may be applied to the surface of the ulcer with a camel-hair brush. Dip the brush into the *Tincture of Perchloride of Iron*, and just touch the surface of the ulcer ; leave it for a moment or two, and then tell the patient to wash out his mouth with water. But it is better to mix the iron with glycerine. Equal parts of *pure Glycerine* and *Tincture* or *Solution of Perchloride of Iron* make a very valuable application. This may be applied, as I have recommended, with a camel-hair brush, or one teaspoonful may be mixed with half a tumbler of water or more, and the mixture used frequently (every two or three hours) as a gargle or as a wash for the mouth. The patient should rinse the mouth with a little tepid water afterwards, for the frequent application of iron without due care causes temporary discoloration of the teeth. The glycerine assists the adhesive properties of the solution, and the morbid changes taking place are interfered with, the low vegetable organisms destroyed, and healthy action is soon reëstablished.

Another very useful local remedy is *Nitrate of Silver*. The stick of fused nitrate of silver is lightly applied to the spots, or a strong solution (ten grains to an ounce of distilled water) may be applied with a brush every day until the cure is effected.

The *Thrush* of infants usually yields to increased care in feeding. A very mild laxative is sometimes required, and oftentimes a little lime-water mixed with the milk is of great use. A little of the *Mel Boracis* may be put into the infant's mouth from time to time. My friend, the Professor of the Diseases of Women and Children, will give you better advice on these matters than I can do, and I must not trench further upon his department.

Offensive Breath.—I will now briefly refer to a derangement which occurs sometimes in connection with deranged gland action, and which gives people extreme annoyance. This is the emission of a very offensive odorous compound in the breath. It comes partly from the glands connected with the upper part of the respiratory and alimentary mucous membrane of the mouth and throat, and partly probably from the blood as it traverses the pulmonary capillaries. Even the individual himself is greatly annoyed by the smell which he exhales.

The odor is not by any means the same in all cases, though I cannot tell whether chemical substances of different kinds are really produced. The odorous material is, I believe, however, formed in a great many cases by the glands of the mucous membrane of the air passages of the throat and of the mouth.   I think these glands secrete the material which ought to be removed in another form by excretory glands in other parts of the body, the action of which is much lessened or stopped in these cases.

As offensive breath depends upon the excretion of a peculiar organic matter from the system, in order to effectually get rid of the tendency you must try to render more active the process of secretion elsewhere. The offensive material may thus be got rid of by another channel. In fact we must endeavor to get it, or the material which yields it, separated from the blood by other glands, particularly those which discharge their secretion into a more convenient emunctory. You will generally find that if you excite the action of the ordinary glands, whose office it is to separate odoriferous compounds from the blood, and discharge them into the bowel, the disagreeable smell of the breath will soon cease. In short, if you can only excite the liver, the largest gland in the body, and the solitary and other excreting glands of the small and large intestines to a little increased action, and keep up the action for a time, the patient will cease to be vexed with the derangement. Sometimes he is afraid to go into society, or be much in the company of other people, for fear of annoying them, as much as he is himself annoyed by the smell and taste of the air he expires.

Acting upon this view, the first remedies to be tried in such cases will be purgatives, diuretics, sudorifics. In all cases antiseptic substances may be used to wash out the mouth frequently. *Charcoal Powder* mixed with water as a wash for the mouth. A teaspoonful of *Tincture* of *Myrrh* in half a tumbler of water is also a good wash. *Carbolic Acid* is useful in such cases. A weak solution of carbolic acid (one part to two hundred of water) may be taken internally, and the mouth may be rinsed out frequently with a stronger solution. Weak carbolic acid spray may also be tried (see p. 69). Condy's fluid is another useful remedy. The mouth may be washed out several times daily with a solution consisting of half a teaspoonful of the red Condy in a tumbler of water.

But to effect any lasting relief, you must be particularly careful to regulate the patient's diet. Many of those who suffer from trouble of this kind are too fond of rich sapid substances, and perhaps take too much beer or porter, and upon inquiry you will find perhaps that they habitually eat more than a not very vigorous stomach can properly digest. The excess of all the good things taken is imperfectly oxidized, and the chemical compounds formed clog the emunctories, and are in too considerable proportion to be got rid of by the various glands whose business it is to remove them from the body. Certain materials remain in the blood, and instead of being discharged from the bowels are eliminated in a crude form by the skin, by the glands of the mucous membrane, and in part by the lungs. Thus the expired air becomes contaminated. It is most important that people who suffer in this way should not overeat, should not take more of anything than is required for nutrition, and the work of the body. As a matter of fact, almost every one does eat more, and many very much more, than is required to keep the body in health. In some people, perhaps, in consequence of the liver being less active than it should be, the excess of food, instead of being excreted

7

in an altered form in the usual way by the solitary and other glands of the bowels, undergoes exceptional chemical change, and odoriferous compounds are formed in large amount, and persistently, to the patient's great distress. As I have suggested, the way to remedy this great annoyance is to encourage the more free action of the glands, whose ordinary office it is to separate this class of substances from the organism. Try and transfer the action from the surface of the gastric and respiratory mucous membrane to that of the large bowels.

For persons who have long suffered, besides giving occasional doses of calomel, blue pill, or gray powder, you must prescribe some mild, harmless purgative, and of this frequent doses may be taken. You must, in fact, take care that the bowels act freely, and that the excreting glands do their work efficiently.

Almost any purgative will have a good effect in many cases:— Different preparations of *Colocynth, Aloes, Podophyllin, Scammony, Rhubarb, Jalap, Senna*, have all been prescribed with benefit. Several other purgatives have been recommended by different authorities. As a general rule, it is better not to give large doses, as it is necessary not only to excite the action of the intestinal glands, but to keep it up—to help the glands from day to day to do their work—to give them just a little artificial stimulus, and no more. From three to five grains of the *Pilula Colocynthidis et Hyoscyami*, or the same amount of *Pilula Rhei Composita* may be ordered, or you may add half a grain or less of the *Extractum Aloes Barbadensis*, or one fifth or less of a grain of *Podophyllin* to half the quantity of either of the pills mentioned. At first the pill should be taken every night, or just before dinner ; and when it begins to act, every other day, or once in every three or four days. Our object is to so regulate the bowels as to cause a daily action. With some persons *Scammony* acts admirably. One or two grains of Resin of Scammony, *Scammoniæ Resina*, may be added to two or three of the *Compound Colocynth Pill*, which, as you know, contains a certain proportion. A patient of mine, who died at the age of ninety-five, had taken Scammony two or three times a week, for many years, with the greatest benefit ; but neither this nor Podophyllin, nor any purgative that I know of, acts equally well upon all. You must be well acquainted with a number of purgatives, and must be able to combine them in many ways. With this knowledge you will often be able to hit upon the right thing for particular patients. Our predecessors were more skilled in prescribing combinations of remedies than we are. There is not the smallest doubt that we may often succeed with a combination, although we may quite fail to effect the desired object with a single drug.

Use of Mercury.—Although I must not tire you with mentioning a multitude of remedies for a condition which sometimes resists all our efforts to relieve, there is yet one thing which, as already stated, is of the greatest service, if given with judgment and due care. This is mercury, which, as you know, has the credit, and deservedly, of acting specially on the liver, but which also causes increased action of most of the glands connected with the alimentary, and probably also the absorbent system. Mercury is one of the remedies upon which our forefathers relied more implicitly than we do. I think they often gave it too frequently and in unnecessarily large doses, but nowadays I think we err in an opposite direction, and some practitioners not only do not prescribe mercury in cases where immediate relief would follow its administration, but refuse to prescribe it altogether, and encourage the prejudice needlessly excited in the minds of patients against its use. Many a mother, who seems to be shocked at the very name of calomel, nevertheless frequently gives it to her darlings in some patent powder which she has used for years, and which she will tell you is a most excellent remedy for every complaint of infancy and childhood.

In many instances in which the patient suffers from offensive breath, with a dirty tongue, and a disagreeable taste in the mouth, and defective secretion of saliva, with perhaps slight nausea, and fulness or discomfort about the pit of the stomach, you may effect a cure and earn the gratitude of your patient by prescribing a few small doses of blue pill, gray powder, or calomel. The medicine should be given with a little rhubarb, compound colocynth pill, or some other purgative, every third or fourth night, three or four doses in all being ordered, though often one or two only will be required. With some persons, however, no compound of mercury will agree, and in these very exceptional cases you must employ other purgatives, and give various salines to act on the bowels, the liver, and kidneys, especially the *Nitrate of Potash, Potassæ Nitras*, and the *Chloride of Ammonium, Ammonii Chloridum;* five to ten grains of the first and twenty grains of the last, dissolved in two or three ounces of water on rising and on going to bed.

Impaired Appetite, Loss of Appetite.—Next let me say a few words about loss of appetite, a grievous complaint in the opinion of many people, who will tell you with dismay and astonishment that they have ceased to enjoy their food. They never feel hungry, and never eat with appetite. Sometimes this lack of inclination for food is due to the circumstance that the complainants ordinarily eat too frequently, and perhaps also eat too much. There is, however, unquestionably, a form of loss of appetite, or impaired appetite, concerning which you will be consulted from time to time. This ailment is learnedly known as *Anorexia*, the scientific term for loss of appetite, the word being derived from the Greek α, priv., ὀρεξις, appetite.

Loss of appetite in some cases is rather advantageous and conservative. Many a man who boasts of always enjoying an excellent appetite would be more fortunate if he lost it from time to time. It is in truth a misfortune to have too good an appetite unless you have great self-command; for the temptation to satisfy it is considerable, particularly in the case of those who are well off, and are obliged, owing to their social position, to keep good cooks. Many such persons are doomed to suffer, as they get older, from having eaten too much at an earlier period of life. He who wants to keep himself in a state of health must learn to care little about eating, and must not only sit down to his meals with an appetite, but will take care that he leaves off before he is satisfied.

Loss of appetite very frequently depends upon a state of the mucous membrane of the stomach approaching to inflammation. After chronic inflammation has existed for a considerable time, degeneration of the gastric glands and other tissues takes place, and, just as occurs sometimes in old age and after prolonged exhausting diseases, digestion becomes permanently weak, and in many such cases there is loss of appetite. In treating many of these cases, it is necessary to help digestion artificially, as I shall explain more fully in another lecture. But in persons whose stomach is fairly healthy, you will observe that anything which induces a state of the system in which the nerves become weak, great fatigue, over-much brain work, anxiety, mental emotions, fear, or joy may give rise to impaired appetite.

In cases in which the loss of appetite depends merely upon some temporary derangement of the mucous membrane of the stomach, many of the remedies useful in weak digestion will afford relief. *See* p. 101. Very often a change of diet for a few days will effect a cure. Advise the patient to take nothing but milk and beef-tea, with a little stale bread, or corn flour or lentil flour properly cooked. But where the loss of appetite depends upon undue wear and tear of the nervous system and is associated with mental depression, general weakness, inability to exert body or mind, a thorough change is required—a complete alteration in the general habits of life, an abandonment for a time of the general daily routine whatever it may be. Some of the cases in which the appetite becomes gradually reduced, or completely lost, are very curious and difficult to relieve. They occur commonly in the so-called hysterical *diathesis* (disposition, constitution, from δια and τιθημι, I place, I dispose). In many instances there certainly is no structural alteration either in the stomach or in any part of the nervous system. The affection is no doubt due to some deranged nerve action, which lasts for a time and then passes off without leaving any actual lesion. Hysterical (ὑστέρα, the uterus, because the condition is often associated with uterine derangement) girls and women are very apt to lose their appetite for a time. At first having little desire to eat, they yield to the impulse, and gradually bring themselves to refuse all ordinary food. If pampered and pitied and regarded as interesting objects, they become worse and soon glory in refusing to eat. Occasionally we do meet with people in a state almost of starvation in consequence of having given way to this feeling of want of appetite. From there being no desire for food there is soon acquired an actual distaste, dislike, aversion. People often tell us that the mere smell of food at once causes all desire for it to disappear. There may be danger of actual starvation if the patient is not managed with judgment; but in such cases, when a fatal result occurs, death more commonly depends, not upon actual inanition, but upon the development of some intercurrent malady when the body is in an excessively weak and exhausted state.

Some of those remarkable "fasting" celebrities have commenced by degrees as above suggested. The fasting tendency has developed itself after loss of appetite, occasioned by a weak state of the digestive process, due to imperfect action of the secreting glands of the mucous membrane of the stomach, or of the nerves which excite these glands to form and discharge their secretion, and which has existed for some time. Fasting becomes a passion. The patients are pitied and patronized by the people about them, who humor them in every conceivable way, and encourage them in the belief that they are peculiar beings, who, unlike common folk, can actually live without eating. This gradually leads on to deceiving. They systematically refuse anything that is brought to them, and are soon looked upon as mysterious persons. Most of them surreptitiously obtain a little, and in this way may live in a weak, emaciated state for a great length of time. They lose weight very slowly, and then become stationary, which fact of itself is proof that nourishment is somehow introduced into the body. An excellent account of one of the most remarkable of these cases, together with much matter of importance in connection with the general subject of starvation, has been published by my friend Dr. Robert Fowler, who investigated the evidence in the most thorough manner. I strongly recommend all who are interested in the physiological, moral, and legal aspects of fasting cases, to study " A Complete History of the Case of the Welsh Fasting Girl (Sarah Jacob), with Comments thereon; and Observations on Death from Starvation," by Robert Fowler, M.D.

Voracious Appetite.—Occasionally we are consulted about an inordinate appetite. The patient is never satisfied. He eats a pound of beefsteak or more, and stills feels hungry. In some persons this great desire for food can hardly be considered as a disease or even an ailment. Children are occasionally the subjects of it. No doubt the state is often induced by injudicious management.

Remarkable voracity is, however, not uncommonly associated with morbid states. In certain forms of mental disease it is a prominent symptom, and in *Diabetes* (δια, through, and βαίνω, I pass), a condition characterized by the formation and elimination of an enormous quantity

7 *

of sugar from the system, the appetite is very frequently, but by no means constantly, enormous. Many a diabetic can consume one pound, or even two pounds, of rump steak at a sitting, and, what is more remarkable, thoroughly digest it. Children and adults who suffer from worms have often a very large appetite, and it will be well for you to bear in mind this circumstance. Get rid of the worms and the child again eats moderately.

Inordinate appetite is spoken of as Bulimia. This word, like many others I have referred to, is derived from the Greek. You must have been struck with the great number of medical terms, and particularly the names of diseases, which are Greek. Those among you who have been taught Greek at school enjoy an advantage over those who are ignorant of it, inasmuch as the meaning of a vast number of words will be at once apparent. It is somewhat unfortunate for all who are going into the profession that for some time past there should have been a dead set against Greek, for no one can learn Medicine without at the same time learning the meaning of a number of Greek words. The word *Bulimia*, I learn, comes from βοῦς, an ox, or βοῦ, the augmentative particle, and λιμός, hunger. Bulimia, or voracious appetite, is a condition which I suppose may be due to a very irritable state of the nerves of the stomach. Not unfrequently the affection is associated with vomiting, the stomach rejecting its contents as soon as they have accumulated up to a certain point.

The voracious appetite, as we see it existing in children and young people, usually comes from undue encouragement. The greater the desire for food the more food the individual eats, and so he goes on until he succeeds in consuming several times as much food as his system requires. Thus is thrown upon important organs the task of eliminating a quantity of useless material which ought not to have been taken. Sad mistakes are frequently made by parents in this matter. A child perhaps is rather thin, and therefore encouraged to stuff, and by degrees the habit of taking enormous quantities of food is acquired, with the not uncommon result to the patient of getting thinner, instead of gaining in weight.

Many of the railway navigators, and very strong laborers who have heavy work to perform, suffer from this affection, in consequence partly of yielding to desires which their high wages enable them to gratify, and partly because they act upon the generally received theory propounded by some popular philosophers, that the more you consume in the way of food the more work will your machinery perform—a principle which may to slight extent apply to machines, but is altogether inapplicable to any form of living organism, and very inaccurate as regards the work performed by man, for oftentimes the man who works the hardest and does the most is he who eats very little. The railway navigators are fine, strong men, many from 5 feet 10 to 6 feet high, and some of them certainly do consume an enormous amount of animal food, probably three times as much as is required for the performance of their work, and very much more than would be a most liberal allowance for them. The excess, of course, must be somehow excreted, and before it can be excreted, must be acted upon by the secretions of various organs, especially the liver. This and many other glands in the body are thus called upon to do an excess of work, and, as a general rule, they get damaged by over action, before the man reaches the age of forty, and in not a few cases the organs completely break down from overstrain, passing into various states of disease which soon lead to death. Indeed, we seldom see one of these men as old as forty. The great majority break down before that age is attained. The model navvy has unquestionably to work very hard indeed. His wages depend upon the amount he can lift, and the rapidity with which he can move heavy weights, so that he is encouraged to exert himself to the utmost. The more work he can do in the time, the more money he earns. Like the popular philosopher, he adopts the absurd theory that the more he eats the more work he will be able to do, and unfortunately acts upon it, squandering his money in beef and beer that strain his organs of digestion, assimilation, and secretion, and ruin his health and shorten his life. There is no one to teach him better, so he acts upon unscientific dogmas, adopts the prejudices of his order, and follows his own inclinations.

If these men exercised common sense, and consumed about one-fourth of the food and beer many of them indulge in, they would have a chance of living to the ordinary period of life ; and if they did not do quite so much work in the time, they would work for many years longer. Many men who belong to the middle and upper working classes, and who have lived moderately, are often very strong and vigorous, and able to endure a considerable amount of bodily fatigue at the age of sixty-five or seventy, and there are many hard-workers who have passed the last age.

It need scarcely be said that, as regards the treatment of these cases of inordinate appetite, it is a matter of the first importance to carefully regulate the diet. Small doses (three to five minims) of Hydrocyanic or Prussic Acid, *Acidum Hydrocyanicum dilutum*, and fifteen or twenty grains of Carbonate of Soda in an ounce of water, half an hour before meals, is often useful. Liquor Potassæ, Bismuth, Tincture of Hop, Tincture of Henbane, and preparations of Opium given with caution in small doses, with several other medicines, may be prescribed to allay the feeling of hunger in cases in which it depends upon unusual irritability of the nerves of the stomach.

Nausea.—Some persons suffer frequently from nausea, and a most unpleasant sensation it is to experience. You must, however, take care to distinguish between *nausea* and vomiting—actual sickness. People often tell you they are often sick, although they never reject the contents of the stomach. This feeling of nausea is a very common one, and is met with in various degrees; sometimes being very slight, just a little qualmishness, which as often as not passes off soon after food is taken; sometimes so severe that the patient feels as if he must vomit. The nausea, perhaps, comes on as soon as he wakes, and lasts for some hours, and possibly may not entirely disappear for many days at a time. Nausea prevents people from eating, or at any rate makes them careless whether they eat or not, and entirely takes away what some people highly appreciate, the enjoyment of tasting, masticating, and swallowing food. There are, however, persons who, instead of always having a good appetite, hardly know what it is to feel hungry. They eat as a duty, but would quite as soon go without food. The feeling of being moderately hungry,—looking forward to and desiring food, undoubtedly is a pleasant sensation, especially if there is a prospect of its being gratified within a reasonable time.

Nausea may be brought on by very many circumstances. If you were to take but a 1-4th, or even the 1-6th, of a grain of *Tartar Emetic, Antimonium Tartaratum*, a drug much in vogue fifty years ago, but now seldom prescribed, you would soon learn what the feeling of nausea is like, if you had not already experienced nausea otherwise caused. Those who go a short journey by sea often suffer from nausea, or something worse. The very few among you who have never learned to smoke may easily study the phenomena of nausea, and will afterwards remember what is meant by the term if you smoke a portion of a cigar for the first time. If the feeling should be so unpleasant as to make you determine not to repeat the experiment, perhaps, upon the whole, it will be so much the better, for smoking wastes a great deal of time which might be better employed.

Slight nausea is no doubt dependent in the ordinary way upon a somewhat disturbed state of the mucous membrane of the stomach or a deranged condition of the liver, or upon both. The sensation may be relieved in many ways. Pepper and various pungent substances, which excite the secretion of the stomach, are often useful. Cayenne pepper and Curry powder are well known remedies. But nausea seems to be due in many cases to some slightly impeded circulation in the vessels of the mucous membrane of the stomach, and those of the liver. The latter gland is sometimes much enlarged in consequence of the large quantity of blood which accumulates in it. After a few days, especially if the patient rests, it regains its usual volume without having undergone any permanent alteration, and without being in any way damaged. Nausea, dependent upon temporary vascular congestion, may be removed by promoting a more free flow of blood through the vessels of these organs. A warm bath, or a Turkish bath, will very often effect a cure, particularly in the case of those whose habits are too sedentary. Plenty of fresh air, and but little food for a day or two, will sometimes alone cause the discomfort to cease. If these means fail, a mercurial purgative should be tried. See p. 75.

Many healthy persons who suffer from time to time from nausea depending upon over-sensitiveness of the stomach, liver, and other glands, discover not only how to cure themselves in a very simple way, but also how to keep themselves well. They find it necessary from time to time to give their stomachs rest for from twelve to twenty-four hours, and then they get well. The prejudice that exists against going without one's dinner now and then is really most absurd. An occasional fast is almost necessary for many who live even moderately well, and some, especially ladies who are little out of doors, and take little exercise, would be in much better health, and would feel in better spirits, stronger and more capable of moving about if they would not dine quite every day, as well as take a good lunch. It is also advantageous to take fish and no meat twice a week. People who suffer from nausea or biliousness and want of appetite,—and there are not a few who are habitually ailing in this way, who seldom indeed during a long life have felt really well,—often find out for themselves, or they are told by too officious friends, that a little alcohol just before a meal will give relief. Brandy, gin, bitters of various forms, pick-me-ups, etc., are taken for this purpose, and a worse system has never been carried out. That bad habit of taking now and then ginger brandy, cherry brandy, or the worse one of frequently imbibing strong sherry for relieving nausea, a sensation of hollowness, or faintness, or fulness, or all-overishness, or what not, has been the ruin of thousands. Having once acquired it, many find it far more difficult to give up this vicious practice than would be supposed.

Bad indeed is the fashion of taking just before dinner a small dose of brandy, or ginger brandy, or dry sherry, or some other strong alcoholic stimulant, just to excite the appetite in order that justice may be done to the repast—that is, that people may swallow more than is good for them, and more than they can easily digest. If a man cannot eat his dinner without first taking a stimulant, he had better go without it. He might wait a few hours, and then he would probably be able to take simple food without the help of condiments or stimulants. The habit of taking alcohol too frequently and too regularly often comes from this most objectionable practice of taking a little stimulant before dinner. The unfortunate person who is regarded as the "life of the party" cannot help himself, for he must be sprightly and entertaining from the beginning to the end of the feast.

Doctors are often accused of teaching and encouraging people to

F

"tipple," because in certain morbid conditions they have found it necessary to prescribe stimulating doses of alcohol. For one person, however, recommended to take alcohol by us, how many thousands who have never consulted a doctor in their lives, take it on other grounds,—take it because they like it, or because they see others take it, or because they like the sensation it produces? Many will admit that they began when they suffered from a "sinking sensation," or from nausea, or uneasiness about the stomach, and after having been troubled from time to time, discovered that the unpleasant feeling was invariably relieved if they swallowed a little brandy. The little brandy gradually increases in amount. Nausea and other unpleasant sensations instead of occurring once or twice in the day, occurred a great many times, and the victim will tell you that he was, after a time, obliged to resort to the remedy in order to do his work. Of those who allow themselves to act thus not a few become slaves to alcohol, and then a more deplorable phase is soon reached. They are no longer able to abstain, all self-command is lost, and the unfortunate people are no longer able to control themselves in any way, while few will submit to be influenced and controlled by others. This state may last for a time, and then a new and very remarkable phenomenon is occasionally developed. The intemperate individual abstains entirely, and hates alcohol even more than he loved it before. He despises himself, is overwhelmed with remorse. In a little time he gives up the *rôle* of sinner and adopts that of saint, and saint of the most despotic and uncompromising kind. For a long time he was quite unable to govern himself, but now he is determined to govern others, and in a very decided manner. He expresses virtuous indignation against all who take or sell or produce alcohol, and thinks it very hard that he is not able to punish every one who prefers wine to water, and who dares even to look at a stimulant. We have the curious spectacle of a very small minority who, by their own confession, for some time could not keep themselves within the bounds of reason, now seeking to impose their arbitrary veto upon the very large majority who have never had the slightest difficulty in either taking a little, much, or abstaining altogether, as seemed to be the best for their organisms at the time. With as much reason might power be given to convalescent lunatics to put all the sane people in straight waistcoats, or shut them up in padded rooms.

The unfortunate people who cannot taste a certain fluid without making themselves worse than animals, will sometimes come to you and crave advice. You may be of some use to them by ordering certain medicines which will act, to some extent, like alcohol, but which are not open to the objections pertaining to that substance. Ammonia is often of use. You may order a teaspoonful of Salvolatile, *Spiritus Ammoniæ Aromaticus*, with twice as much Compound Tincture of

Cardamoms, *Tinctura Cardamomi Composita*, in a wineglassful of
water every three or four hours, for a few days or a week.   Tincture of
Hop, *Tinctura Lupuli*, Tincture of Orange, *Tinctura Aurantii*, or Syrup
of Orange, *Syrupus Aurantii*, are good additions to improve the flavor
of the dose.

As regards medicines for the relief of nausea, you will find that from
one to three or four drops of *Hydrocyanic acid, Acidum Hydrocyanicum
dilutum*, in two tablespoonfuls of water, or with a little *Bicarbonate of
Soda* or *Potash*, or in half a tumbler of Soda or Potash water before
food, will be useful.   In some cases three or four drops of *Solution of
Ammonia, Liquor Ammoniæ*, in a wineglassful of water, when the feeling of nausea is most troublesome, may cure the ailment.   A small dose
of blue pill or calomel will sometimes cure very obstinate nausea,
although many other remedies may have failed.   In not a few instances
counter-irritation is also of use.   A mustard poultice may be applied
over the region of the stomach and liver for twenty minutes every third
or fourth day.   Or a wet rag, covered with oiled silk, or a piece of
Spongio-piline, wetted with warm water, and worn for an hour or two,
will frequently be found efficacious.   See also the treatment of Indigestion, p. 97.

Thirst.—It is probable that thirst is less dependent on the state of
the stomach than is the feeling of hunger, though it is quite true that
thirst may be excited by Cayenne pepper, and irritating matters introduced into the stomach.   It often occurs in connection with certain
forms of indigestion, and is almost always experienced an hour or two
after a good meal, during which little fluid has been taken.   The fact
that thirst is relieved by injecting fluid into the blood, and by the
absorption of fluid from the general surface,—that it is present in all
febrile states, and comes on after diarrhœa, after the action of ordinary
purgatives, and after free perspiration, however excited,—would seem to
indicate that the feeling is somehow due to the reduction of water in the
blood.   The sensation of thirst seems to be experienced principally
in the back of the mouth and fauces.   Considering this part of the
mucous membrane very readily gets dry even in health, it is probable
that very fine nerve-fibres, close to the capillary network of wide
capillaries having an unusual number of bioplasts in their walls, are
afferent fibres, and take part in the initiation of the phenomena which
constitute what we know as thirst.   The capillaries and nerve-fibres
referred to in that part of the mucous membrane which covers the
convex surface of the epiglottis, and which is admirably situated for
the detection and registration of varying degrees of moisture of the
mucous membrane, are represented in pl. XCIII. of "How to Work
with the Microscope," 5th edition.

No rigid rules can be laid down as to the exact quantity of fluid that should be taken per diem, for the proper amount varies in individual cases. It should undoubtedly bear a certain relation to the solids taken, but in practice it is impossible to say precisely what this relation should be. One man finds he digests better, and feels better, if he takes from two to three pints of fluid daily. Another taking about the same amount of solid food or more, finds that half as much fluid suits him best. When in practice, you will find that some people are habitually taking too much to drink, and some too little. You will meet with cases of greatly impaired digestion, general weakness, and feeble health, evidently due to the habitual introduction of too much liquid with the food, the patients nevertheless always feeling thirsty. On the other hand, not a few persons complaining of muscular and nerve pains in various parts of the body, who are evidently suffering from a tendency to gouty and rheumatic affections, may be completely cured by a course of water-drinking, three or four pints or more of water being taken during the twenty-four hours. By ordering this plan to be continued for two or three weeks at a time, three or four times in the year, we may succeed in washing out the tissues thoroughly, and keeping them in a healthy condition.

INDIGESTION: ITS NATURE AND TREATMENT.

Indigestion—Dyspepsia.—Many lectures might be devoted to the consideration of dyspepsia, but I shall only attempt here to give you an imperfect outline of the subject, with a few suggestions concerning points of treatment which seem to me of some importance. The process of digestion, when it occurs naturally, goes on without the slightest disturbance, and without our being aware of what is taking place. Those of you who are in perfect health probably do not know, from any feelings you experience, that you possess such an organ as a stomach, with five and twenty feet or more of small intestine beyond it. Many come to study medicine without knowing what a stomach is like, until they see one in the dissecting-room, so little can we learn concerning the structure and action of our own organs from sensations experienced, or from the contemplation of what is going on in our bodies. But there are some unfortunate persons who, without being actually ill, hardly swallow anything without soon afterwards being made painfully conscious of the existence of their stomach, and its exact whereabouts. They cannot define its precise limits, but they very frequently suffer from uneasiness, or actual pain, which is referred to the neighborhood of the stomach, and seems to be situated in structures some distance beneath the surface of the skin. This discomfort usually comes on after taking food, but in certain forms of indigestion the pain precedes the introduction of solids or fluids, and when this is the case it may be relieved by food. When pain or uneasiness comes on some time after food has been taken it may continue as long as the process of digestion lasts, but then the pain subsides, and does not usually return until after the next meal has been taken. Indigestion is learnedly spoken of as dyspepsia, which comes from two Greek words, δὺς, with difficulty, and πέπτειν, to concoct or digest.

The pain or discomfort consequent upon slow or imperfect digestion, or indigestion, may be induced by many different circumstances. There may be some deranged action of the mucous membrane of the stomach, and hyper-sensitiveness (ὑπέρ, over, or above); or severe pain may be occasioned by an altered state of the circulation, caused directly or indirectly (by reflected action) influencing the nerves of the stomach. Very many times one comes across cases of what may be called ordinary indigestion, where there is no actual disease, but still where a troublesome and almost constant fixed pain, aching, heaviness, or sense of weight, or fulness, or of pressure is complained of, so wearying to the patient that it deters him from taking food. In consequence he gets thin and pale, and perhaps loses heart and becomes weak and despondent, and is much out of health.

If we could see the mucous membrane in many cases of indigestion, we should no doubt find it unduly vascular. There would be a state approaching to inflammation over a limited area only, possibly over a portion of mucous membrane not larger than a sixpence. Here the vessels would be seen distended, the blood moving very slowly along the capillary tubes, and some exudation from the vessels would very likely be found in the surrounding tissue. The nerves distributed to the mucous membrane would have undergone those changes which result in their being unduly excitable. Their bioplasts and those of all the tissues in the neighborhood would be found enlarged. Partly from this last circumstance, and partly from the pressure upon them exerted by the undue distention of the vessels, the sensitive nerve-fibres would transmit impressions of a painful character. The state of the mucous membrane I have just referred to may soon give place to the normal condition, or it may persist and lead on to a state of things which may result in the formation of an ulcer, the nature and symptoms of which disease I shall have to refer to in another part of my course.

Of Pain, and of the Arrangement of the Finest Nerve-fibres in the Stomach and Intestines.—The whole question of pain is one of great interest and importance, and as the pain in indigestion and other derangements of the digestive organs is experienced through the instrumentality of nerves which in the normal state transmit impressions only of which we are not cognizant, it will be worth while to consider the arrangement of the nerve-fibres concerned, and discuss their probable action. Nor can disorders of the intestinal canal be understood without the knowledge of the way in which healthy action is governed

8

and carried out. Although the bowels in every part are very freely supplied with nerve-fibres, so long as the functions are properly discharged we remain quite unconscious of the existence of any exquisitely sensitive tissues in connection with the alimentary canal. Fortunate are all who pass through life without discovering that sensitive nerves are distributed to the intestines. We know nothing of the changes taking place in the stomach and bowels until something interferes with their due performance. Then indeed we become aware of the contrast between ease and certain forms of dis-ease as it affects these wonderful structures.

The whole of the intestinal tissues are most abundantly supplied with nerves. You will find in some of the older anatomical books, descriptions given which would give you a very imperfect notion either of the number or arrangement of the nerve-fibres. In fact, the most important and most extensive portion of these nerve-fibres is known to few anatomists even now, and only a few years ago it would have been impossible for us to form a conception of the true arrangement of the nerve-fibres of the digestive tract, or of the actual phenomena going on during life in any part of it. All the tissues entering into the formation of every part of the intestinal canal are most abundantly supplied with very fine nerve-fibres, although you might read much that would lead you to infer that the mucous membrane and muscular coat of the stomach and intestines received very few nerves. It used to be supposed that the contraction of involuntary muscular tissue resulted from direct irritation or stimulation. And even now little attention is given to the highly important part played by the nerves and nerve-centres which influence every action and every movement connected with every part of the digestive process. In every part of the digestive apparatus, from the mouth to the anus, the secreting and absorbing as well as the muscular apparatus receives an abundant supply of nerve-fibres.

The muscular fibres which are distributed around the stomach and intestine, as well as those situated just beneath the mucous membrane, are frequently, though not constantly, in active movement, each fibre alternately shortening and lengthening—undergoing contraction and relaxation,—actions which occur at different times in different parts of the alimentary canal, and in all alternate probably, with comparatively long periods of rest or quiescence. But invariably the contraction of the muscular tissue, like that of every form of voluntary and involuntary muscle, takes place under the influence of the nerves.

Besides the nerves distributed in networks and plexuses to the mucous membrane and muscles in great number, there is a highly complex system of ganglia or nerve-centres little appreciated, and indeed hardly known to more than a few observers. You all know, of course, what multitudes of ganglia help to constitute the sympathetic system

Many of the large ones you see in the course of your work in the dissecting-room, and the more skilfully you dissect, the more ganglia will you find. You are also well aware of the complex interlacement of coarse nerve-fibres and trunks in many parts of the abdominal sympathetic system, but from the most perfect ordinary dissection that can be made, you will form but a very imperfect idea of the vast number of minute ganglia and ganglion cells connected with what seem to be excessively fine nerve threads.

If, now, from a piece of small intestine pinned out upon a strip of wood or cork, you will detach carefully the mucous membrane from the muscular coat, and soak it for a few days in equal parts of glycerine and water, replacing the solution from time to time with fresh fluid, and then gradually add stronger glycerine, you will find the tissue will assume a state favorable for the demonstration of the ganglia. Small pieces of the submucous tissue are to be snipped off, placed on a glass slide, and after being gently teased out with pins or needle points, and moistened with fresh glycerine, covered with thin glass. If you examine such a specimen under an inch object-glass, you will have no difficulty in demonstrating a vast network of ganglia and nerve-fibres. You will observe hundreds of little microscopic ganglia on different planes, and these you will discover are all connected with one another by numerous intercommunicating bundles of nerve-fibres, constituting quite a network or plexus of fibres and ganglia. The ganglia in question were discovered some years ago by Meissner; Auerbach had some years previously described plexuses and ganglia close to the muscular coat. But of course these observations were contradicted by some and ignored by others, and long papers were written by great authorities to prove that the nerves, ganglia, and plexuses were really vessels, the points of divergence of which, in their opinion, had been mistaken for ganglia. There is, however, no difficulty in demonstrating these ganglia most conclusively. I have many times shown in connection with the course of physiological anatomy which I used to give in this college, the cells composing them, with the bioplasm of the nerve-cells and fibres artificially stained with carmine, and I can assure you, with the greatest confidence, that the cells are true nerve-cells, and that fine nerve-fibres pass from them to supply with nerve-fibres the tissues of the mucous membrane, as well as the thick layers of muscular tissue which encircle the intestinal canal. So numerous are the fine nerve-fibres that there is not a portion of tissue the one five-hundredth of an inch in width which does not receive an abundant supply.

Every villus of the intestinal canal is supplied with nerve-fibres, and the action of each of its several component tissues is presided over by nerve-cells. Every gastric gland as well as every intestinal follicle is also abundantly supplied. Its structural connection with the nerve-fibres is a nerve-centre, or rather a group of ganglia by which nerve action is regulated, the changes resulting in the secretion of gastric juice and intestinal fluid governed, and actions emanating from other nerve-centres or groups harmonized. The nerves have also much to do with the simultaneous discharge of the secretion upon the surface of the mucous membrane from thousands of microscopic glands.

But in spite of this marvellous nerve supply, as long as things go on rightly, you are not cognizant of any of the changes which are taking place. The intestinal tube is sometimes full and distended, sometimes relaxed, sometimes contracted, and yet all these alterations in volume, all this stretching and contraction, take place for the most part without our knowing anything about it. If, however, these same phenomena occur in an exaggerated way, or if anything interferes with their due performance, we very soon become conscious that things are not as they should be. We cannot always say exactly what part of the intestine is in fault, or what sets of ganglia are disturbed in their action, but we experience discomfort if not actual pain, and almost instinctively we so act as to give the whole digestive system little to do. We let it rest for a time. We take no food or confine ourselves to small quantities of easily digested slops, and in the course of a short time things generally right themselves.

But surely it is very remarkable, seeing how unconscious we are in the healthy state, at least as far as feeling is concerned, of the existence of the intestinal canal, that when its action is much deranged, the pain experienced should be so very severe, and so difficult to bear, as is the particular pain which is developed at the peripheral distribution of the sympathetic nerve-fibres, the ordinary actions of which go on quietly and almost incessantly, but quite unconsciously.

The peritoneum (περί, around, and τείνω, to extend) or thin membrane external to the muscular coat of the intestine, which is supplied with nerves from these same ganglia, and which in the healthy state is always sliding smoothly in contact with the moistened surface of another layer of the same delicate tissue, becomes exquisitely sensitive in inflammation. The pain of peritonitis (περί, around, τείνω, to extend, and ιτης, rash, the suffix itis denoting inflammation) is one of the most terrible forms of pain that any human being can have to bear, and yet these same nerve-fibres which are concerned in the causation of most horrible suffering, act as a general rule quite unconsciously, do their work without our knowing anything of them, or of the action of the apparatus they govern.

Pain-conducting Nerve-fibres.—The nerve-fibres concerned in the transmission of the sensation we call pain, are not, I think, those which have been regarded as special sensitive nerves, but the fine fibres which were first demonstrated by me close to the capillary vessels, and so situated that any change in vascular turgescence would affect them. As is well known, the pain of a bad sore throat is much less severe than the pain experienced in pleurisy, pericarditis, or peritonitis, and yet the number of sensitive nerve-fibres distributed over a given area of tissue is many times greater in the mucous than in the serous membrane. When the tonsil is inflamed the pain is very great, but it depends less upon the tension of the mucous membrane covering it than upon stretching of the vessels and nerve-fibres in its substance. Again, the pain we suffer from in rheumatism originates in tissues which are rich neither in nerves nor vessels, and yet it is more severe than many kinds of pain, the seat of origin of which is in parts more highly vascular. The pain in the lungs when pulmonary capillaries are congested, even if they be seriously damaged, is slight as compared with that which results when the capillaries of the pleura are involved. Nerve-fibres of the same kind are not only distributed close to the capillaries, but in many tissues, as for instance the cornea, are situated at some distance from any vessel ; but these nerve-fibres belong to the same order as those distributed to capillaries, and act as afferent nerves to centres, the efferent nerves of which are distributed to the muscular fibres of the little arteries. It is, I believe, when these afferent fibres are made to act violently, that *pain* is experienced.

The pain associated with circumscribed inflammation of various kinds is due partly to the stretching and pressure to which the fibres of these nerves are subjected, and partly to the increased nutrition which proceeds in the nerve bioplasts, in consequence of the increased amount of nutrient pabulum which bathes them, and which has transuded through the vascular wall.

Gastrodynia.—If the vessels of even a small part of the mucous membrane of the stomach become unduly distended from any cause, discomfort results. If there is too much action of the glands or insufficient action, pain in the stomach, learnedly called *Gastrodynia* (γαστήρ, the stomach, and ὀδίνη, pain), or *Gastralgia* (ἄλγος, pain), is occasioned.

If the food we take does not digest, that is, if it does not gradually dissolve after it reaches the stomach, as it should do, but remains there, being moved round and round by the muscular action of the organ, we experience pain—and sometimes extreme pain. If you take rich, improper food, and drink a quantity of bad champagne, more especially if your dinner comprises tough beef and concludes with a good supply of heavy pudding or pastry, you will probably learn what is meant by an attack of *gastrodynia*, unless you happen to have an unusually vigorous digestion. You will at the same time be thoroughly convinced of the existence of a vast number of extremely sensitive nerves in connection with the walls of your stomach. Not only so, but in all probability the action of the whole intestinal canal will soon be violently disturbed, and you will be fortunate if you get off with a sharp attack of vomiting and

8 *

active diarrhœa : for in this way you may perhaps find a short cut to returning health. But thousands who eat moderately, and some even who eat immoderately, go on from year to year without the slightest discomfort of any kind in any part of the intestinal canal, and without discovering from any sensations they experience that they possess one.

Indigestion may be due to altered gastric juice, or to the secretion being too acid or not sufficiently acid ; or the active dissolving substance, the pepsin, may be in insufficient quantity or imperfectly formed ; or, on the other hand, the derangement may depend upon the pouring into the stomach of a considerable quantity of alkaline fluid, which probably neutralizes the action of the gastric juice, and in other ways impedes digestion and interferes with the changes taking place in the stomach. Strange to say, two fluids of opposite qualities are secreted by glands in different parts of the stomach.

Heartburn, Pyrosis, or Waterbrash.—There are certain glands at the cardiac extremity, near the point where the Œsophagus opens into the stomach, and called by some The Cardiac Glands, the secretion of which possesses an alkaline reaction. It seems that these glands in certain cases secrete a great quantity of a clear, somewhat viscid, alkaline fluid. Few of us are aware of the existence of the secretion of these cardiac glands in our own organisms, nor have we any actual experience of the formation of a fluid of the characters just mentioned. As is well known, the contents of the stomach, under ordinary circumstances, are extremely acid, and many suffer from the regurgitation from time to time of a small quantity of highly acid fluid into the pharynx, when its distinctly acid taste is experienced. Chalk or Magnesia is taken for the relief of the *Heartburn*, which, when physicians thought very much of hard words, was known as Ardor Ventriculi, or Cardialgia (καρδιαάλγος, pain). The acid fluid will effervesce freely if bicarbonate of potash or soda be added to it. A similar action occurs if chalk is mixed with it, but as it is more slow the effervescence is not so easily observed.

Some of the Dispensary patients of the Hospital will tell you that they frequently reject from the stomach a large quantity of clear liquid, which you will find will cause the blue color of reddened litmus to return. It is, therefore, of alkaline, not acid, reaction. This alkaline fluid is vomited or rejected in certain cases, which are termed *Waterbrash or Pyrosis* (πίρωσις, burning, from πῦρ, fire, *Fer Chaud* in French). The affection is very common in Scotland, and in England there are many old women who suffer from it. Patients sometimes bring us a few ounces or even half a pint or more of alkaline fluid. Sometimes they say the fluid burns them as it comes up. In other cases it is described as slightly salt, or mawkish, or tasteless. The secretion when very alkaline neutralizes the acid of the gastric juice if it is not rejected soon after its secretion, and greatly impairs the digestion of albuminous matters.

With regard to the acid which gives its reaction to the gastric juice. Although this consists principally of Hydrochloric acid, it must be borne in mind that it is by no means the only substance present having an acid reaction. We may divide the acids found in the stomach into two classes :—1. The acids formed or, at any rate, secreted there ; the acid of the gastric juice, probably hydrochloric acid, phosphoric acid, and lactic acid ; and, 2. Acids which are formed, and sometimes in large quantity, too, in the contents of the stomach, and which are detrimental to the process of ordinary digestion, and interfere with the conversion of albuminous matter into peptones. Valerianic and Acetic acids, Formic acid, Butyric acid, and a number of other organic acids, seem to be produced in cases in which digestion is much deranged ; and it is astonishing, when once these chemical changes have been initiated, with what persistence they continue, in spite of alterations in diet and various remedial measures.

Waterbrash is often difficult to cure. The diet must be carefully regulated, so that the work of the stomach may be uniformly the same for each meal. Purgatives, and especially preparations of Rhubarb, are often useful. Magnesia, Bismuth, and Ginger, and small doses of Opium have also been advocated. Astringents, such as Catechu and Kino, sometimes do good, and bitter infusions, particularly Calumba, have been given with advantage. Valerian, Assafœtida, and Galbanum are in the catalogue of medicines that may be prescribed in pyrosis, but I shall presently have to refer to the treatment of dyspepsia, and shall bring these and some other medicines under your notice.

In many of the cases of persistent Heartburn and Indigestion, too, much food has been taken and has been allowed to accumulate in the stomach. As it is not possible to neutralize organic acids which are formed by the decomposition of the food, without at the same time neutralizing the acid of the gastric juice, it is often useless to give alkalies. Sometimes, it is true, benefit does result from the use of this class of medicines. By more than neutralizing all the acids present, an increased secretion of gastric juice may be excited, but in many cases the pathological state persists, and in consequence of the continuance of the processes of fermentation and decomposition, fresh quantities of the organic acids referred to are set free. The patient gets thin, because the greater part of what he eats is resolved into compounds which fail to nourish him, many of which indeed cannot be absorbed. In the management of these cases an almost forgotten proceeding is obviously the right one. First, clear out the stomach. Give an emetic. Vomiting is the natural way of curing many cases where a quantity of unusual organic acids is formed. Any food undergoing chemical decomposition in the stomach, renders healthy digestion for a time impossible. The normal action of the stomach may become completely impeded, for decomposition may be excited in every form of nutrient matter introduced by the decomposing substances already present. People may suffer for months from a state of things which in former days would have been cured in a week or two by the aid of emetics and purgatives. Remember, then, that a patient may actually increase in weight if you cause him to reject the contents of his stomach once or twice a week. Clear out the stomach from time to time, put him on a carefully regulated diet for a week or two, and his sufferings will very soon cease.

Next, as to the emetic you should employ. *Warm water* will answer in many cases. You tell the patient to take two or three or more glasses of lukewarm water one after the other. The stomach gets distended, nausea is experienced, and in a few minutes the greatest relief is afforded by vomiting an amount of acid fermenting matter which astonishes the patient and convinces him that the proper treatment has been adopted. Some persons can vomit without even taking warm water, by a simple effort of the will; others have to tickle the fauces and the soft palate with the finger. *Mustard* also may be used to excite vomiting. A dessert-spoonful of the ordinary flour of mustard, mixed with half a pint of water, will make most persons sick in a very few minutes. *Ipecacuanha* is one of the least disagreeable of emetics. You suspend 20 grains of powdered Ipecacuanha in half a tumbler of water, and direct the patient to drink freely of lukewarm water afterwards. In the course of twenty minutes free vomiting will occur, and the whole of the contents of the stomach will be rejected without pain or discomfort. For a few hours after the emetic, the stomach may be allowed to rest. Perhaps some desire for food will be manifested, and then it will be found that the mucous membrane has resumed its normal condition, and that a supply of healthy gastric juice has been formed by the stomach glands.

Flatulence, Wind in the Stomach.—I must say a few words about flatulence or wind in the stomach—a somewhat disagreeable digestive derangement which depends in some cases upon unusual decomposition going on in the food, and in some cases probably upon the actual separation of gases from the blood, or their secretion into the stomach or other part of the alimentary canal by some of the glands of the mucous membrane. Some unfortunate persons seem to have a baneful predisposition to inflation, and are habitually troubled with an enormous quantity of gas in the stomach. The organ is invariably greatly distended, and I am sure, in some of the cases that have come under my notice, the stomach must have frequently contained two or three quarts of gas besides more solid contents, and this not now and then, but constantly for weeks or months, this state of distention being in fact the general condition.

It has been supposed that the peculiar knocks and taps characteristic of certain spiritual manifestations may be due to the movement of gas from one part of the stomach to another, or from the stomach into the intestines. But if in few instances these flatulent croakings are under the influence of spirits or take place in obedience to the will, there is no doubt that in the great majority of instances they occur in spite of the strongest voluntary efforts to restrain them. The gas is moved about in the stomach and intestinal canal by the action of the muscular fibres, and in the most capricious manner. Borborygmi ($\beta o \rho \beta o \rho v \zeta \omega$, I make a dull noise) are a serious annoyance, and on occasions a misfortune, as, for instance, when they trouble the sufferer in a select company during a pause in general conversation. It is a very common ailment, and people often complain that they have wind in the stomach or bowels, and much desire to be relieved. You must, therefore, pay attention to the matter, and study the circumstances favorable to the development of the unpleasant phenomenon, and the methods by the help of which you may be able to give relief. Sometimes by setting right the process of digestion, you may cure the patient. Pepsine alone continued for a week or two sometimes relieves. In very obstinate cases, occurring in people who live too freely, it may be necessary to begin with an emetic, followed up by a restricted diet for some weeks. Sometimes a single emetic will effect a complete cure.

Another very valuable remedial measure consists in purgation. You give a smart purge, say a three-grain *Calomel pill*, at night, and on the following morning a black draught or some *Sulphate* and *Carbonate* of *Magnesia* in *Peppermint water* with a little ginger. In this way the contents of the alimentary canal are got rid of. After careful dieting for a time the patient completely recovers. In not a few cases you may relieve these symptoms by mitigated starvation. Of course, if a patient came to you and you advised him to starve himself, you would never see him again. But there are many ways of inculcating good advice without shocking the nerves of sensitive people who suppose that abstinence from food for a few hours means death. Tell your patient not to take any solid food for a week. Order him a little beef-tea three times a day. Towards evening he may take with it a biscuit or a little dry toast. If very hungry you may permit him to have a little bread and butter, but a cup of lentil gruel will be better for him, and will be found more satisfying. By a little exercise of ingenuity you may suggest various things to take that will satisfy him, but which altogether will not amount to much. In this way, in the course of a few days, the effect desired will have been accomplished. You permit as little matter as possible to pass into the alimentary canal for a time. Some prefer to be ordered to have nothing but oatmeal or lentil gruel for a few days.   The last is a really valuable thing.   It is nutritious, satisfying, and acts as a sort of soothing poultice to the stomach and intestinal canal.   Tell the patient to live on this or on Revalenta Arabica if he prefers it for three or four days, and in this way you will probably get the action of the stomach and bowels right, and completely relieve all dyspeptic symptoms.   The flatus from which the patient had long been suffering will be no more generated.

General Observations on the Treatment of Ordinary Forms of Indigestion.—I shall not pretend to discuss this large subject exhaustively, but endeavor rather to direct your attention to some general remedial measures which you will find useful in your practice.   Sometimes there is actual discomfort when the stomach does not digest the food as rapidly as it ought to do.   The patient feels full and uneasy for several hours after a meal has been taken.   Very commonly under these circumstances sleep is disturbed, or perhaps cannot be obtained.   Those who dine too late in the evening often find that the stomach does not work well.   The food in consequence long remains in the organ in an undigested state.   It is being continually moved about and worked up by the unceasing contraction of the muscular coat of the stomach, but still its volume is but little changed, and the stomach remains much distended.   A feeling of general discomfort results, which interferes with sleep.   This, in fact, is a very common cause of wakefulness.   The patient in consequence soon becomes weak, feels fagged, and unable to work.   The sense of lassitude, and failure, and sometimes extreme despondency, suggests to him the need of "support."   Friends advise him to partake more freely of nutritious food.   Port wine, turtle and oxtail soup, and other highly nutritious delicacies are wasted upon him ; for instead of improving he gets worse, and feels more ill and unfit for business than ever.   Knowing the importance of rest he flies to soporifics, takes *Chlorodyne, Nepenthe,* or *Chloral* and thus possibly, in addition to his many troubles, experiences a terrible headache, tremor of muscles, general "nervousness" which never before troubled him, and dread of impending failure of health.   He tells you that he really feels very ill indeed.   But a few inquiries and a little consideration on your part enable you to afford speedy relief.   A mercurial purge, followed by a few doses of some gentle laxative, will soon cause all the more serious symptoms to disappear, and then you must attend to the digestive process.   Diet the patient carefully, only allowing easily digestible substances, and in very moderate quantity for a week.   A single purgative dose may not suffice.   You must bear in mind that in many of these cases the muscular action of the stomach and small intestines, or the sensitive surface which plays an important part in the reflex action, is at fault, and medicines which encourage the muscular contraction and the driving down of the intestinal contents may be required.   Castor oil, Rhubarb, iu powdei or in pills, Colocynth, Podophyllin, are often of great use in some of these cases; but as I shall have to consider their action under the head of purgatives, I need not say more here. Advise the patient to take small doses of Dilute Hydrochloric acid (fifteen or twenty drops, in two tablespoonfuls of water), half an hour before food, and his digestion will soon be restored. Hydrochloric acid is, as you know, the natural acid of the gastric juice, and if you continue to give it for some time, you will find great improvement, not only in the digestive power of the stomach, but in the performance of their function by other parts of the alimentary canal. You must not forget that from ten to twenty drops of this acid in water before meals is also of great use in treating very many cases of weak digestion. And *Acids* of various kinds are valuable in many forms of dyspepsia. The dilute Hydrochloric acid, *Acidum Hydrochloricum dilutum*, and the Nitro-hydrochloric acid, *Acidum Nitrohydrochloricum dilutum*, are most useful, and by their aid you may cure many a patient. There is more than one distinguished physician in London, whose reputation, it may almost be said, has been gained by ordering acids. There can be no doubt of the efficacy of these medicines. Phosphoric acid, the *Acidum Phosphoricum dilutum*, in doses of twenty drops in water, seems to suit some people better than the other mineral acids. Lactic acid has also been described; but upon the whole I think you will find the acids first mentioned very efficacious. If you give from fifteen to twenty minims of the dilute Nitro-hydro-chloric acid, with half a drachm of Tincture of Orange, *Tinctura Aurantii*, a like quantity of the Syrup of Lemon, *Syrupus Limonis*, and perhaps ten drops of Chloric Ether, *Spiritus Chloroformi*, with an ounce, or an ounce and a half of water,—you will prescribe a dose which will please your patients, and will be of great service to them. The mixture should be taken twenty minutes or half an hour before food twice or three times a day. In some cases it is well to add ten drops of Tincture of Ginger. I have known people continue a mixture of this sort for six or seven months at a time, and with great benefit. It is well to encourage them to give it up now and then for a week or so, but if they persist, it can do no harm, and may possibly deter them from indulging in alcohol. Lemon juice, Citric Acid, the Acid Tartrate of Potash, *Potassæ Tartras Acida*, and other organic acids and acid salts, have also been found of great use in the treatment of these cases.

If decomposition take place in some of the constituents of the food after it has been some time in the stomach, instead of the ordinary solvent action proceeding until complete solution is effected, as I have already said, a large quantity of fetid gas may be generated. In these cases you will sometimes find benefit will result from an opposite plan of treatment—from alkalies instead of acids. The alkali is usually given after food, but I have found that in some instances where gas is generated in quantity after food is taken, it is advantageous to give it about ten minutes before food. You may order twenty drops of Liquor Potassæ and ten drops of Tincture of Ginger in water. Sometimes you will find that five minims of Liquor Ammoniæ will answer better than the Liquor Potassæ. It is probable that the alkali acts by exciting the secretion of an excess of acid which at once exerts a solvent action upon the meat and allied substances. The condition we are speaking of may sometimes be relieved by taking a stimulant remedy which excites a free secretion of gastric juice, such as brandy, or ginger, or pepper, without giving alkali at all.

In some obstinate cases the plan of giving Hydrochloric acid before meals, and Carbonate of Soda, or Potash, or Liquor Potassæ, or Liquor Ammoniæ after meals, has succeeded after many other modes of treatment had completely failed. If I want to give an ordinary alkali, I often prescribe twenty grains or more of Bicarbonate of Soda, *Sodæ Bicarbonas,* in an ounce of water. You may order Peppermint, or Pimento, or Cinnamon water, *Aqua Menthæ Piperitæ, Aqua Pimentæ, Aqua Cinnamomi,* as you may think best, and you will find that two or three drops of Dilute Hydrocyanic Acid, *Acidum Hydrocyanicum dilutum,* and a few drops of Tincture of Ginger, *Tinctura Zingiberis,* will improve the dose. Some physicians prefer Bicarbonate of Potash, but Liquor Potassæ is, in my opinion, better than either, at least in many cases, and *Liquor Ammoniæ* may be of use in cases in which other alkaline remedies do not agree.

Preparations of Bismuth, too, are often very useful. You may order from five to twenty grains of the old Nitrate of Bismuth, *Bismuthi Subnitras* of our Pharmacopœia, or about the same quantity of the Carbonate of Bismuth, *Bismuthi Carbonas,* suspended in an ounce of water by the help of a little mucilage, and flavored with Ginger, Peppermint, or some such substance. Or you may choose one of the more elegant preparations of Bismuth, of which so many are now made. We have a solution of Citrate of Bismuth and Ammonia, *Liquor Bismuthi et Ammoniæ Citratis,* in the Pharmacopœia, which contains three grains of Oxide of Bismuth in a drachm, and of which a dose of from half a drachm to a drachm may be given in a diluted state. Many other solutions of Bismuth supposed to be improvements upon this have been recommended. Bismuth lozenges, *Trochisci* (τροχος, a wheel) *Bismuthi,* are also a convenient form in which to give this remedy.

Preparations of Iron, Arsenic, and Zinc in small doses are of value in some instances, and when the mucous membrane is unduly sensitive and irritable, you will find that small doses of Conium, Hyoscyamus, Morphia, or Opium will do more good than anything; but of these I shall have to speak in another place.

External applications are sometimes beneficial. Stimulating liniments may be gently rubbed on the skin over the region of the stomach. Sedative applications externally are also often recommended. A Belladonna or Opium plaster will cure some persons, while others derive more benefit from ordinary counter-irritants. A mustard poultice, a poultice consisting of equal parts of mustard flour and linseed meal, or a mustard leaf, a piece of wet writing paper being interposed between the mustard and the skin, is often tried with advantage. And you must not forget the very simple and efficacious measure of applying wet rag covered with oiled silk, or a piece of Spongio-piline, moistened and worn over the upper part of the abdomen for two or three hours daily. This is pleasant to wear. It is soothing, and often useful.

In cases of very obstinate flatulent indigestion accompanied by unpleasant explosions and croakings (Borborygmi), advantage may result from the use of pungent substances, like Horseradish, Peppers of various kinds, as well as Ginger. The Compound Spirits of Horse-radish, the *Spiritus Armoraciæ Compositus* of the Pharmacopœia, is not used now as it used to be; but it is well to bear it in mind, for it is a very useful preparation. You may order half a drachm or more in an alkaline or acid mixture, or with one of the preparations of bismuth above mentioned.

As to condiments generally, I would remark that if taken with judgment, and only occasionally, they do no harm, and most persons as they advance in years indulge in them more or less, but it is bad in many ways for a patient to get into the habit of taking very strong peppers, for after a time the stomach fails to work without its artificial stimulus, and may become very weak indeed. Unquestionably, as regards children and young people, we may be quite sure that " Fames condimentum optimum est; " but as we get older and gradually become more dominated by the customs indulged in by the more fortunate of our friends and approved by the rest, our appetite becomes less, and perhaps we almost forget what it is to feel hungry. We begin to appreciate delicate flavors, and to learn to like sauces. Sapid materials are desired, and often too freely indulged in, until we arrive at that high pitch of degradation, liking and longing for delicate viands,— desirous of dining daily, and giving our hearts to friends who are rich enough to possess a skilful cook and an extensive larder.

Few men are more injudicious in the management of their digestive organs than well-to-do Englishmen. Not a few who go to India and other hot climates, in defiance of reason, actually live as they have been accustomed to live here. They tell you they must daily have their good meat meal, or would certainly lose strength. They cannot digest as much meat as they like to swallow, so they get into the way of taking large quantities of pepper. Curry, which is a mixture of pungent seeds and peppers ground very fine, is very popular. No doubt it is appetizing, and the flavor of a well-made curry is certainly pleasant to the palate of most persons—even to those who have no pretension to be considered epicures, or good judges of delicacies. But this mixture, curry, has become a very favorite dish with Europeans who live in India and other hot climates on account of its stimulating action, and because it helps the stomach to digest a greater quantity of meat than could be properly dissolved and absorbed without its aid. Our system of dining off a number of rich meats, as many do day after day, is bad enough, and damaging to the organism in this cold, damp, changeable climate, but in the hot parts of the world the practice is disastrous. There, diet should be light, and should consist principally of vegetable matter. Too many consider that if they do not take much meat they must take much beer, and not a few will insist on damaging their stomachs with liqueurs or brandy and brandied wines. Derangement is soon followed by serious illness. The liver, kidneys, and all parts of the alimentary canal become highly congested, and weeks or months of rest and carefully regulated very moderate diet are necessary to gain for the patient a valetudinarian existence. Every one going to a hot climate should study physiology sufficiently to understand the importance of living according to reason, and the penalties that must be paid for indulgence. Let him draw conclusions from what he observes concerning the food of the people around him. He may take fruits and vegetables, farinaceous matter of various kinds, milk and eggs, and just meat enough to satisfy his prejudices in favor of that kind of food. But he will be very unwise if he allow himself to get into the way of constantly stimulating the gastric and other glands by strong peppers in order that the undue action required for the digestion of considerable quantities of meat may be established.

Those who come from a hot to a temperate or cold climate will do well to modify their diet. They should consume more butter, or cream, and milk than they would desire or find agreeable in a warm climate; the quantity of meat may be increased, and possibly some will find benefit from taking a little alcohol. Alcohol, though apparently desirable in the case of some persons living in cold climates, is very deleterious in hot ones. It is a remedy which is often employed in certain forms of dyspepsia, but it is a dangerous one. Drinking habits are easily acquired, and although a little alcohol will often remove discomfort and assist digestion, many find that after a time they cannot digest without it, and not only so, but gradually increasing doses are taken as they find the small ones fail to have the desired effect. It is far better to suffer slight indigestion and discomfort than by imbibing too much alcohol to run the risk of bringing on a worse form of dyspepsia due to structural changes in the stomach and liver, which lead to far wider and more serious morbid changes in various tissues.

Although in winter digestion is often very good, and not un-commonly weak stomachs work better in cold than they do in hot weather, there can be no doubt that some of the most obstinate forms of indigestion arise from the body not being sufficiently protected. Those who adopt light clothing in an ungenial climate are very likely to suffer, and I feel pretty confident that, next to injudicious eating and drinking, injudicious clothing is the commonest cause of various disorders, among which are some of the most serious we have to treat. The fear people express of being too thickly clad in this climate would be ludicrous if the consequences were not often so serious. The young of both sexes are the chief offenders in this particular, and many an attack of rheumatic fever, of bronchitis, of pneumonia, and of other serious maladies, has been due to light clothing. Now, although I admit that woollen material of the thickness suitable for those who live in such a climate as this, is uncomfortable, nay, disagreeable, for perhaps a fortnight or three weeks in some summers, I have never known any illness brought on by the practice. To be bathed in perspiration from morning to night and from night to morning is not pleasant, but neither is it dangerous, and it is better to endure such discomfort during our short summer than run the risk of taking cold in consequence of a change in the weather finding us insufficiently protected. Not a summer passes but we have to treat a number of cases of illness brought on by insufficient clothing, and among them will be a few cases of phthisis and other affections which after a time destroy life. Depend upon it, people had better clothe very warmly in winter and not change their clothing in the summer, than be insufficiently protected during the chilly days which occur even during the hottest period of the year. I should say woollen should be always worn next the skin by all, though in the hottest weather it may be somewhat thinner than in the winter. Of course you do find exceptional people who do not need this, just as you find people who eat and drink enormously without paying any penalty for their excesses; but we must advise persons as if they were average organisms—not remarkable exceptions. In strongly recommending a very decided additional protection to the delicate nerves and vessels of the skin to that afforded by the thin epidermis (ἐπί, upon, δέρμα, the skin), which forms a very essential and absolutely necessary part of us, I confess to one considerable difficulty, and this is to name the material which may be worn by every one without discomfort. It is curious that with all the ingenuity exhibited in the woollen manufacture no texture has yet been invented to wear next the skin which is wholly satisfactory and cheap. Nothing I believe is yet to be obtained better than good flannel, but it is practically difficult to get flannel garments made to fit comfortably; and unless great care be taken to shrink the flannel thoroughly before it is used, uncomfortable diminution in all directions will soon be manifest, and will progress to a degree which is most inconvenient. The ordinary woven goods are still worse in this respect, and those who purchase things to fit them find in the course of a few months that they are so small as to be unwearable. Nevertheless, you must advise your patients of both sexes to wear woollen of some kind next the skin. For the weak and sensitive this protection is absolutely necessary, and the strong and healthy will, by adopting this course, escape many small derangements. Wash leather has been recommended. It is comfortable, but too warm during the greater part of the year. Like silk, it is very expensive, and there are other objections to its use which I need not describe in detail. Upon the whole, as I have said, good soft flannel is probably the best texture yet made for wearing next the skin, but if people absolutely object to flannel, you must advise them to wear silk, or some very thin, unirritating material under the flannel. Those who wear woollen under-clothes may go out in all weathers, and will not require the very heavy and oppressive overcoats which are such an encumbrance in walking.

Indigestion from Failing Glands, as in Old Age.—But there are cases in which the stomach loses its power. The action becomes weaker. The glands require some artificial stimulus to excite them to discharge the proper amount of work. As we get older we become more particular as regards the flavor and other characters of what we eat and drink, and many cease to feel that desire for food, that pleasant feeling of hunger, which is worth more than perfection in cibo-critical powers. As a general rule, you notice that gentlemen over forty are more particular as regards their dinners than gentlemen of twenty-one, while even working-men of fifty or sixty years of age look upon a quiet good dinner as a very important and not unpleasant portion of the daily round of life. A boy or a young man in perfect health and vigor digests without knowing that he possesses digestive organs, but if the stomach becomes weak its owner gets particular, and the food he eats must be nicer as well as more digestible. And so it comes about that increased interest is taken in cookery, and the cook becomes a person of the highest consequence. In old age the stomach often becomes so weak that only certain well-cooked and very delicate things can be digested. Sometimes the stomach fails altogether, and we have to adopt various expedients in feeding, if we are to succeed in keeping old patients alive.

You must also bear in mind that a very common cause of indigestion in advanced age, and in but too many instances long before, is the failure to perform their office on the part of the natural comminutors of the food. The teeth, from defective formation and growth during the early period of life, have nearly worn away, or they have decayed, or perchance the gum has altered in structure and the teeth have dropped out. The consequence is that practically there is no proper mastication, the food is very imperfectly subdivided, and far too little saliva is mixed with it. Often it is bolted, and the large hard masses which reach the stomach cannot be properly acted upon. It is often necessary to ask a patient whether he is able to bite.

If, as sometimes happens, the food passes into the stomach in boluses of considerable size, but a small portion, in fact, only the surface of each mass can be subject to the action of the gastric juice, and if the meal is a large one, a very small portion only will be properly digested. The rest gradually passes onwards in a state not fit for absorption, or it remains in the stomach until the next meal is taken, and increases the confusion and disturbance. Do not forget that many cases of imperfect digestion depend upon the bad state of the teeth. If you do not find this out you may go on prescribing a number of useless remedies, to the disappointment of your patient and to the loss of your credit. There are people even under thirty who are incompetent, from a dental point of view. Happily the condition is a remediable one, and the new organs which can be supplied by art, are in some cases superior to those developed by nature operating under the sad disadvantages needlessly imposed by the ignorance and wickedness of man. A patient may be provided with artificial teeth which will work better than his own, though he may have to suffer some unpleasant twinges before his mouth is set right for mastication under the new circumstances. When, therefore, you are consulted about difficult or weak digestion, or indigestion, it is very necessary to examine the mouth with the view of ascertaining the general state of the teeth, and of determining whether the patient can or cannot properly masticate.

And now let me revert to those cases where the digestive power of the stomach becomes weak because the gastric glands have gradually wasted, and are perhaps shrivelled and incapable of secreting gastric juice either good in quality or sufficient in quantity. When one considers the immense quantity, amounting perhaps to ten or more pounds, of gastric juice formed during every period of twenty-four hours, one cannot wonder that the secretion should diminish as the vigor of life becomes impaired and reduced. As age advances the action of the gland-cells gets more feeble and the secretion is more slowly formed. The glands participate in the general shrinking and wasting and change into connective tissue, which goes on in other organs and interferes with the due discharge of their functions.

If digestion is impaired, the proper amount of nourishment absorbed will be less than is required, and persons who suffer for some time gradually become weak. The muscles lose their vigor and the tissues generally suffer. Much of their substance is absorbed, and in some cases there is considerable wasting. Patients frequently get perceptibly thinner,

9 *

and become unable to properly discharge their usual duties. In too many instances, in consequence of such phenomena going on for a considerable time, the organism loses its power of resistance to adverse circumstances, and the patient becomes liable to special morbid changes, affecting lungs, liver, or kidneys, and may suffer from intercurrent maladies, which may cut short life. A state of weak health may be engendered, the blood becoming much altered in quality; and not unfrequently morbid conditions are developed, which are known to be due to an unhealthy state of the circulating fluid. The blood may coagulate in capillary vessels and small veins; and in the changes resulting from the stagnation, substances are formed which, re-entering the blood, may poison or otherwise damage the system. In short, the most complex changes, and serious forms of disease, may be dependent upon long-continued imperfect action of the stomach and upper part of the bowels.

You may often improve digestion by giving those acids which I have before referred to. Even where there is a gouty tendency, and you would be disposed to prefer alkaline to acid remedies, you will not unfrequently find in practice that mineral acids before meals will greatly benefit the patient. In some of these gouty cases, in which many different plans of treatment have entirely failed, I have found advantage from giving mineral acids before, and a dose of alkali after, meals. You will also discover, in the course of your practice, that half a grain or a grain of Calomel, or two grains or less of Gray Powder (*Hydrargyrum cum Cretâ*) with three or four grains of compound Colocynth pill (*Pilula Colocynthidis Composita*) once or twice a week, will be of immense service in many cases where the liver is congested or sluggish, as well as the stomach out of order. The following mixture half an hour after breakfast, lunch, and dinner is often of great use to those who have any tendency to the state of system which precedes the development of gout. Fifteen or twenty minims of *Liquor Potassæ*, five grains of *Nitrate of Potash* (*Potassæ Nitras*), ten minims of *Tincture of Ginger* (*Tinctura Zingiberis*), a drachm of *Tincture of Hop* (*Tinctura Lupuli*) and one ounce of *water*. There is, however, one remedy which often succeeds in cases in which other plans of treatment have completely failed. The remedy to which I refer is Pepsine.

Of Pepsine and its Uses.—Pepsine has been introduced into medicine for some thirty years or more, but a certain number of medical advisers during every portion of this time have confidently pronounced it a worthless remedy, and one that, if it acts at all, acts by pleasing the fancy of the patient. Not a few have condemned it as a ridiculous thing altogether, as a substance that has no action whatever and does not relieve. But if pepsine were really useless, like hundreds of other things which have been introduced, become fashionable and fallen into disrepute, it would have been before this time entirely discarded, if not forgotten. But what is the fact? In spite of many adverse circumstances, pepsine is probably more used than ever, and is now made and prescribed in every part of the world. Many different preparations of pepsine are sold to the public. Some are extensively advertised and their value extolled in superlative expressions. Large sums of money must be annually devoted to the purchase of different preparations stated to be composed of pepsine. Some persons have no doubt found out that at least certain of these preparations are of real use. They speak highly of them to their friends, and thus the demand increases. At this time there is not only a vast number of different forms of pepsine to be had, but you may obtain the remedy in many different forms. There is pepsine in powder, pepsine in pills, pepsine in lozenges, pilules of pepsine, pepsine wine, and pepsine in glycerine. It is certain that a great number of people have found it of use to them. The demand thus created for a really valuable remedy has led to the supply, not only of the real thing, but to the production of a number of cheap and worthless substitutes. Some preparations indeed exist which have been proved to possess little or no solvent action. He who recommends pepsine, or takes it, ought to be quite sure that the material is really what it purports to be. Although it is very easy to adulterate this substance or to pass off something else in its stead, it is fortunately also very easy to ascertain whether the pepsine possesses the proper degree of digestive efficacy. One grain of good pepsine ought to thoroughly digest one hundred grains of boiled white of egg in three or four hours at a temperature of 100° F.

In order to test the value of any particular specimen of pepsine you may proceed as follows :—One hundred grains of hard-boiled white of egg cut into thin slices may be placed in a wide-mouthed bottle or flask with one ounce of water, and twenty drops of dilute hydrochloric acid (*Acidum Hydrochloricum dilutum*). One grain of pepsine powder is to be added, and the mixture placed before a fire, at a temperature of about 100° F. The flask is to be shaken from time to time. In about an hour the white of egg begins to look transparent at the edges, and in about four hours it will be completely dissolved if the pepsine is good. Pepsine will dissolve white of egg at ordinary temperatures if a longer time (from twelve to twenty-four hours) be allowed for the action.

Now, since less than one single grain of good pepsine will digest 100 grains of white egg, two or three grains ought to digest as much meat as would be found in the "eye" of a small mutton-chop. Three or four grains, therefore, of good pepsine is a sufficient dose, and will enable a patient to digest a small meal of meat even if the stomach secretes hardly any of the active substance, but, as a general rule, pepsine is only required to set the digestive process going, and probably much more than the amount of meat which an invalid would require would be dissolved by the dose of pepsine taken. You may obtain different preparations of pepsine and ascertain whether they really possess the power of digesting white of egg, and you may be sure that those preparations which will not artificially digest the albumen in the flask will not digest food in the stomach, and therefore ought not to be prescribed.

You may not only easily ascertain whether the pepsine you purchase is good or not, but if you choose to take a little trouble you may make your own pepsine. There is no difficulty or uncertainty in the process if a little care is taken. When I held the Professorship of Physiology and of General and Morbid Anatomy, I used to show to the class, as my predecessors had taught me to do, the action of the gastric juice upon different kinds of food. But we always found it most difficult to prepare a satisfactory digestive solution. We used to make an infusion by soaking for a time in tepid water pieces of the fourth or true digestive stomach of the calf. A little hydrochloric acid was then added, and the viscid mixture was strained through muslin. But it was often difficult to strain it properly, and at best we had a thick ropy mass which was by no means clear and transparent, and could not be made so by filtration. Many of the students of those days were sceptical, and probably concluded that I had carefully rounded off the edges of the albumen so as to make it appear as if digestion had commenced, and some were not satisfied that the viscid opalescent mixture really possessed the solvent action I attributed to it. I was, therefore, induced to try whether I could not obtain a digestive solution as clear as water, in which every stage of change occurring in substances placed in it could be watched from first to last. In my first attempts I followed the instructions given by scientific chemists, and after conducting a number of complex chemical operations, with the invariable result of losing the greater part of the pepsine I was in search of, from decomposition in the chemical operations to which the mixture was subjected, and finding that the processes for isolating the pepsine turned out so very unfortunately, I determined to try to find some new method of getting a clear solution possessing active digestive properties. As usually happens, after adopting somewhat complicated plans of proceeding, one slowly comes to adopt more and more simple methods, and at last an efficient plan which can be readily practised is perhaps discovered.

I taught myself to prepare an artificial digestive fluid by a process so simple and obvious that one wonders no one had employed it before, though up to the time I put it into practice, 1856–7, no one seems to have thought of the process. While considering the digestive process as carried out in different animals, it occurred to me that there was one domestic animal whose diet coincided more nearly with that of the human race than any other. The sheep and the ox were evidently less likely to possess a potent digestive material adapted for dissolving albuminous and allied substances than the pig. There is, I believe, no kind of animal food that the pig will not easily digest, and very quickly, too. A pig's diet contains animal as well as vegetable matter, and I need not tell you of the extraordinary quantity of nutritious substances of all kinds that a pig will consume and digest without difficulty. It seemed, therefore, not improbable that the best and strongest gastric juice would be found in the gastric glands of the stomach of the pig.

I procured some fresh pigs' stomachs, and, after having slit them open and removed the contents, I dissected the mucous membrane away from the muscular coat. This must be done, because the mucous membrane will be found in the stomach of the animal to be thrown up into a number of thick folds, and it is required to be laid out smoothly on a flat board. When the thick mucous membrane is thus spread out, a little water is allowed to run over it so as to remove much of the dirty mucus, and the remains of the food,—and pigs' food, as you well know, is not of the nicest character. You have then before you a soft, tolerably clean, smooth mucous membrane, which, in its entire thickness, consists of hundreds of thousands of pepsine-producing glands. But these gland-tubes are very minute. How are we to get the modicum of secretion which each contains? The mouths of the little glands, as is well known, open on the free surface of the mucous membrane. It occurred to me that, if I could only squeeze these glands, I might be able to press from the tube the active digestive substance which each contains, and before any chemical change of the nature of decomposition could even have commenced in it. I took a paper-knife, and by firmly scraping the surface in one direction, I succeeded in squeezing out the little drops of mucus from the gastric glands, without any difficulty whatever. In this way I sometimes obtained as much as three or four teaspoonfuls of thick viscid mucus from a single stomach. But this substance is not a very manageable material for experiment. It will not dissolve in water, though it may be diffused through it. The mixture will be very viscid, and it will not pass through filtering paper, while it very quickly passes into a state of decomposition. Few things could be less suitable for delicate experiments.

Having then obtained the potent material in the active state in which it exists, as formed in the body of the animal, I thought that, in order to prevent decomposition, the plan would be to dry it as soon as possible. I therefore spread the mucus in a very thin layer over the surface of a piece of clean glass about a foot square. The glass, with the mucus, was next quickly dried, at a temperature of 100°, before the fire, a current of air being allowed to play freely over it. In from twenty minutes to half an hour the mucus became perfectly dry, and could then be easily

scraped off the glass.   Being powdered in a mortar, it formed a tolerably
fine powder, which had scarcely any smell, but tasted a little salt.   If I
took a pinch of this dry mucus and mixed it with a little tepid water, I
no longer got a ropy mass, but a mixture which, by filtration, yielded a perfectly clear fluid.   You may, indeed, without difficulty, make a perfectly
clear acid infusion of the mucus from the pig's stomach, by adding to
the dried mucus and water a few drops of dilute hydrochloric acid.   You
will then have a very potent digestive fluid, which, after standing for an
hour or so with occasional stirring, will be found to readily pass through
the pores of the filter.   If all the operations have been successfully performed, the filtrate will be as clear as the purest water; indeed, you
would not from its appearance know it from water.   If you perform the
experiment with white of egg, as described in page 103, and place the flask
at a temperature of 100°, you will find that the clear solution possesses
active digestive properties.   You may try various experiments, for the
fluid being so clear you can watch the changes which take place, and
study the process of digestion with facility.

Having obtained this dried powder from the mucus secreted by the
gastric glands of the pig's stomach, and found that such excellent artificial digestive fluids could be easily prepared with its aid, it seemed
desirable to try it medicinally as an aid to digestion, as it was evidently
more efficient than many of the preparations of pepsine at that time in
vogue.   So I put it to the test in my own body, and swallowed some of
the dried powder.   It did me no harm.   Then I made some into three
grain pills, and took one before each meal for several successive days.
Infusions were prepared, which I drank, and no inconvenience whatever
resulted from their use.   After a time I prescribed the medicine for
others, and soon found that it was really useful in assisting digestion.
It relieved the uneasiness accompanying the process in many cases,
slightly encouraged the action of the bowels, and prevented the development of flatus in many instances in which inconvenience and suffering
had resulted from this circumstance.   Indeed, there could be no doubt
that this would be a useful remedy in many cases where the digestive
power of the stomach was impaired.   Mixed with the food of infants,
the powder assists digestion in many cases, and in old age it is invaluable.   Many old people whose digestion is greatly impaired may,
indeed, prolong their lives if the process of digestion be assisted by
mixing with the food, or by administering just before meals, a little of
the powdered mucus from the pig's stomach.

By careful microscopic examination I satisfied myself that there
were no substances in the powder likely to do harm, and though I have
examined the mucus from the pig's stomach in very many cases, I never
once discovered an entozoon of any kind, or an ovum of an entozoon.
When one considers how quickly the epithelial surface is formed, and

cast off in the discharge of function, one is not surprised at this. Indeed, though of course the possibility of such objectionable bodies being present in the mucus occurred to me at the outset, and has doubtless suggested itself to others, the facts of the case render it most improbable, and any objections under this head to the method of preparing pepsine powder rest on no foundation in fact. I therefore had no hesitation in taking and recommending the remedy. The next thing to do seemed to be to try and get some one to prepare this pepsine in quantity, so that the profession might prescribe it, and patients have the advantage of its use. I therefore spoke to Mr. Bullock, of the firm of Bullock and Co., whom I had known for many years as a scientific chemist of the highest character, and begged him to try my plan of preparation, and see if he could arrange for a sufficient supply of pigs' stomachs to make the powder in quantity. This was more than twenty-five years ago, and the remedy is now made in large amounts both here and in America, and it is used in every part of the world. The process I adopted for making it was described in the first volume of the "Archives of Medicine," page 269. Mr. Bullock has, I believe, made some improvements in the details of the process of preparing the material, and by great care and rapid drying at a low temperature the proper degree of activity of the solvent matter has been insured, and maintained at a given standard in every specimen that is made. Any of you can test the action of the *Pepsina Porci* in the simple manner I have described in page 103. You will find that a single grain, in point of fact 8-10ths of a grain, will completely digest one hundred grains of the white of egg. It is interesting to watch, in a common bottle before an ordinary fire, the opaque albumen becoming gradually translucent, and then the transparent albumen gradually breaking down until a complete solution, a peptone, is formed. In this way you may get what is known as albumen peptone.*

Mr. J. R. James, of the firm of Bullock and Co., has lately been studying the properties of the so-called "Ostrich Pepsine" ("Pharmaceutical Journal," February 20th, 1880). This substance, of which

---

* The only objection made to the process I have recommended is the very strange one, urged by Mr. Squire, who remarks that the pepsine made according to the plan above described contains epithelium, and that if exposed to a damp atmosphere "it becomes putrid more or less, and acquires a most repulsive odor." But who would think of placing pepsine or other organic substances of any kind in a damp atmosphere? Does Mr. Squire mean to suggest that the pepsine made by him, or any pepsine in the world, will not *putrefy and acquire a most repulsive odor if placed in a damp atmosphere?* The substance that does not change under these circumstances cannot be pepsine. I regret to have to comment upon such criticisms as the above. The test of pepsine is, of course, its solvent power, and the dried mucus of the pig's stomach is in this respect so potent that 8-10ths of a grain will dissolve 100 grains of coagulated albumen.

there is a specimen in the Museum of the Pharmaceutical Society, is thus described ("Medical Times and Gazette") by M. Ebelot:— "The stomach of the ostrich is celebrated for its incredible power of digestion. The abundance of pepsine, to which it owes this faculty, has created among the Indians a curious commercial fraud. They dry it, and sell it literally for its weight in gold. It is used for the purpose of restoring worn-out stomachs." A correspondent to the "Pharmaceutical Journal" says:—"In the Argentine Republic, ostrich pepsine is prescribed by medical men, and known by the public as 'pepsina nostra.' A good wine is made by digesting the stomachs in wine. I consider this a useful article ; but being a rough preparation our pepsine is preferable."

Beyond these loose statements no experimental results have been published, so far as I know. A fair and impartial trial should, of course, be given to this substance by those who have the means at their disposal of testing it, but care must be taken that a worthless preparation should not receive credit for performing a service which it is incapable of rendering.

Mr. James says:—"Whilst conducting my experiments upon ostrich pepsine my attention was drawn to another preparation, called 'Ingluvin,' thus described in the 'Medical Times and Gazette' for May 10, 1879: 'This is a new remedy, prepared by Warner and Co. from the *ventriculus callosus gallinaceus*. It is said to be superior to pepsine as a remedy for feeble, painful, and imperfect digestion, and may be prescribed in the same manner, dose, and combinations. . . . Ingluvin prepared from the gizzard of the chicken is the nearest approach to ostrich pepsine that can be obtained in Europe, we suppose.' Naturally, I felt a little curious to test this preparation, and applied for some to the agents, who most readily supplied me. Below I have tabulated the results obtained.

"Fresh eggs were kept in boiling water for one hour, and then allowed to get quite cold ; after depriving them of their shells the whites were cut into the thinnest possible slices—not minced, as it is easier to observe the progress of the digestion of albumen if it be sliced than if it be minced—and care was taken to reject any portion of yolk. Fifty grains of coagulated albumen thus prepared were placed in each wide-mouthed bottle and covered with five drachms of distilled water, containing 1 per cent. of hydrochloric acid, specific gravity 1·16. The quantity of pepsine was then weighed out and added to the mixture of albumen and dilute hydrochloric acid. The bottles and their contents were then placed in a water-bath and kept at a temperature of 98° to 102° F. for four hours, when digestion was regarded as complete.

Kind of pepsine employed.	Weight of pepsine employed.	Result.
Pig Pepsine	½ grain.........	Digested.
Ostrich Pepsine ...	2½ grains	Not Digested.
" " ...	5 "	"
" " ...	10 "	"
Ingluvin	2½ "	"
"	5 "	"
"	10 "	"

" From the results detailed in the foregoing table, and illustrated in the bottles shown, it will be seen *that the albumen is scarcely acted upon at all, and that both ostrich pepsine and ingluvin are destitute of the power of digestion.*" Much larger quantities of "Ostrich pepsine" and "Ingluvin" might have been taken with probably no difference in results.

" In the stomach of the river crayfish is found a plentiful supply of a yellowish-brown, feebly acid juice, which possesses an energetic, fermenting power, and rapidly dissolves fibrin, but the *addition* of a few drops of a dilute hydrochloric acid solution stops the action. Also, a somewhat similar ferment to pepsine, discovered by Fick and Murisier, in the stomachs of frogs, pikes, and trout, differs from it (pepsine) in being more active at a low.temperature, as at 20° F., while it loses its digestive power at the temperature of the blood (96° to 98° F.)."

Besides indigestion and weak digestion, there is another class of cases in which pepsine is of the greatest service, in which you must not neglect to employ it. In fever the action of the stomach is more or less disturbed. Indeed, in all fevers the process of digestion seems to be greatly deranged. When the feverish state is induced in one's own organism, one of the first points noticed is loss of appetite. The feverish patient does not feel the ordinary desire for food. When mealtime arrives, he is disinclined to eat. If, therefore, you find a patient who, perhaps, has been suffering from fever for many weeks, especially if emaciation is extreme, and the strength almost exhausted, it will be well to adopt the practice I have long acted upon, and add pepsine to the milk and beef-tea in the proportion of three or four grains to a pint. Milk will be coagulated at first, but soon afterwards it will become partially digested, and the curd may be easily broken up into very small pieces. Both the whey and curd will be in a state favorable for digestion, and for being rapidly absorbed and appropriated by the bioplasm or living matter of the tissues and organs.

If the feverish attack is of a kind which may continue severe for a considerable period of time, the body may lose very much in weight, the patient becoming excessively weak, and his life, perhaps, for some time in jeopardy. Under such circumstances it is of the first import-

10

ance to support the strength to the utmost. By mixing a little pepsine with the food you will greatly assist the digestive process. It may be during a most critical period of the malady, that the nutriment is given in the form of a peptone, and in a state fit to be immediately taken up by the vessels, and converted into blood constituents, and thus by this expedient life may be actually saved. I have lately (1878) had under my care a poor girl who became excessively emaciated in a prolonged attack of typhoid, the temperature varying from 102° to 105° during a period of six weeks. About the first week distention of the stomach and bowels by gas became considerable, and added much to the distress. I gave six grains of pepsine daily, with a little hydrochloric acid in the beef-tea, and kept this up during the whole period of the illness. The distention diminished after a few days, and I think that this simple plan had much to do with recovery in this instance. In the case of beef-tea you may with advantage add a little hydrochloric acid, and place the mixture before the fire at a temperature of 100°, for an hour or two before the patient takes it. He will not dislike it, and to some the acid beef-tea seems even pleasant. But generally when patients are as ill from fever as I am supposing, the taste is very much impaired, and practically there is no difficulty in getting persons to swallow the easily digestible peptones in the form of beef-tea. Peptonized fluid meat was first made in quantity some years ago by Mr. Darby. This useful preparation may now be obtained ready for use, in small pots or bottles in a form in which it will keep good for some time, of Messrs. Savory and Moore, 143, New Bond Street, London. Do not, therefore, forget this hint as regards the treatment of very bad cases of fever, and of prolonged exhausting disease. Whenever too little nutriment is absorbed for the support of the patient in consequence of the imperfect action of the stomach, the remedy will be useful, and now and then I have no doubt a life may be saved by the practice I have described.

Another plan based on the same principle may be adopted. Instead of giving strong beef-tea or soup containing pepsine, you may make a sort of meat jam. Underdone or perfectly raw mutton or tender beef may be cut up into small pieces, put into a mortar and well beaten with the pestle until it forms a soft pulpy mass. A small quantity of salt may be added to make it palatable. Pepsine in the proportion of ten grains of the powder to an ounce of meat is then to be beaten up with it, when a drachm or more of dilute hydrochloric acid is to be poured in, and the whole thoroughly mixed together. If you choose you may further add a little sugar instead of salt to the mass. This panada or paste may be spread upon bread and butter, or it may be diffused through beef-tea or soup. Children, and many invalids, will often take a compound of this sort when it is difficult to persuade them to take ordinary meat food at all.

In some cases of illness we are unable to feed the patient by the mouth, and in fevers it sometimes happens that everything that touches the mucous membrane of the stomach immediately excites the most violent vomiting, and occasionally this state lasts for so long a time that there is danger of the patient perishing from inanition. In these, as well as in those bad cases where there is a physical impediment to the entrance of food into the stomach, or to its escape from the organ into the duodenum, we may keep the patient alive for many months by injecting nutrient substances in small quantities (an ounce to three or four ounces) at a time into the lower part of the bowel. The nutritious matter dissolved, or suspended in some mucilaginous substance like boiled starch, is introduced into a small elastic syringe made for the purpose, and slowly injected into the rectum, the operation being repeated every three or four hours. To the beef-tea employed for this purpose it is well to add two grains of pepsine to the ounce. The rate of its absorption is increased, and it is more easily assimilated and taken up by the vessels of the mucous membrane.

You will find in the memoirs of Dr. W. Roberts, published in the "Transactions" and "Proceedings of the Royal Society," and in his Lectures at the Royal College of Physicians, many new points in connection with the question of the action of the gastric juice, pancreatic, and other secretions concerned in stomach and intestinal digestion, as well as instructions for applying the principles deduced from scientific investigation to the treatment of disease.

OF CONSTIPATION.

We must now consider a very important and almost universal accompaniment of the most common forms of deranged digestion and indigestion, and of which the majority of persons at some time or other have to complain. Constipation, a condition which varies greatly in degree, would, perhaps, be more correctly described as imperfect or insufficient action of the bowels. Probably nearly every one of us has suffered more or less from this trouble. And those who are accustomed to sedentary pursuits and intellectual work have usually a more extended experience of sluggish action of the bowels than those who take a good deal of exercise, and those who have to live by bodily labor. But I suppose there is hardly one who follows any walk of life whatever, or who follows no walk at all, who has entirely escaped this derangement. The most idle, as well as the most industrious, often have to complain of constipation, and the condition may afflict people of all ages and of all classes and in all climates. It is probably one of the most common of the slight derangements to which civilized man is subject. Whether savages suffer from it I do not know, but unquestionably the majority of persons forming a civilized community experience the discomfort.

The word "*constipation*" comes from the Latin "*constipare,* to crowd together." Generally speaking, people attribute constipation to the accumulation of fæces in the large bowel, and infer that it is invariably to be relieved by purgatives. But you will see, as I go on, that in cases of constipation a number of points have to be considered, and that many cases, so far from being relieved by the frequent administration of purgatives, are aggravated by that proceeding.

Most persons empty the lower part of the large intestine, or at any rate partially empty it, once during each period of twenty-four hours. But some persons' bowels have a habit of not being relieved oftener than every other day; some have an evacuation once in two or three or four days, and a few females maintain that once a week is enough to empty their bowels. Nay, I have heard it asserted that an action once in a fortnight was sufficient, and I am bound to admit that there are instances in which habitual constipation is not associated with derangement of the health, although, as a general rule, this sluggish state of the bowels brings about general disturbance of the health, and sometimes leads to very distressing results. Of course, in cases in which fæcal accumulation goes on for many days, the lower part of the large bowel gradually attains enormous dimensions, and considerable increase in its capacity and stretching of its walls must ensue before it is sufficiently large to hold the excrementitious matter formed, as well as all the refuse material of the food which accumulates during the considerable periods of time just mentioned. I need scarcely say that this is a very unsatisfactory state of things, and if allowed to persist for years, is likely to lead to disastrous consequences as age advances. There is no doubt, that if the large bowel, and indeed the intestinal canal generally, is to retain its healthy state, and to be preserved in good working order for sixty or seventy years, or more, its contents ought to be expelled, as I have before stated, once in every period of twenty-four hours.

Many of the physiological processes of the body, like this one, occur periodically and uniformly at about the same time during each period of twenty-four hours. Regularity as regards time much assists the daily evacuation of the bowels, and it is very desirable that every one should do all he can to acquire the habit. I do not think it matters much whether the bowels act the first thing in the morning, after breakfast, or the last thing at night, so that the habit is acquired and a fixed time kept. Even in the case of animals, at least domestic ones, this operation is usually performed with the greatest regularity at a particular hour. If you have a pet cat or dog, you will find it convenient to teach it to evacuate its bowels at a given time, and it will prove more than inconvenient if the creature should be unteachable in this respect. An unmanageable disposition, or disobedience in this respect, renders an otherwise valuable animal almost worthless.

You must impress upon all patients the importance of regular habits, which are, in fact, easily acquired, and ought never to be broken through. Many small ailments and troubles of various kinds will almost certainly result from carelessness in this particular, and serious maladies are not unfrequently the consequence of disregarding advice.

Having referred to the desirability of regular action, I must now try to impress upon you the equal importance of complete, or nearly complete, evacuation of the lower part of the large bowel, for what is called regular action may be associated with very imperfect removal of the contents. Although a small quantity of fæcal matter is daily discharged, this bears so small a proportion to the quantity formed, that there is a constantly increasing residue, which goes on accumulating, to the great discomfort of the patient, and the derangement of his health. In not a few cases this is no doubt due to the weak muscular contraction and imperfect action of the parts above, so that too small a quantity is sent down to the rectum to excite that part of the tube to sufficiently vigorous contractile action. As regards efficient action, a good deal usually depends upon the rectal contents. If a person lives upon highly nutritious diet, such as very strong soup or potted meat, he may find that his bowels will soon get obstinately constipated. If now he adds to this highly nutritive diet a quantity of amylaceous and soft fibro-cellular vegetable matter, which in itself possesses very little nutritive value, and of which comparatively little may be absorbed, he will find that the bulk of excrementitious material will be augmented, and the action of the bowels will become more satisfactory. In fact, if we are to be in good health, we have to take a certain quantity of material with the food which is not in any way of use to the nutritive operations. The proportion of nutriment in bread and potatoes is small as compared with that existing in fat meat. To obtain an equal amount of nutritious matter, a comparatively large quantity of bread must be taken, and of potatoes many pounds daily must be swallowed, if this is the only article of diet. Up to a certain point the admixture with the really nutritive materials of a large amount of innutritious dross is advantageous, and even in the case of vegetable feeders this matter has to be considered. A horse does not do so well upon pure corn as upon corn and hay. Chaff is of far more value than you would be led to suppose from its chemical constituents. Many of us indeed require a certain amount of chaff to keep ourselves in fair health. Brown bread is very dear, because it contains so much valueless material, and is a rougher kind of bread than white bread. If you examine brown bread, you will find that it contains a large percentage of the testa of the wheat, which is quite indigestible. Oatmeal is useful in the same way. All these things help to increase the bulk of the evacuation, and in this respect are of great use and do good. Unless there is a certain bulk to excite the fine nerve network of

10 * H

the mucous membrane of the intestine, the reflex action upon which the expelling action of the muscular fibres entirely depends, is not brought about, or is only very feebly and inadequately performed.

Lastly, the action may be perfectly regular, and the contractile powers of the bowels sufficient to expel the contents, but, owing to the formation of a very insufficient quantity of excrementitious matter, the bowel is seldom excited to act, and the patient suffers perhaps through the greater part of his life with the most troublesome form of "constipation." If the formation of fæcal matter is insufficient, many of the most important functions of the organism get out of order. You will find that people who suffer from this condition, though they may have a regular, but quantitatively deficient action, complain of certain unpleasant sensations. There is no organic disease. Indeed, if you examined every part of such person you would not find the least indication of the slightest structural change. Nevertheless, the almost constant discomfort many of these people have to endure is really great ; and not only so, but various more or less serious conditions may result from this state of things. It is in this way that unpleasant condition known as Hypochondriasis in the male, and as a form of Hysteria in the female, very often commences. There is even the possibility that a condition of disease bordering upon insanity may be brought about by long-continued defective formation of fæces and improper action of the bowels. Patients will often come to you complaining of very great discomfort. They tell you they feel more or less oppressed, and heavy and overwhelmed. Some complain of an unpleasant sensation all over the surface of the abdomen. Instead of the food which they have taken gradually disappearing, it seems as if it went on accumulating and distending the stomach ; the patient is blown up with wind, and the distress is great. Many persons who suffer in this way soon lose their healthy complexion and become more or less sallow and pasty. Indeed, it is quite extraordinary how many different derangements of the health may result from imperfect action or a torpid state of the secreting and expelling structures of the large bowel. There may be violent and persistent nerve pains referred to the back, or hip, or groin, and certain other symptoms which lead pessimist practitioners excelling in the discovery of neuroses to diagnose structural changes in some part of the spinal cord, or the antecedent state which is supposed to lead to them. Certain remediable forms of Sciatica are undoubtedly due to this cause, and violent lumbar pain is also not unfrequently occasioned by imperfect action of the excreting functions of the lower part of the alimentary canal.

There are many craftsmen peculiarly subject to constipation ; shoemakers and tailors, for example, suffer greatly. Undoubtedly many of them live to get old, and most of them are extremely intelligent, thoughtful people, but, nevertheless, they do not pay attention to the action of the colon. Literary men, teachers, male and female, professional men generally, who take little exercise, more especially if they live and work in small, badly-ventilated rooms, are great sufferers. You seldom see a shoemaker or a tailor with a good color ; and the same remark applies to many more whose habits are too sedentary. Nevertheless, it will be remarked that pasty, sallow complexions often characterize men having high mental endowments. Shoemakers are renowned for intelligence, energy, patience, endurance, and cogitative power. Organisms of this class, moreover, frequently have great resisting capacity, and often live to be old. Many are excellent lives to insure. Such persons may suffer much, and, in consequence, are often neither happy nor contented. They are, perhaps, very despondent or excessively irritable, and are not always very pleasant companions. Some of them who are so unfortunate as not to have to work for their living, spend too much time in thinking of themselves, their aches, and pains. Sufferers often complain of slight nausea, and of some discomfort about the stomach, with a sense of fulness of the head. An indescribable feeling of depression is sometimes described as being so severe as to render the patient almost unable to control his actions. Persons who suffer from constipation get very tired after slight exertion, or feel tired without having exerted themselves at all. They tell you they are unable to walk ; or, if they walk a little way, they get so tired and exhausted that they are obliged to come back and lie down. Very commonly, as I have mentioned, there is uneasiness, and not unfrequently actual pain. Almost invariably in this disorder there is a feeling of lassitude, an indescribable malaise, a disinclination to exertion of every kind, and frequently the patient is discontented with the position in which he happens to be placed, though the discontent is shown rather by frequent grumbling than by any active attempts to change his surroundings. He does not make any effort to place himself elsewhere, in order that he may be better pleased and happier. The only way to help such people is to allow them to growl, and then try to persuade them to take steps to relieve the troubles from which they suffer, and in this effort you will generally meet with at least partial success. They perhaps find fault with you and with everybody about them. You may meet with individuals belonging to this class who seem inclined to pick small quarrels with almost any one, and cannot, or will not, control their discontent. Successful critics are often of this disposition, and many a severe article would never have seen the light if the glands of the critic's large bowel had been in good order at the time. This troublesome ailment then has its advantages. It brings profit to editors, proprietors, and that important section of a civilized community which delights in finding fault, and flourishes according to the skill it displays in reviling. Any of you who desire to excel in this department of literature cannot do better than cultivate indigestion and imperfect action of the bowels, and a condition to which I shall presently have to refer, under the head of biliousness. A constipated, bilious dyspeptic is the sort of person soon to become a first-class critic, and his articles will command high remuneration, and be read by every one who is dissatisfied with his environment.

Constipation with Impaction of Fæcal Matter in the Large Intestine.—As the tissues get old their action becomes less vigorous, and the nerves respond more and more slowly and less readily to their wonted stimulus. The muscular fibres of the bowel become weak and lose much of their contractile power. Particularly the muscular tissue of the large intestine, like that of the bladder, becomes more or less feeble, and the viscus is unable to expel its contents. The collection of fæces therein may give rise to serious trouble. In old age some artificial stimulus is required from time to time to excite the weakened muscular fibres to contract with sufficient vigor to cause the bowel to empty itself. In old age fæcal matter often goes on accumulating for a long period of time. The collection is so gradual that the patient may not be conscious of it. By putting your hand over the belly, and particularly over those parts in which the large bowel is situated, you may often feel the colon for a considerable portion of its extent much distended by an accumulation of hard fæcal matter. At the same time you may ascertain whether there is also wind in the large bowel. If you place one or two fingers of the left hand over the surface and strike the back of one finger sharply with the tip of the finger of the right hand, you will be able to decide at once according to the note elicited by percussion. A dull sound indicates solid matter, while a hollow, drum-like note (tympanitic) indicates air in the bowel beneath.

Constipation has caused death. I recollect seeing an old lady who had been bedridden for years, and was in fact dying when she came under my observation, whose abdomen had increased to an enormous size. To my great astonishment, when I came to examine it, I found the swelling due to an enormous accumulation of hard fæcal matter. There was no fluid, and very little gas; but the whole abdomen seemed occupied by a huge mass of hardened fæces—I should think amounting in weight to 30 or 40 pounds. Unfortunately, I only saw the patient a few hours before death, when she was reduced to the last state of exhaustion, and when it was impossible to interfere. In this case fæces had probably been gradually accumulating in the intestines without attracting notice. The patient being bedridden, the circumstance seems to have escaped observation. Probably, if a medical practitioner had been allowed to interfere some six months before, the patient might have been saved. Injections might have been given, and the contents of the bowel thus removed before any harm to it had resulted.

Influence of the Reabsorption of Fluid by the Intestinal Surface in causing Constipation.—In many cases of constipation you find that the fæcal matter is too dry to pass freely along its wonted channel. It would seem that in many persons there is too rapid absorption of fluid by the intestinal surface. If the vessels of the large intestine take up too much of the fluid which is associated with the fæcal matter, the bulk may be so much reduced that the peristaltic action of the bowels is not so readily excited, and it may be insufficient to drive on the contents fast enough. The consistence of the excrement is no doubt a matter of some importance as regards the action of the large bowel and the process of defecation. In different animals the character of the fæces varies greatly, and we meet with every degree of difference from the extreme of dryness and firmness to the very opposite condition. For example, the fæces of the rabbit are hard, and are almost dry before they are expelled from the bowel. The same, too, is the case with the sheep. But in many other vegetable feeders the contents of the large intestine, instead of becoming inspissated before their expulsion, are very largely diluted with water. The fæces of oxen contain much fluid, while those of the horse contain comparatively little. Such facts are, of course, "explained" by evolutionists, according to their "laws" of evolution, and their "laws" of the correlation of secretion, excretion, and growth.

The too rapid absorption of fluid should doubtless be regarded as one of the circumstances concerned in the production of constipation. But the quantity of liquid swallowed may be defective, and the undue inspissation dependent upon actual deficiency of fluid in the organism instead of reabsorption. Some persons habitually take too much liquid, others too little. In the last, the fluid part of the blood is probably too highly concentrated for the quick removal of many of its constituents by the secreting cells engaged in the process. The various chemical changes under such circumstances are interfered with, or do not take place with due rapidity. In some persons many of the secretions of the body are formed in too large a quantity, and in too great a degree of concentration, and cannot be thoroughly dissolved and washed away by the proportion of water present.

After constipation has lasted for some time, as I have already remarked, various constituents, out of which fæcal matter is ordinarily formed, unduly accumulate in the blood, and cause disturbance in many of the physiological actions. Derangement of the general health of the organism follows. There may be suppression as regards the formation of excrementitious matters, or of the substances out of which these are elaborated by gland-bioplasm agency, as well as the mere retention or accumulation of these after they have been fully formed. After a person has been living long in town, in close rooms, too much indoors, taking too little exercise, and especially if he has been in the habit of eating too much, it may happen that the blood is constantly only imperfectly aerated, and the chemical changes which end in the production of compounds to be separated by various glands, and at last removed altogether from the organism, have not taken place at the proper rate nor to the full extent that is desirable. The excretory processes may have been for a long while only imperfectly performed. Much matter which ought to have been removed will have accumulated in the blood and tissues of the system, and may have done harm to tissues and organs. Gout, rheumatism, or other ailment may in consequence have been developed. In the reduced action of the excreting apparatus the intestinal glands participate. Too little fæcal matter is formed, and of the amount formed, as I have already explained, only a portion is expelled on account of the sluggish state of the nerves and muscles of the bowel. Moreover, reabsorption of soluble matters from the large intestine proceeds, and the materials taken up add to the accumulation of excrementitious matters in the blood, the serum of which is in consequence often actually changed in color as well as in composition. The general health soon suffers, the clear, florid complexion of health disappears, and the patient becomes sallow. The color of the skin generally is dusky, the capillary circulation through the tissues miserably sluggish, the intellect dull. There is an indisposition to exertion of every kind, and the nervous and muscular systems do not act or respond to a stimulus as vigorously and as quickly as they ought to do. People suffering thus may go on with their work, and as a fact numbers do so—but their work is performed, as it were, against the grain, and as though the workers were heavily weighted.

If, now, for a time the conditions under which existence is carried on be modified, it is wonderful how great a change will take place. Perhaps for the first few days, even in the best of climates and amid the most beautiful scenery, the interest will not be excited or the despondency shaken off. Sleep may not be sound, and the patient on rising in the morning not refreshed. The muscles of many parts of the body ache; some, and particularly those in the front of the leg, may feel sore, and after much walking become actually painful. The patient is conscious of a certain stiffness in his movements, and generally the elasticity both of mind and body seem to be for the time impaired. But, before long, a change takes place. The appetite improves and the sensation of hunger returns. Towards evening a tired feeling is experienced, soon succeeded by a desire for rest. Many hours of sound refreshing sleep succeed, and the patient gets up a different man. His spirits rise, he is seized with a desire to see, to walk, to do. The mental and bodily lassitude no longer troubles him. The complexion becomes ruddy, the skin smooth, and moist, and healthy. The bowels begin to act freely,.

and in three or four days the excretory glands separate from the blood, and the excretory channels discharge in twenty-four hours more than had previously been removed in a week. In this way the blood is soon depurated and changed for the better, and I have no doubt that, at least in many cases, the improvement in mental action is consequent upon the restoration of the blood to its normal healthy state. There is another fact which may be adduced in favor of the conclusion that in constipation, or imperfect action of the bowels, the blood becomes altered in character. If you happen to have any little scratch or abrasion on any part of the body, it will look more or less "angry" if the excretory processes should not be going on freely, and wounds will not heal. Instead of healing in the course of twenty-four hours, a scratch will discharge altered and sometimes irritating liquor sanguinis from its surface. Healing under these circumstances goes on very slowly, if, indeed, the process is not altogether entirely interfered with for a time. If you happen to be troubled with any little cracks about the margin of the mouth, you will find that they will gape and give you pain. They will not heal, but will remain open for several days, until free action of the bowels occurs, and then they soon improve and gradually get well. This angry state of scratches, or wounds, or little cracks or sores on the lips or margin of the tongue, depends, I think, upon an altered state of the blood, which is gradually brought about by constipation.

There is yet another matter to which I must direct attention, because it is of the greatest importance in connection with the views I have advanced concerning the state of the blood in these cases. You will often meet with cases in which, a few hours after a surgical operation, the temperature of the blood rises three or four degrees, and the patient becomes feverish. The pulse increases in frequency. There may be some wandering at night or actual delirium, with a hot, dry skin, and indeed the patient's state may be such as to cause his attendant considerable anxiety. The surgeon examines the wound and finds that instead of progressing favorably, it looks more or less angry, and the discharge on its surface is changed in character, losing its viscidity and becoming thin and watery, with perhaps a little softened and discolored, broken-down blood clot mixed with it. Now, if when things are in this state you give a purgative which will act freely upon the bowels, you will perhaps find within four hours after the purgative has been taken, and even before it begins to act, all the grave symptoms are mitigated, and the patient from that moment will progress favorably. I have many times watched with interest the fall in temperature in such cases —a fall of some three or four degrees of Fahrenheit's scale, in the course of a few hours, from the action of a purgative.

Phenomena of the same general nature may be frequently observed in young children. Many troublesome ailments occurring in childhood are due solely to the imperfect action of the bowels. When you get into practice, oftentimes you will be called to see a child who seems extremely ill, is irritable, sleepless, and feverish, perhaps wanders somewhat and screams at night, perhaps is even delirious. Such symptoms necessarily cause grave anxiety to the parents. And yet serious as they appear, all these untoward symptoms will very probably be completely relieved as soon as the bowels have been made to act freely.

The facts I have just briefly reviewed prove conclusively that the imperfect action of the large bowel may derange some of the most important physiological changes going on in the system, and disturb some of the most important organic actions. By affecting the composition of the blood, constipation may occasion derangement in the action of many secreting organs and seriously interfere with the due performance of many of the most important nervous actions and impair for the time the intellectual powers, as well as disturb the temper.

Moreover, you will find that the particular remedies which act most advantageously in these cases of derangement, depending upon constipation or imperfect muscular and excretory action of the bowels, are those which possess the special property of exciting various secreting organs to increased action. Among these perhaps the most useful are preparations of mercury, though sudorifics and diuretics not unfrequently exert a beneficial effect without any purgation whatever being produced. And I am sure that you will not fail to acknowledge that this fact also lends support to the view that the composition of the blood is modified by persistent constipation, and that excrementitious matters which ought to be quickly excreted, accumulate in it, nutritive operations being in consequence deranged. Lastly, you must bear in mind that the blood can be brought back to its normal state and health restored, by the action of those remedies which have the property of exciting the excreting action of the glands of the intestine and other parts to act very freely, and thus eliminate from the blood the accumulation of deleterious excrementitious matters.

Piles or Hæmorrhoids.—In many instances constipation is associated with *piles* or *hæmorrhoids* (αιμα, blood, ρεω, to flow), as they are termed, which consist of troublesome little nodules about the orifice of the anus. Sometimes pendulous papillæ form on the mucous membrane, half an inch or more above the orifice. These *internal piles* gradually enlarge and occasion pain and inconvenience. Each includes one or more loops of vein, with a number of dilated capillaries. They frequently bleed, and sometimes a considerable quantity of blood may be lost in this way. An ordinary pile or hæmorrhoid is a small growth, which may vary much in shape, but which depends from the general surface. The subcutaneous or submucous areolar tissue is

thickened, and the small vessels dilated. Little irregular varicose dila-
tations of the veins can be seen in well-prepared sections, and the outer
coat of the vein is more or less thickened from successive attacks of
inflammation. Dilated veins of the mucous membrane or skin near or
above the anus often exist around and between the actual hæmorrhoidal
swellings. Sometimes the pile consists of spongy tissue, almost like
that of the placenta, and undergoes great alteration in volume, like an
erectile tissue. There may be a number of small hæmorrhoids around
or within the anus, each gradually increasing in size until it is as large
as the top of the finger, when great inconvenience results. Walking is
accompanied by much suffering, and every now and then the vessels
become more congested and the swelling increases in size. The
tissues around the dilated vein become inflamed ; cracks and little ulcers
form, and severe pain, necessitating complete rest in the recumbent
posture for a time, is the result. Gradually this inflammation ceases.
The swelling subsides again to its usual dimensions, and perhaps some
time may pass before another acute attack comes on.

Not unfrequently, clots form in the little venous pouches and irregular
cavities. The fibrin of the clot gradually contracts and thus very
hard nodules result. These remain for weeks without undergoing
much change, but gradually the coagula are absorbed and the patient
considers himself cured, or nearly so. But soon another attack occurs.
Coagula again form and he is as bad as before. A pile or hæmorrhoid
which attains the size of a pea is seldom cured without removal. A
little surgical operation is necessary, and then the patient goes on
perhaps perfectly well for the rest of his life. In many instances there
is reason to think the development of piles might be prevented if the
bowels had been made to act pretty freely and the intestinal canal kept
in a healthy state from an early period of life. It is, however, sometimes impossible to do this owing to hereditary tendency to constipation, or to structural changes in glands occurring at a very early age.
You may prevent them from enlarging rapidly and giving trouble, by
making the patient frequently take moderate laxatives and attend carefully to his diet, especially as regards animal food, of which only a small
portion should be taken. Most persons eat far too much meat in this
country, and thereby induce many slight or serious derangements of
the health.

Primarily the condition is probably due partly to original weakness
of vessels and to a relaxed state of tissues, to the so-called scrofulous
diathesis, in which there is too rapid formation as well as imperfect
hardening and condensation of tissue, and in part to an altered state of
blood which interferes with the formation of healthy texture having the
due property of resistance. The dilatation and other changes in the
coats of the veins are in many cases general and not restricted to the

hæmorrhoidal veins. Want of exercise, defective oxygenation, and generally that state of blood which favors the development of the gouty and a certain form of the rheumatic state, seem to predispose to the formation of "piles" in various parts of the superficial venous system. Not a few cases of "phlebitis" belong to this category. In constipation or imperfect action of the bowels, the vessels of the walls of the intestinal canal generally are somewhat distended, the capillaries almost constantly unduly distended with blood, and the capillary circulation slow and impeded. The blood accumulates in the veins which unite to form the large portal vein. The flow of blood through the liver is affected, and the portal capillaries in the lobule become habitually distended with blood, and the action of the liver itself is of course much disturbed. The undue tension of the walls of the portal vessels is oftentimes temporarily relieved by the flow of fluid into the intestinal canal, as occurs in diarrhœa, or after the administration of certain purgatives; and if at the same time very little food is taken, so as to allow the organs loaded with inspissated blood to rest for a while, complete recovery may take place. If the diet be regulated and the general mode of living be corrected in cases in which it has been injudicious, the blood, and through the blood the various tissues and organs, may soon regain their normal state. Sometimes, as I have said, relief is afforded by actual hæmorrhage from the distended veins, and occasionally the capillaries of the surface or the mucous membrane give way, and thus the tension is relieved.

Among many proximate causes of hæmorrhoids, I believe congestion or impeded circulation of the blood in the portal capillaries of the liver is not an uncommon one. In many persons the liver often seems to act sluggishly, and for days together the circulation through it is much impeded. The whole organ temporarily increases in size in consequence of its vessels being distended with blood. The practitioner, under these circumstances, directs his attention to relieving the congestion and increasing the action of this important organ, as I shall describe further on.

An astringent ointment, like the old Compound Gall Ointment, *Unguentem Gallæ Compositum*, applied at night, is certainly useful in the early stage of formation. Attacks of congestion, and the accumulation of blood in the vessels which are productive of pain, may often be prevented, or if not very severe, at once relieved by proper treatment, particularly by paying attention to the action of the liver and bowels.

For the sore state of the skin and mucous membrane between or over the hæmorrhoids, as well as for healing the fissures that so commonly form, there is no remedy like Vaseline; but you must be careful to recommend your patients to ask for the *pure colorless Vaseline*, for the

ordinary substance contains irritating matters which do harm, and sometimes interfere with the healing process.

Of the Action of Enemata.—You must not forget that, as was shown
by Marshall Hall, defecation is a reflex action, and is dependent upon
the contraction of the muscular fibres caused by a current transmitted
along efferent nerve-fibres emerging from the nerve-centre which receives
the sensitive or afferent branches. The excitation beginning in the
peripheral nerves of the mucous membrane of the large bowel being carried to the nerve-centre by the afferent fibres, changes are produced in
the centre which result in the transmission of an impulse to movement
being conducted by efferent fibres and which causes contraction of the
muscular fibres. The afferent nerves in the mucous membrane, like
many special fibres in other parts, seem to be generally in a quiescent
state. They do not instantly respond to very slight stimulus, like certain
other nerve-fibres, as for example those spread out on the conjunctiva,
but decided and somewhat prolonged pressure or other form of irritation seems to be necessary to throw them into full action. In many
cases of constipation, the ordinary stimulus of the fæcal matter present
is not sufficient, and if contraction is to be produced, additional excitation must be brought about. It is upon this principle that the practice
of introducing purgative enemata into the rectum is founded. Ordinary
water may be gradually injected, and in this way the contents of the
lower part of the bowel are much increased, until having reached
a certain volume, powerful reflex action occurs, and fæces and injection
are forcibly expelled together. Do not, however, suppose that the
response takes place immediately. A certain interval, perhaps five or
ten minutes or a quarter of an hour, may elapse before the bowel
contracts, and generally it is better that the contraction should not
occur too quickly, for then only partial expulsion of the contents may
be effected.

In administering an injection you should direct that the fluid should
be introduced very slowly, the operator stopping for a time whenever
the patient feels contraction coming on. If the bowel is only gradually
distended, you will often find that a pint and a half of fluid or more
may be introduced before reflex action is excited. This simple operation, which is known as giving a *Clyster*, or *Injection*, or *Lavement*, is
a practice which is very commonly adopted, and some people are in the
habit of resorting to it very frequently. Some of the French ladies, I
am told, never get an action without injecting water into the bowel, and
have to carry out the practice daily or every other day. The lavement
is an efficient but rather troublesome measure to resort to daily, and
probably few English people could be persuaded to take so much
trouble.

Of enema syringes there are numbers constructed upon different principles and made of different forms. The simplest are made of vulcanized India-rubber. The most ingenious and most perfect I have seen is about to be brought out. It serves more than one purpose, and will be of the greatest service both to practitioners and patients.

Purgative Enemata.—Instead of injecting ordinary water, you may employ water containing various purgative medicines, such as *Colocynth*, *Aloes*, *Castor Oil*, or some others dissolved or suspended in weak gruel or in *Soap and Water*.

In making a purgative enema you may use from a half to an ounce of soft or ordinary yellow soap to a pint of warm water ; with this two ounces of castor oil or olive oil, or half an ounce of turpentine, may be mixed. Gruel is better than soap and water. If you require to give an aloes or colocynth enema, half a drachm of the first or the same quantity of a drachm of the compound extract of colocynth may be well rubbed down in a mortar with a little water or syrup, and then mixed with a pint of gruel. Two or three drachms of the Confection of Rue, in the proportion of three drachms to a pint, is a good addition in cases where there is much flatus in the bowel.

Sometimes the accumulation of fæcal matter in the large intestine is so considerable that the bowel becomes almost paralyzed, and the individual cannot expel anything by the strongest efforts he can make. Under these circumstances you may inject some gruel, or plain water, or soap and water, or castor oil and soap and water, into the bowel, and in considerable quantity, without succeeding in exciting reflex action. The fæces remain as it were impacted, and cannot be dislodged by such means. This condition is sometimes spoken of as *impaction*. You may occasionally find the lower part of the large bowel of an old person so full and choked by impacted fæcal matter that it overflows as it were, although there is not the slightest effort on the part of the bowel to empty itself.

As the bowel does not contract, and has indeed nearly lost its con-tractile power, the fæcal accumulation must be removed. A sort of scoop, or paper-knife, or the handle of a spoon, or any other convenient instrument of the proper shape and with rounded edges so as not to cut the parts, may be used to remove the hard fæcal matter. The operation is always a disagreeable one, and sometimes it is very difficult to perform, but it must be undertaken, and we must be prepared to interfere in this way many times in the course of our practice. Those of you who may by-and-by be engaged in country practice are sure to meet with such cases from time to time, particularly amongst the inmates of asylums for the aged, and in poor-houses, and you must be ready to afford the only relief that is possible.

THE HYGIENIC AND DIETETIC TREATMENT OF CONSTIPATION.

There are certain methods of preventing and treating ordinary constipation with which every one ought to be acquainted. By having recourse to some of them persons who have suffered may not only obtain relief, but may succeed in preventing the recurrence of the trouble.

Exercise, we are often told, is a great preventive of constipation, and sometimes will cure it when established. Many practitioners are very confident on this point, and invariably assure those who suffer that if only they will take sufficient exercise, they will be cured. Some obedient patients at once adopt the system of a regular constitutional. But here and there the plan completely fails. A man regularly walks his six or seven miles or more daily, but so far from his constipation being cured, he may perhaps find it even worse than before. Exercise, it is perfectly true, is advantageous within certain limits. But if a person takes more exercise than is good for him he may actually encourage and increase this derangement instead of curing it. Nor is walking exercise so necessary or advantageous to all persons as is generally supposed. Individuals differ from one another extremely in this respect. One cannot keep himself in health without his long dreary daily constitutional, while another enjoys excellent health though he may not walk a mile a week. Not only so, but it is a fact that many persons, particularly women, who have taken little active exercise at any period of life, have nevertheless enjoyed excellent health and have lived to be very old. In advocating exercise in constipation and in other slight ailments, you must be careful in the case of those who have not been accustomed to long walks to recommend moderate distances, at a quiet pace, or your means of cure may have the effect of doing harm. Two or three miles a day will probably be enough for most persons. The man who is engaged in hard intellectual work will, as a rule, require little exercise. During a holiday you may engage in a greater amount of muscular labor than you could advantageously perform if you were studying hard. And I have known several instances of persons getting thoroughly out of health in consequence of acting upon the mistaken notion that such exercise is required at the same time that intellectual work is carried on. When you are working for an examination, and reading several hours day after day, you will find that a gentle walk for an hour or so in the afternoon, or spending one or two hours in the open air, will be more conducive to your progress than a long walk. Fast walking, running, and all violent athletic exercises should, like dinners and high living generally, be avoided by those who are preparing themselves for examination.

The Cold Bath is commonly said to be of use in the treatment of constipation. People tell us that if we indulge in cold tub every

11 *

morning or plunge into cold water, the bowels will act properly and
without artificial help of any kind. This system again is excellent
for some, but the daily use of cold water will not suit all equally well.
With some persons it disagrees and causes them to feel chilly and
uncomfortable. On cold foggy mornings at this time of the year
(November) it requires some strength of mind to cover oneself with cold
water just after turning out of a warm bed. Still, many Englishmen
declare that it not only suits them, but affords them delight and keen
enjoyment. Those with whom the cold bath agrees experience a
pleasant glow all over the body, and feel warm and in good spirits for
some time afterwards. When this is the case, you may advise that the
cold bath should be continued. But if, on the other hand, the patient
feels chilly, miserable, and uncomfortable, with slight headache and
chilliness of hands and feet, and especially if his skin should get cold
and bluish, and he comes down to breakfast without an appetite, you
should tell him that cold tub in the early morning is not suitable for
him, and suggest that he should take his bath tepid or even warm.

Rubbing.—Another good general remedy, and one that is not open
to any objection, is rubbing. I believe this method is very little employed, and that its value is much underrated. There are many who, if
instead of taking a cold bath would simply rub themselves well with a
rough towel, using strong muscular efforts in doing so, would find a
gentle glow come over the skin, and experience a far more comfortable
sensation than is afforded by a cold bath, while an equal amount of old
epithelium would be removed from the cuticular surface. The beneficial
effects of rubbing the surface are probably due to movement of the
blood in the cutaneous capillaries, caused by the pressure exerted.
This movement of the blood in cases where there is a tendency to its
stagnation in the capillaries of the tissues and organs is of the greatest
consequence, and must be borne in mind as an important principle
which must not be lost sight of in the treatment of many derangements
and diseases.

Moist Application to the Abdomen.—Persons who suffer from torpid
bowels are often much relieved by the application of a wet compress
over the stomach. This is a very old remedy. You may apply a moist
rag or towel, folded into four, to the surface of the belly, or a piece of
moistened spongio-piline may be used. It matters not whether the
water be cold, tepid, or warm. If applied cold it soon becomes warm,
and I am not aware that any benefit results from the, to many
persons, very unpleasant application of a cold rag to the warm skin.
Care must be taken that the compress or other application is not
too wet when applied. It may be worn for two or three hours daily,
and in this way relief is often obtained, without the use of any medicine
whatever.

Of Kneading the Bowels.—Another very simple way of assisting the action of the large bowel is to press or knead the abdomen with the hands. Any one can do this for himself. The two hands should be moved upwards and downwards over the surface of the belly, and the large bowel pressed backwards in different places. Those who have studied anatomy know the course taken by the colon round the abdomen, and should press or knead it in a direction from its commencement in the cæcum in the right iliac region, upwards, and across the upper part of the belly to the left, and then downwards, following the *ascending, transverse, and descending colon* towards its termination, in the rectum. This kneading encourages the contraction of the large bowel, and is certainly in many cases useful.

Diet.—There can be no doubt that diet has very much to do with the regular and efficient action of the bowels. A liberal allowance of meat and a too highly nutritious diet favor constipation. On the other hand, various kinds of fruit and many vegetables cooked and uncooked, as lettuces, water-cresses, and mustard and cress, tend to prevent and relieve constipation.

Bread.—The bread that we eat should not be made of very fine white flour, from which all the bran has been carefully separated, and with which a certain proportion of alum—itself possessing astringent and constipating properties—has been added, to make it appear perfectly white. The best bread for keeping us in health is not the whitest. As regards pleasant taste and nutritive qualities, the sort of bread you eat at farm-houses, and which is by no means white, is much to be preferred. *Brown bread,* such as we get in London, is good, but it ought to be made of flour from which the branny particles have not been separated before being finely ground. I fancy that a good deal of brown bread is made by adding coarse particles of bran to ordinary flour. Brown bread taken from time to time will certainly help to excite the action of the bowels. The whole meal bread now so much recommended is doubtless the best form of bread to take.

Indian corn flour is one of the most wholesome and nutritious forms of food, but it is at present far too dear to be used as staple food ; it is much to be desired that this substance should be brought into ordinary use.

Oatmeal, again, is another good and very desirable kind of food. It is taken by many, particularly by Scotch people, who well understand how to live cheaply. The best oatmeal is the Scotch, made into "stirabout." It may be cooked in many ways. Milk may be added, or it may be formed into thin cakes, which can be dried. These may be toasted when required, and eaten with butter. Oatmeal sometimes proves a good remedy in certain forms of constipation. In it all matters required to form the staple of ordinary diet are found, and it is a good substitute for bread. Some persons, however, dislike it, and with some it disagrees.

Coffee.—A small cup of sweetened black coffee (*Café noir*) before rising sometimes acts as a purgative. Some persons gain the same advantage by drinking a cup of tea.

Fruit.—There can be no doubt that fruit is a very useful article of diet. This will be freely acknowledged, but many are unable to indulge in fruit in the winter season. In a climate like ours, except for a very short period in the height of summer, fruit is a rather expensive luxury. However, though few can afford to obtain as much fresh fruit as they could eat, very good substitutes are within the reach of all, even of the poor, though few English people take advantage of the opportunity they enjoy of being able to purchase excellent dried and preserved fruit, apples, plums, and other kinds of fruit, at a very cheap rate. Oranges and lemons are also to be had during the greater part of the year.

French Prunes and Apples.—Prunes may be bought for a few cents a pound, and a pound of prunes will last for many days. If properly prepared, cooked prunes are very good. The French and the Germans use prunes very generally. They stew them and add some syrup, and eat them with the meat at dinner almost daily. If you determine to try them, you may have to turn cook for a time, for you will find few British cooks disposed to follow your directions. Should the cook be exceptionally amiable and willing to learn, you may suggest to her some such plan of proceeding as the following :—The prunes may be soaked in cold water for several hours, perhaps twelve hours or longer. When they are found to have swollen up, and to have become quite soft, in consequence of imbibing much cold water, they may be stewed in the ordinary way, and sugar added. If properly cooked, they will be perfectly soft and of a very pleasant flavor. In this way you can all provide yourselves with perfectly good fruit all the winter. You may also recommend French plums, which are nicer than ordinary prunes, but more expensive.

Lenitive Electuary (*Confectio Sennæ composita*) contains prunes. Although this is a very good purgative, you will find that some people do not like it. Children will often take stewed prunes, although it is a most difficult matter to give them any form of medicine. You may increase the purgative properties of stewed prunes in a very simple way —and the hint I shall give you is a useful one to bear in mind in the management of children. Suggest that a teaspoonful of *Senna leaves* be tied up in a small muslin bag and soaked for an hour in the water in which a pound of prunes is stewed. In this way you add a little infusion of Senna to the prunes, and, although you hardly alter their taste, you considerably increase their purgative action.

Apples dried.—Another fruit you can always get is dried apples. They are ordinarily sold now at all the grocers. These you will find to be an agreeable change, and may take the place of the prunes. They must be soaked in water for a few hours, and then stewed in the ordinary way. A pound of these will be sufficient for several dishes. Of late apples have been introduced in a new form. Thin shavings of apples dried in the sun, retain their flavor so thoroughly that when moistened and cooked you could not distinguish them from fresh apples.

Another dried fruit, which is now very cheap and to be obtained in good order all the winter, is the dried fig. Figs are now brought over in large quantities, and are very cheap. The purgative action is increased by soaking in water over night. The fig, in a state of soft pulp, may be eaten on the following morning.

Of Taking Fluid.—The quantity of fluid taken has some influence upon the action of the bowels. Many people are seldom thirsty, and more object, and with good reason, to drinking water. Tea is often discarded on the supposition that it causes indigestion. If tea and coffee and alkaline and effervescing waters, and all forms of alcohol, are objected to by the medical adviser, as not uncommonly happens, the unfortunate patient will, in his efforts to comply with very unreasonable advice, probably take too little fluid in the twenty-four hours, and thus disturb many of the chemical changes going on in his body. One cup of tea or milk and water, at breakfast, half a pint of beer in the middle of the day, and perhaps another half a pint of beer, or wine in water at dinner, will scarcely amount to a sufficient quantity of fluid to keep the body in health, especially if the appetite is good, and a fair amount of solid food is consumed. People who are never thirsty will occasionally suffer from constipation, as well as from other derangements, which will be referred to in their proper place.

When you have reason to think that a patient is suffering in health from taking too little fluid, you may suggest to him the propriety of taking a certain quantity of water at fixed times. You recommend him to drink a glass of ordinary water on rising, another about eleven o'clock, and another at bed-time. Or you may suggest that at dinner he should take hock and seltzer water, and an hour after dinner, or at bedtime, another glass of seltzer, or some other effervescing water. In some cases you may recommend cider or perry to be taken at dinner. You may advise that broth should form part of the most important meal of the day, and, generally, you suggest various things—milk, whey, more tea, linseed tea, or barley water, etc.—with the object of getting more fluid into the body.

I

In general it does not do to advise the patient to take ordinary water, for in the first place, few would adopt your prescription, and, secondly, there is the real and serious objection that ordinary water may be bad and, though not disagreeable to the taste, may contain typhoid fever or other disease germs. All objections to ordinary water are, however, removed, if it be boiled. Some do not dislike taking warm tea or warm water with their meals. Either often suits the stomach far better than cold fluid, which sometimes checks digestion. In cold weather I have long been in the habit of taking warm water, and have recommended the practice to others, but many object and prefer to let the water get quite cold before they drink it. Householders should make a rule that every morning a kettle of water that has been boiled for ten minutes or longer should be allowed to cool, and then poured on the filter. The boiling renders the water perfectly safe, for it destroys every living organism as well as any animal poisons that may be suspended in it.

Most practitioners recommend their patients to drink special aerated waters, and there is no doubt that some of these are more pleasant to the taste than is ordinary water, but the rapidity with which waters of particular kinds come into favor and are forgotten, and give place to others, is sufficient to show that the water is, after all, the active and efficient ingredient. The patient who goes to some celebrated spa is no sceptic, and according to the instruction he has received from his teacher, attributes the beneficial effects he experiences, not to the ingredients dissolved in the water, but to some mysterious properties which these substances are supposed to have somehow acquired as they were dissolved, or while the solution was being forced upwards through the soil to the surface of the ground. The potash and soda, etc., accordingly are not ordinary potash and soda, with the ordinary properties of the molecules, but are imbued with some very remarkable powers somehow communicated to them in the bowels of the earth. Fashion and caprice sanction and demonstrate the universal healing powers of this or that spring, and then a new fashion decrees its impotence and transfers infallible potencies to some newly-discovered water. The self-denying supplicant who determines to devote himself for a few weeks to the worship of Hygeia must turn out at about five A. M., and, according to the established rites of the place, may have to walk a certain distance, and drink a definite quantity of water, before he is permitted to enjoy the frugal breakfast, at which even butter is often proscribed. More drinking and more walking follow in due course, in obedience to well-defined rules. The simple midday meal is succeeded by more walking, more air, and more water. Improvement is soon manifested. The bowels act, the appetite returns, the spirits rise, and due credit is given to the mysterious agencies communicated to some of the chemical ingredients of the water during their solution or afterwards. The air, the simple, wholesome, and restricted diet, the substitution of water for alcohol, the exercise, the rest enjoyed, and peace of mind are the mere accidents attending the curative action of the special water. But those who drink good water in London, and live according to reason, may work hard and enjoy all the year round the advantages which some go so far, and at great expense and inconvenience, to try to find during what they call their holiday.

Smoking Tobacco.—Other unfortunate individuals, slaves to a bad habit, tell you they never can get their bowels to act without smoking the accustomed cigar or pipe. Whether it be the force of habit, or whether the nicotine, the active principle of the tobacco, actually gets into the blood and excites the bowel to act through the nerve-centres, I do not know, but we are often assured that smoking does exert a purgative influence. Tobacco smoking in moderation certainly does no harm whatever, and he who finds that it is followed by the desirable consequences referred to, will be wise to smoke.

THE MEDICINAL TREATMENT OF CONSTIPATION.

Of Purgatives in Constipation.—As I have shown, in cases of prolonged insufficient action of the bowels, the general health is impaired, the blood becomes altered in composition, many substances remaining in it, and circulating with it through the vessels, which ought to have been eliminated, and the action of many secreting and other organs is, in consequence, more or less disturbed. This after a time may lead to structural change, and result in disease.

It may be necessary to advise the patient who has been suffering from deranged health, resulting from a prolonged state of constipation, to submit to systematic medical treatment. In some instances the condition may be relieved by attending to the state of the secreting organs without giving any medicines having purgative properties. The character of the urine and other secretions is often much altered. Deposits of considerable quantities of urates are formed, and the urine itself may be of very high specific gravity, and in other respects may have departed, more or less, from the healthy state. In such cases a few doses of Bicarbonate of Potash (*Potassæ Bicarbonas*) will set everything to rights in a day or two, without any purgative action being excited.

In many cases of constipation in which the blood is in such a state that any little wounds or scratches do not quickly heal, an ordinary purgative that acts on the alimentary canal will not suffice, but you must select one which, besides producing purgation, also acts upon the secreting glands, particularly those which discharge their secretions at once into the alimentary canal. As soon as the medicine begins to act, and that is oftentimes hours before any purgative effect is experienced, the red and angry appearance of the wounds and scratches will subside, and the healing process will be proceeding satisfactorily within twenty-four hours after the dose has been swallowed.

Where constipation has existed for a considerable period of time, and the general health has in consequence become considerably deranged, you must not expect that the patient is to be at once cured, and indeed generally you will find that purgatives administered from time to time, in moderate doses, act more favorably than a smart purge administered once only. Very free purgation is often followed by constipation, and the patient, instead of being permanently benefited, is only relieved for a very few days. You will often find it necessary to give moderate doses of certain purgative medicines at short intervals for a time, taking care, however, not to carry this system too far, so as to worry and irritate the alimentary canal, and give the patient much pain and discomfort. Again, it not unfrequently happens that an ordinary purgative will not properly act, or it acts only very slightly, without affording the relief which is expected. In such a case it may be advisable to repeat the medicine two or three days running, but sometimes it is better to wait for a few days, and then repeat the dose. The same observation has been made as regards many other medicines. Bicarbonate of Soda or Potash often fails to relieve if given in single doses, though they be large, while if fifteen or twenty grains be taken three times a day, and continued for three or four days a week, a very distinct and highly satisfactory effect is produced.

The same medicine administered to a person in precisely the same dose will sometimes act freely and sometimes will not act at all. The state of the bowel varies greatly as regards secretion, and its response to stimulants to secretion and muscular contractility. No doubt this depends to some extent on the appetite, and the kind and amount of food taken, but not entirely so, for sometimes after a person has lived sparingly for some time, a moderate purge will produce a very free action. The action of the intestinal, like that of other glands, is not uniform within corresponding periods of time, but sometimes it is very free, sometimes almost suspended for a while. If we can just hit upon the time when the glands are about to act freely, for the administration of the purgative, the effect will be exactly what is desired. Most glands form and discharge their secretions, and then rest for a while. It is, therefore, wrong in principle to be continually trying to excite them to action by giving remedies which excite free action, day after day, for a considerable period. This injudicious and unreasonable practice, which was much in favor fifty years ago, did weak people a good deal of harm, and to it we are indebted for the present unreasonable opposition to the employment of one of the most valuable medicines (mercury) known to us.

When the constipation depends upon sluggish action of the large bowel only, the daily or almost daily administration of a mild purge, containing Rhubarb, Aloes, Senna, Colocynth, or Podophyllin, is un-objectionable, and by adopting this practice, which has been solemnly condemned by some authorities, you will sometimes enable a patient to get through a great deal of work which otherwise he could not perform, and you will now and then succeed in transforming a thoroughly miserable and discontented person into a happy one. See also the remarks on the use of mercury under the "Treatment of Sick-headache."

One is often assured by a patient in answer to inquiries that his bowels are "regular," that is, that an action occurs every day, and he will perhaps tell you that he is quite confident no purgative medicine is required. Although from the first you suspect that he requires a purge, according to his wish you try various remedies to relieve the symptoms of which he complains, but without effect. He may go from doctor to doctor, and at last he is ordered to take a purgative, and gets almost immediate relief. Oftentimes it is necessary to order a mild purgative pill to be taken daily before dinner, for a week or longer, and the patient is not unfrequently quite astonished at the effect. Up to that time he had felt convinced that his colon was clear, although, in fact, fæcal matter had been very gradually accumulating in it for a considerable time.

You will often find small doses of purgatives, given just after food for several days in succession, of great use in imperfect action of the bowels, from which many persons engaged in sedentary pursuits in towns very commonly suffer. From three to ten grains of Rhubarb, with or without Carbonate of Soda, or five grains of Compound Rhubarb pill, will be sufficient. You must teach people to experiment a little on themselves, in order that they may find out the least quantity required to produce the effect desired. As before remarked, fruit taken daily is of use in such cases, but many persons do not try the plan long enough to obtain success. The digestive organs which act sluggishly require a good deal of humoring, so to say. Violent purgatives are worse than useless, and in such cases a moderate purge is often followed by a headache and general upset, lasting perhaps for many days, and succeeded by the sluggish, torpid, imperfectly acting state. There is no difficulty in managing those who eat well and take plenty of exercise, but those who live very moderately, and whose work is intellectual rather than muscular, will require some thought and the exercise of a little ingenuity on your part to get them right, and to regain for them the much desired feeling of contentment dependent upon healthy intestinal action.

As regards the doses of purgatives, you must be very careful, for you may order a patient a dose that will certainly clear out the whole

12

intestinal canal, but which will also gripe him very severely, and make
him for a time very weak and miserable ; while a dose which you might
perhaps hardly believe would have any purgative action at all, would
have been quite sufficient to effect the desired end, and without producing the slightest pain or discomfort. You must vary the doses of
the drugs you prescribe, according to the state of the patient, and
according to the sort of organism you have to treat. If you are prescribing for a highly nervous, anxious, excitable person, who thinks he
has got all sorts of ailments of a very serious character, you must, as a
rule, not give very violent purgatives, for, if you do, you may bring on
pain and sickness, and much increase the intensity of the suffering you
have been asked to alleviate. On the other hand, if you are treating a
robust laboring man, accustomed to work hard and feed well, and in
the habit of drinking three or four pints of beer a day, and more when
he can get it—who has a florid complexion and great muscular vigor, it
would be foolish to order him a gentle pill or mild draught. To such a
person two or three grains of Colocynth pill would be perfectly useless,
and ten grains might be required to act at all, and if you were to add to
these two or three grains of Calomel, the patient would probably feel the
more grateful to you. Many of the chemists, in town and country, sell
good strong pills, and which are most useful for those for whom they are
prepared, though they would not suit many of your patients. This necessity for varying the doses of medicines according to the individual patient,
ought to convince all of the importance of each practitioner learning how
to prescribe, and mix, and combine medicines, instead of exclusively
relying upon the pills and mixtures prepared for the profession in
enormous quantities by large firms, and to be purchased by the gross and
by the gallon, but which cannot be altered to suit individual patients, and
combined so as to agree with peculiar temperaments. Moreover, there
is no doubt that many extracts and pill constituents lose much of their
virtue by being kept for a considerable time. Practitioners have, from
time to time, discovered certain combinations of things which are very
valuable, and the receipt for many a useful pill or mixture has been
handed down from generation to generation. In these days, not only
do we neglect to use many of the old prescriptions, but we no longer
suggest new ones, and many combinations of drugs of tried value and in
frequent use in former days, will soon be altogether forgotten. The old
system of teaching such elementary but practically important matters
has been entirely abandoned, and many a wrinkle of the greatest importance in practice, instead of being preserved and transmitted as
formerly from master to pupil, has been lost. Let me advise you
never to neglect an opportunity of picking up from old practitioners
any receipts for medicines they are willing to give you, and not to

despise their teaching, especially as regards the treatment of many slight ailments difficult to manage and to cure. Do not receive with contemptuous indifference their suggestions for the treatment of functional disorders, the exact nature of which they may be unable to adequately explain.

Castor-Oil, Oleum Ricini, which is the oily substance expressed from the seeds of the *Ricinus communis,* is one of the best and most frequently used of purgative medicines, and were it not for its nauseous flavor would be yet more popular. It is at the same time one of the mildest and most certain of purgatives, and is suitable to persons of all ages. You may give it to the infant as well as to the most infirm and delicate. It is usually given by the mouth. But Castor-oil may also be employed in enemata. It is one of the few purgatives that act upon every part of the intestinal canal, from the stomach downwards, but its action commences in the upper part, and it is efficient in driving down imperfectly digested and other matters that may be irritating the mucous membrane and causing pain. The dose varies from a few drops to half an ounce or more, but most persons take more Castor-oil than is really necessary to produce the required effect. One teaspoonful is often sufficient for an adult, and sometimes acts as well as a larger dose. Not the least advantage of prescribing the smallest dose that will be useful is that it is so much easier to take. There are many receipts for taking Castor-oil so as to avoid tasting it. Upon the whole I think you will find the following one of the most efficient plans. You direct that a teaspoonful or more of " black coffee," that is, coffee without milk, be poured into a wineglass, the whole of the interior of which, including the lip, has been well wetted with the coffee. A teaspoonful or a little more of the oil is then to be steadily poured on the surface of the coffee, when it will form a large globule lying perfectly free and not in actual contact with any part of the glass, because the latter has been well wetted with the adhering coffee. The patient then opens his mouth wide and pours the oil and coffee down his throat, swallowing the whole in one gulp. If the operation has been successfully conducted, he will not have tasted the oil in the slightest degree. Tea, a little Ginger or Orange Wine and water, or Peppermint, Camphor or Orange-flower water, or Brandy and water may be used instead,—but strong spirit being lighter than the oil will not do. Some strongly recommend that the dose of Castor-oil should be well shaken up in a bottle with twice its quantity of milk, and when well incorporated poured into a cup or glass and quickly swallowed.

Rhubarb, Rhei Radix, Pulvis Rhei is one of the best of purgatives, and its virtues are very widely known. It has been a popular remedy for more than two centuries, and is one of the best purgatives for children. Mixed with Carbonate of Soda, *Sodæ Bicarbonas,* it is very

useful in derangements of digestion.   From five to twenty grains of
Rhubarb with twice as much Bicarbonate of Soda, will often give great
relief.   The dose may be repeated once every other day after food for a
week or two in cases of constipation or imperfect action of the bowels.
See also pp. 139, 141.

   Pulvis Rhei Compositus, formerly known as *Gregory's Powder*, consists of Rhubarb, 2, Light Magnesia, 6, and powdered Ginger, 1.   It
is an excellent and safe remedy and may be given in doses of from ten
grains to a drachm, in water.

   *Ordinary Compound Rhubarb Pill, Pilula Rhei Composita, and
Compound Colocynth Pill, Pilula Colocynthidis Composita,* suit most
persons very well.   You may order three to eight grains of either of
these pills, and it is better to combine with them a grain or two of the
Extract of Hyoscyamus or Henbane, *Extractum Hyoscyami,* which will
prevent any griping or discomfort.   Three or four grains of either of
the above pills with a grain of Extract of Henbane may be made into
a pill, and one may be taken every night or every other night for a
week or two, in many cases with great advantage.   In this way the
bowels may be thoroughly relieved and got into the way of working
regularly.

   One of the great advantages of giving purgative medicines in the
form of pills is that the particles of the drug are thoroughly comminuted
and diluted, as it were, by less active ingredients.   The importance of
the minute division of active substances was known even to the ancients.
A smaller quantity of the active material is sufficient, and it is far less
likely to do harm, while its action is sure to be more moderate and
equable, if intimately mixed with a quantity of inert or slightly active
material, than if administered in a pure state.   Many pills and powders
have been compounded on this principle.   Compound Ipecacuanha
powder, *Pulvis Ipecacuanhæ Compositus,* Compound Jalap powder,
Pulvis Jalapæ Compositus, and Compound Rhubarb powder, *Pulvis
Rhei Compositus,* are examples.   If there be much flatulence, or if you
desire to give a little stimulus to the secretion of the gastric juice, you
may add to the pill or pills half a grain or a grain of Capsicum, *Capsici
Fructus,* or ordinary Cayenne Pepper, with advantage.

   You must recollect in administering pills not to order more than
five, or at the most six grains in one pill, or you will astonish your
patient by the size of the bolus you have ordered him to take.   Five
grains form a moderate-sized pill, but if blue pill or calomel should be
one of the ingredients, the pill will be small, because a grain of these
mercurial preparations occupies very little space.   This matter of the
size of pills must be borne in mind, for some people think it an insult
to receive a large pill, and many will tell you they cannot swallow one
of even moderate size.   The professed inability to swallow a pill is often

mere affectation or determination on the part of the patient not to attempt to do so; but some persons have a real difficulty. For them the pill may be silvered or gilt, or covered with a tasteless starch coating, and if neither of these plans will please, tell them to pack the pill up in a small piece of moistened "pastry-cooks' paper," when the whole will slip down whether the patient will swallow it or not. This pastry-cooks' paper can now be obtained at many of the large chemists, and is an excellent thing in which to give powders to children. Little capsules of this material have been prepared and made in separate halves. The powder or pill is placed in one and the cover applied, the edges being slightly moistened, the two halves adhere, and the little parcel with the included medicine can be swallowed without any difficulty.

Nux Vomica is another remedy which may be given, by itself or combined with a purgative, in cases of imperfect action of the bowels. It is useful by giving tone to the bowel and stimulating, probably through its action on the nerves, the muscular coat of the intestine. It is now frequently prescribed. It comes from the plant which yields Strychnine, *Strychnos Nux Vomica.* You may give of the Extract of Nux Vomica, *Extractum Nucis Vomicæ,* from a quarter of a grain to a grain. If added to a purgative pill, it helps the action of the large bowel. The Tincture of Nux Vomica, *Tinctura Nucis Vomicæ,* may be prescribed in doses of from five to twenty minims with some Compound Tincture of Bark or other tonic. Decoction of Aloes, *Decoctum Aloes Compositum,* Tincture of Senna, Tincture of Rhubarb, are simple remedies which are often prescribed in doses of from a drachm to half an ounce.

Scammony, *Scammonium,* a gum resin from the root of Convolvulus Scammonia, is a component of many purgative pills, and is a very active purgative. For children suffering from intestinal worms, Scammony is one of the best remedies. It may be given in doses of one or two grains, or from three to five grains of the Compound Scammony Powder, *Pulvis Scammoniæ Compositus,* which consists of Scammony, 4; Jalap, 3; and Ginger, 1, may be ordered instead of the pure drug. It may be taken in a little milk. Probably many patent purgative medicines contain Scammony. It is a rather searching purgative, which clears out the bowel well, expelling any hardened fæces and wind that may have collected.

Compound Licorice Powder is now in the Pharmacopœia. The preparation is much used in Germany and Russia, and is certainly one of the best and safest of ordinary purgative medicines. The *Pulvis Glycyrrhizæ Compositus* of the British Pharmacopœia contains two ounces of finely powdered Senna and the same quantity of powdered Licorice root, with six ounces of powdered sugar; but the German preparation is made as follows:—" Powdered Senna, powdered Licorice, of each 2; powdered Fennel, Sulphur, of each 1; white sugar, 6: mix."

12 *

The dose of the powder is a teaspoonful, carefully mixed in a little water.

Aloes is another purgative which has the property of acting upon the large bowel. It probably irritates the mucous membrane, and excites its glands to secrete; but also, by reflex nervous action, it stimulates the action of the muscular coat of the intestine, and excites vigorous contraction both of the circular and longitudinal muscular fibres. It is a very good purgative to give in cases of torpid bowels, but it is important for you to bear in mind that aloes has the effect in some cases of encouraging the formation or increase of hæmorrhoids or piles, see p. 120. It seems to irritate the mucous membrane of the lower bowel, and those who suffer from an irritable state of this part sometimes find their sufferings much increased if they take any of the ordinary preparations of Aloes. There is the Socotrine Aloes, *Aloe Socotrina*, and Barbadoes Aloes, *Aloe Barbadensis*. The Compound Decoction of Aloes, *Decoctum Aloes Compositum*, is ordered to be made of Socotrine Aloes, and contains besides, Myrrh, Saffron, Carbonate of Potash, Licorice, Compound Tincture of Cardamoms, and Distilled Water. This is a very valuable preparation, and enters into the composition of many favorite draughts which used to be prescribed in former days, and which brought gain to the apothecaries of old. That once very fashionable but rather nasty dose called a *Black Draught* was composed of Decoction of Aloes, with Sulphate of Magnesia, Senna, and Licorice. Its composition was modified by different authorities, and some improvements, more nasty still, were made by ingenious physicmongers; but the reputation of the black draught is gone, and, though an excellent purgative, it is seldom prescribed in these days. Forty years ago Dr. Chambers, who was then the fashionable physician in London, and other physicians only a little less fashionable, prescribed blue pills and black draughts for most ailments. It would not be easy now to persuade people to swallow a black draught. However, with a little ingenuity you may make something less nauseous and equally efficacious. The Decoction itself may be taken in doses of from two drachms to an ounce and a half or more.

Probably the best preparation of aloes, to prescribe in the form of pills, is the Watery Extract of Aloes (*Extractum Aloes Socotrina*). This watery extract does not irritate the bowels, and acts very effectually. It may be given in doses varying from the one-sixth of a grain up to a grain or more, but it is better not to order a larger dose than is absolutely requisite, and in prescribing, it is well to bear in mind that Aloes, as well as many other drugs, have their purgative action much improved by being reduced to a state of very minute division, and mixed with other things. If small pieces of Aloes should stick in the mucous membrane of the large bowel, that particular part might be severely irritated, and in consequence the patient would experience great pain and discomfort ; while, if the medicine was very minutely divided and mixed with a quantity of inactive or less active material, there would be no danger of any such deleterious action. When you prescribe aloes, you should always order it to be intimately mixed with other and less active substances. Let the pill contain, say, a quarter of a grain of the *Extractum Aloes Aquosum* with two or three grains of common Extract of Colocynth (*Extractum Colocynthidis Compositum*), and a grain of Extract of Henbane (*Extractum Hyoscyami*). Although in these days it is the fashion to prescribe one remedy only, and I believe some distinguished physicians consider it improper to order more than two drugs in one pill or mixture, there is not the least doubt that, as far as regards the action of the medicine upon the organism, considerable advantage is gained by mixing several remedies together. Medicines, like foods, affect different people in a different way. If you prescribe several different things together, you may influence different idiosyncracies, while it would be almost impossible to determine the particular purgative suitable for each individual patient. I much prefer a pill consisting of a little Compound Colocynth, a little Nux Vomica, a little Henbane, a small quantity of Podophyllin, and perhaps a little of the Watery Extract of Aloes, to a full purgative dose of any one of these preparations by itself. By mixing these things together, you get a less painful and more efficient action than you do from a large dose of either of them separately. If you desire to test the truth of this observation, you may carry out a very instructive experiment on your own organisms. Take, for example, one grain of Podophyllin and see how it affects you, and the next time you require a purgative take three grains of the Watery Extract of Aloes alone. On another occasion try a very small dose (a quarter or the third of a grain) of Podophyllin or Aloes, mixed with three grains of compound Colocynth pill, and notice whether, upon the whole, you do not get a better result with less griping pain than when you took the larger doses of the simple drugs.

Podophyllin has been much used during the last ten years, and was first employed in America. But it is a purgative of somewhat uncertain action, and those who order it should take care how they prescribe it. I remember the case of a child who was almost killed by half a grain of Podophyllin, incautiously ordered by the practitioner, who perhaps up to that time had been employing some weak and inferior preparation ; but this last prescription, being made up by a chemist who used good medicines, a much too powerful dose was administered. The drug varies much in quality, and it is, moreover, one of those things which acts very differently upon different people. I have patients who have been taking a small quantity of Podophyllin for many years, and who say they have never taken anything which acts so satisfactorily.   On the other hand, I every now and then get into disgrace for ordering the same thing to other persons.   The drug sometimes gripes the patient so much that he does not wish to try the remedy again.   You should always order Podophyllin first in small doses, mixed with compound Rhubarb or compound Colocynth pill, and if it causes no discomfort, you can easily increase the dose.   Do not give more than one-quarter or one-third of a grain, unless you know by experience the patient can take larger doses with advantage.

Drastic and Hydragogue Purgatives can hardly be included among the remedies for slight ailments, but a few of them may be prescribed in small doses for ordinary maladies.   Thus Jalap, *Jalapa*, is a very old and useful purgative, which may be taken in doses varying from five to fifteen grains.   It excites the flow of fluid from the blood into the intestine, and when prescribed should be mixed with an equal quantity of Bitartrate, *Potassæ Tartras Acida*, or Sulphate of Potash, *Potassæ Sulphas.*

Jalapine is obtained from ordinary jalap by rectified spirit.   It is the resin, in fact, *Resina Jalapæ*, deprived of its coloring matter by animal charcoal.   A small dose of from one to three grains will be found to act freely.   It may be prescribed in a pill or as a powder, mixed with a few grains of sugar.

Elaterium, Croton-Oil, Gamboge, are all violent purgatives, which are very useful in the treatment of some diseases, but are not required in the management of slight ailments.   They should all be prescribed in very small doses to begin with.   In fact, the practitioner who uses these drugs should always ascertain whether the patient will bear them by ordering in the first instance a very small dose.   Drastic cathartics all excite the pouring out of a large quantity of fluid from the blood through the walls of the capillaries into the bowel.

In this place I ought properly to speak of the action of preparations of Mercury, but as this subject will come under consideration a little further on, I shall postpone what I have to say for the present.

Saline Purgatives are very valuable in many cases of imperfect action of the bowels.   Many of the salts used as purgatives act not only by promoting osmose of fluid from the blood by reason of the higher specific gravity of the saline solution in the intestine than that of the liquor sanguinis, and by their direct influence on the nerves of the mucous membrane, but also in consequence of being first of all absorbed into the blood, and then excreted by the glands and follicles of the mucous membrane of the colon.   At the same time many other substances are removed from the blood with the salt, and in this way the circulating fluid may be freed from certain deleterious constituents which have accumulated in it, and which if they remained would seriously interfere with the action and nutrition of various tissues and organs.   Most salines act partly as purgatives and partly as diuretics, and not a few of them have the effect of increasing the secretion of many, if not of all, of the glands of the digestive system.

There are many salts in the Pharmacopœia which you will find useful. Some of these are very ancient remedies, and well known in all countries. First of all, there is Epsom Salts, Sulphate of Magnesia, *Magnesiæ Sulphas*, and a capital remedy it is. It forms, as it were, the basis of a great many fashionable medicines, and many people frequently take it without knowing from what a common drug they derive relief. It is one of the cheapest of medicines, for a pound of it only costs a few pence. It may be given in doses varying from half a drachm to half an ounce or an ounce, in solution in water. The small dose, especially if dissolved in warm or lukewarm water, will sometimes purge freely and quickly. As a medical author has metaphorically remarked concerning a much advertised water, it is "speedy, sure, and gentle!"

Sulphate of magnesia is not an unpleasant thing to take, especially if you mix it with about one-fourth of its weight of common salt and twenty drops of Aromatic Sulphuric Acid (*Acidum Sulphuricum Aromaticum*), the whole being dissolved in an ounce and a half of lukewarm water. I often order ten minims of dilute Hydrochloric Acid, *Acidum Hydrochloricum dilutum*, and two drachms of Sulphate of Magnesia, to be dissolved in an ounce and a half of Cinnamon Water, Orange Flower Water, *Aqua Aurantii Floris*, common Water, or Infusion of Roses, *Infusum Rosæ Acidum*. The last gives a rather pleasant taste and agreeable color to the draught, which should be taken in the morning before breakfast, or about two hours after that meal. If you consider it desirable to act upon the kidneys at the same time as the bowels, and often it is very important so to do, you may add a few grains of Nitre, *Pulvis Potassæ Nitratis*, and in this way you make a saline draught which many of your patients will find useful. It may be taken day after day for three or four days, or twice or three times a week; but its daily use should not be continued for longer than a fortnight at a time.

Sulphate of Soda, or Glauber's Salt, *Sodæ Sulphas* of the Pharmacopœia, is not so strong in its purgative action as the Sulphate of Magnesia, but it is not nearly so disagreeable in taste. You may give two or more drachms of Sulphate of Soda dissolved in an ounce and a half of water. Or you may prescribe two or three drachms of the Sulphate of Soda with a somewhat less quantity of the Sulphate of Magnesia with five or ten grains of Nitre and a drachm or more of common salt. The addition of common salt you will find advantageous, as it certainly much diminishes the nauseous taste of the Sulphate of Magnesia. Salines generally, like many other medicines, act more powerfully if they are combined than if taken separately, and, as I have already said, their action is expedited and increased if they are dissolved in warm or lukewarm water.

Phosphate of Soda, *Sodæ Phosphas*, is another salt which acts well as a mild purgative in doses of from one drachm to an ounce dissolved in water. It is not disagreeable, and has long been known as "Tasteless Saline Aperient." It is a good saline for children, and may be given dissolved in weak beef-tea or other form of broth or soup.

Soda Tartarata, a Tartrate of Soda and Potash, commonly called Rochelle Salt, used to be a very favorite saline purgative. It also acts on the kidneys. The acid of this salt, like Citric and many other vegetable acids, becomes changed in the system, alkaline carbonates being formed which render the urine alkaline. The dose is from one drachm to half an ounce or more dissolved in water. You may order a mixture containing half a dozen doses, and direct the patient to take an ounce, that is, two tablespoonfuls, with one tablespoonful of hot water. If the dose is taken before breakfast, it will generally act in the course of two or three hours, and many a patient will have good reason to thank you for the advice you have given him.

Many such saline mixtures may be used instead of purgative mineral waters. Their action is much the same, but you will find that not a few of the most prosperous of your patients will decline to take such salines as you can prescribe. They require a more fashionable form of saline in the shape of a purgative mineral water from some wonderful spring warranted to cure all diseases, and patronized by the nobility of Europe. In these days there are, indeed, a number of potent natural mineral waters having purgative properties from which to choose. A few years since, almost every person was advised to take Pullna water. This after a time, like the once famous Epsom and Cheltenham waters, gave place to others. For years *Friedrichshall* has been credited with virtues of surpassing excellence, but now I suppose opinion is divided between this and the unpronounceable Hunyadi Janos bitter water. The latter contains much more of the purgative sulphates than Pullna, Seidlitz, Kissengen, or Friedrichshall, and therefore acts more freely.

Friedrichshall water is a mild purgative saline. Its composition is shown in the following analysis, for which I am indebted to Mr. C. H.

ANALYSIS OF FRIEDRICHSHALL BITTER WATER.

	Grains per gallon.
Sodium	657·5
Potassium	6·1
Magnesium	200·8
Calcium	18·7
Silica	1·7
Chlorine	1003·1
Bromine	0·13
Sulphuric acid (SO_4)	739·2
Carbonic acid not estimated.	

Piesse, Public Analyst, London. It seems to contain Sulphate of Magnesia and Chloride of Sodium.

Mr. Piesse remarks that if the "Chlorine" be calculated into "Chloride of Sodium," and the "Magnesium" into "Sulphate of Magnesia," and the amounts of the salts thus indicated be dissolved in one gallon of ordinary drinking water, we shall have a solution very like the natural Friedrichshall water, especially if the mixture be well charged with carbonic acid.

You may tell the patient to take a wineglass of Friedrichshall or Hunyadi Janos water with as much warm water every morning before breakfast, and in many cases it may with advantage be prescribed with twice as much Carlsbad water made warm, or hot water added. For patients who object to the expense of mineral waters you may easily prescribe a substitute according to the principles already mentioned, page 141. Whether the Sulphate of Magnesia and Sulphate of Soda in the water obtained from a spring is in a state in any way molecularly different from the salts as sold by chemists has not been determined, but certainly the less wealthy seem to derive as much benefit from solutions of ordinary Sulphates of Magnesia and Soda, as the rich do from purgative mineral waters.

Sulphate of Potash, Potassæ Sulphas, is a very old saline aperient. It may be taken in doses of from ten grains to three scruples dissolved in water. It enters into the composition of many of our remedies in the Pharmacopœia.

Effervescing Saline purgative.—But perhaps the pleasantest saline purgative is an effervescing draught. We have an excellent mild purgative in what is now called *Granular Citrate of Magnesia.* I believe that much of what is sold under this name is really Citrate of Potash or Soda. The ingredients are mixed, and the water of crystallization in part driven off by heat, but the preparation is a difficult one to make well. The dose is from one to two teaspoonfuls thrown into a tumbler two-thirds full of water, and the mixture is to be taken during effervescence. The granulated salts must be carefully excluded from damp, but if this be done they keep for a long period of time. Such effervescing draughts are very agreeable in hot climates. It is of course only a very mild form of purgative, but useful in a great many cases when a cooling saline is required. The urine is rendered alkaline by the salt.

Many different forms of granulated effervescing salts are now prepared by chemists, containing Quinine, Strychnine, Pepsine, Bismuth, Lithia, and many other substances. Granulated Effervescing Salts also constitute a very agreeable vehicle for many different kinds of medicine.

In giving purgatives, do not forget that it is a great point to hit the exact time, for a very moderate dose will often produce a full and sufficient effect, although at another time, in the case of the very same

person, a larger dose will have little or no effect, save causing severe
pain.   If the right time can be selected, a mild purgative will be of the
greatest use, and may possibly have the effect of preventing an attack
of illness.   This variability in the action of the same medicine is very
remarkable in the case of mercury, an extremely small quantity of
which has sometimes the most beneficial effect in dissipating symptoms
which for several days may have indicated serious general disturbance
and the derangement of more than one important organ of the body.

DIARRHŒA.

I pass now to the consideration of a condition the very opposite of
constipation.   Diarrhœa (*δια*, through, *ρεω*, I flow), though a common
ailment, is less frequent than constipation, and is seldom habitual and
persistent, lasting perhaps for the greater part of a lifetime, like the
tendency to constipation.   Now and then, however, you do meet with
people who seem to suffer very frequently from a condition to which
the term diarrhœa would be generally applied.   To your inquiry if the
bowels are open the patient will perhaps reply "Too much so."   On
further questioning, you find that the bowels act three or four times
every day.   In some of these cases the patients do not appear to suffer
pain, nor do they necessarily get thin and weak, or appear to be out
of health.   Whether the looseness depends upon a highly irritable
state of the nerves of the mucous membrane, or is due to weak vascular
walls, or to an altered state of the blood, or to a highly nervous disposition, it is often difficult to decide.   In some cases the condition
results from a peculiar habit of body, and undoubtedly there are types
of constitution which are remarkable for the great activity of various
secreting glands, just as there are others as remarkable for slow and
imperfect action.   In neither case is there any structural alteration ; but
one class is characterized by rapid, the other by sluggish, change.

That diarrhœa may be produced through nerve influence only, is
proved by a number of circumstances.   Many nervous people are very
subject to it.   Fright, anxiety, and sudden joy may be immediately
followed by diarrhœa.   Many students who have been exceedingly
anxious concerning examinations, have experienced the influence of
the mind acting through the nervous system upon the secreting glands
which discharge their contents into the intestinal canal.   The action is
due mainly to a relaxation of the muscular fibres of the small vessels,
permitting dilatation and a free discharge of fluid from the blood directly
into the bowels, as well as indirectly into the secreting glands.

To those who suffer from constipation, an occasional attack of
diarrhœa is very advantageous, and is not to be regretted.   Probably
diarrhœa carries off many noxious materials that have accumulated in
the blood, and may therefore be beneficial to some organisms, provided

it only occurs now and then, and does not last for too long a time, and is not allowed to become very severe at a time when there happens to be an epidemic. But you must not forget that an attack of typhoid fever is often ushered in by slight and sometimes by severe diarrhœa. There is usually a very decided rise in temperature, which in many cases will enable you to form an opinion as to the nature of the malady.

There are times when diarrhœa must be guarded against, and, if it occurs, must not be allowed to persist. During an epidemic of cholera, a person suffering from diarrhœa must be very carefully watched, for, if the condition continue unchecked for even a short time, it may become choleraic. In cholera-times what appears to be ordinary diarrhœa may be succeeded in the course of a few hours by the collapse stage of cholera. The disease usually begins with slight purgation, and you cannot tell whether a person is going to have a mild attack of ordinary diarrhœa or actual cholera. It therefore behooves us to be on our guard, and, during the prevalence of a cholera epidemic, it is important to at once check all cases of diarrhœa.

The commonest form of diarrhœa is that which we meet with in hot summers, and often prevails to a great extent in autumn. This is often called summer diarrhœa, and it is hard to say exactly what occasions it. Certain it is that it is more prevalent in hot, dry summers, than it is in cold, wet ones. Some would explain the fact by the superabundance and cheapness of fruit in the former, and its scarcity and high price in the latter. Plums usually get the credit of exciting diarrhœa, but the condition frequently shows itself before plums are obtainable. No doubt bad, unripe fruit, and decaying fruit are very liable to irritate the bowels, and may excite diarrhœa. Neither is there any doubt that decomposing vegetable and animal matter will bring on an attack of diarrhœa; but what the particular organic material may be which exerts the deleterious influence, I do not know. On the other hand, it is quite certain that many of us can eat very considerable quantities of any ordinary fruit without suffering in any way, and even without the ordinary half-constipated habit being relieved. In summer, the intestinal canal of many persons seems to be in an unusually sensitive or irritable state, so that very slight errors in diet are apt to derange its action for a time. Even a little beer that is out of order, or sour milk, will sometimes set up a very troublesome attack of diarrhœa, which may last for days, and require careful treatment to check it.

Concerning the precise changes which occur in severe diarrhœa, little is positively known. It is generally supposed, as I have already remarked, that much of the fluid escapes from the capillary vessels; but at least, in some cases, it is more probable that the condition depends upon increased activity of many of the glands which discharge their contents into the intestinal canal. In sudden diarrhœa, depending upon the presence of some irritating material, I suppose transudation of fluid takes place from

13 K

the vessels, as well as increased secretion from the glands. In many cases, for some time before the attack, it is probable that the blood has been in an unhealthy state, in which case the free discharge of watery matter will be of advantage to the patient, inasmuch as various noxious materials will be eliminated, which would do harm if they were retained in it in a state of solution. Thus by the attack of diarrhœa is the blood depurated, and may, in this way, be soon restored to its normal healthy state. Unquestionably, therefore, in such a case, diarrhœa may be regarded as conservative and advantageous.

Suppose a child has been eating a quantity of unripe fruit,—and it is nothing very unusual for an English baby to eat half a dozen unripe and very uninviting looking apples,—this will soon produce an effect, the stomach and bowels will be irritated, and a sudden, and it may be, violent derangement will follow, often accompanied by feverishness, the temperature in such cases not unfrequently rising to 103° or 104°, with perhaps violent abdominal pain; and these symptoms may be sufficiently severe to excite alarm. If vomiting occurs relief is at once experienced, but more commonly purgation is excited, and may perhaps have existed for a few days before you are called in to see the patient. You must not expect the diarrhœa to cease until the whole of the irritating matter which excited it has been removed, and the sooner this result can be effected the sooner will relief be afforded. All the particles of half-masticated apples containing immature acids and other irritating organic compounds must be removed from the alimentary canal before the diarrhœa will cease. In such cases, therefore, it is bad practice to attempt to check the diarrhœa unless you feel sure that the whole of the irritating substances have been entirely got rid of. It is even desirable to encourage for a time the flow of fluid from the intestinal canal, so that the noxious matters may be thoroughly washed away. For this reason you will often have to administer a mild purgative to expedite the removal of the matter which excited the purgation. You purge to stop purgative action, and you will often find this the best and shortest method of checking the diarrhœa of children. Of all the purgatives that are known to remove irritating matters from the intestinal canal, oily purgatives are the most suitable. Common Olive-oil, *Oleum Olivæ*, will act in this way, and for very young children is quite sufficient, but as a general rule you will find it expedient to give Castor-oil, *Oleum Ricini*, the purgative action of which is more decided. There is an active principle in the Castor-oil which affects the action of the stomach as well as the glands and vessels of the upper part of the alimentary canal. In this way, Castor-oil in its action contrasts with Aloes, Colocynth, and Sulphate of Magnesia, which act mainly upon the lower part of the small intestines and the colon. I suppose Castor-oil excites increased secretion in the stomach, the duodenum, the jejunum, and ileum, causing a quantity of fluid to be quickly poured out from the vessels and glands of the mucous membrane. Thus the alimentary canal is thoroughly flushed in every part; and the action takes place from above down-wards. Any irritating matters that may be present are thus swept away. For this reason, and for the further reason that Castor-oil is a substance which does not irritate the mucous membrane in any undue or uncom-fortable way, it is the best purgative to give in any cases in which you have reason to attribute the diarrhœa to injudicious eating. Particularly in the diarrhœa of infants and young children is Olive-oil or Castor-oil a safe remedy. As a general rule, you will find a much smaller dose of Castor-oil will act than is usually administered. To a child of ten years old you may give half a teaspoonful or a teaspoonful; to an adult, two teaspoonfuls, but a single teaspoonful of Castor-oil will be sufficient for many people. The objection to Castor-oil is its nauseating, disagreeable flavor. I have already referred to the best way of taking it, and have offered some suggestions for disguising the taste. See p. 135.

After diarrhœa has continued for some time, there may be a good deal of severe griping pain all over the stomach, or at least in its upper part. At the same time the patient feels chilly or very cold, and may actually shiver; very generally there is more or less flatulence, with acid eructations, loss of appetite, and occasionally distressing nausea. The tongue is usually furred, and there may be a nasty taste in the mouth, or the mouth may feel clammy and disagreeable. After diarrhœa has lasted for several days, there may be considerable depression of the heart's action; and not unfrequently severe cramp in various muscles increase the distress.

Acid eructations and the rising of acid fluid into the mouth will be relieved by the administration of alkalies and other so-called antacid remedies. You may give alkalies, such as *Potash, Liquor Potassæ,* twenty drops in a wineglass full of water once in three or four hours, or the *Bicarbonate of Potash or Soda.* Preparations of Bismuth are also useful, as the *Carbonate of Bismuth (Bismuthi Carbonas),* or the *Nitrate,* the old *Trisnitrate of Bismuth (Bismuthi Nitras),* from ten to twenty grains for a dose, suspended in water with the help of a little mucilage, or, better, prepared chalk (*Creta præparata*), or precipitated chalk (*Calcis Carbonas precipitata*). But one of the best as well as simplest reme-dies to give in these cases, and particularly in gastric and intestinal de-rangements occurring in infants and very young children, is Lime Water (*Liquor Calcis*). This is an extremely valuable remedy, which is not used as much as it deserves to be. Infants are very subject to diarrhœa, and I fear that many a child has been lost simply from allowing diar-rhœa to continue, which would have been easily checked, if sufficiently early in the attack a few teaspoonful doses of Lime Water in milk, or sweetened Lime Water (*Liquor Calcis Saccharatus*), had been given. Anything of an irritating character will very soon disorder the delicate mucous membrane of the intestinal canal of an infant, and a very simple remedy administered at the proper time will stop it, but if the purging be severe, and it be allowed to continue for a few hours, extreme exhaustion may ensue, and be soon followed by death. In these cases, mothers often make the unfortunate mistake of feeding the child too much. Fearing lest it should be starved, they keep pouring in milk. The secretions, already out of order, get worse, and the milk, instead of being properly digested and assimilated, is either rejected in the form of curd, or the curd formed is passed onwards into the small intestine, where it excites irritation without being taken up and absorbed. Coagulation of the caseine, without subsequent solution, may persist perhaps for many days, sometimes for a week or more, each new portion of milk that is swallowed undergoing the same change. Thus the intestinal canal, in every part of its course, becomes filled with firm white coagula, which, it will be noticed, constitute the greater part of every evacuation. After death from violent diarrhœa it is not uncommon to find the intestines even distended with coagulated and undigested curd.

Cases of diarrhœa in infants may often be relieved at the outset by small doses of Lime Water. A little may be mixed with the milk, in the proportion of a tablespoonful or less of lime water to half a pint of milk. Sometimes Potash Water answers better, and I have used Liquor Potassæ, in the proportion of twenty drops to half a pint of milk. You must not allow the child to take as much milk as it likes. For a day or two, half a pint of milk in the twenty-four hours will be sufficient. It must be obvious that, as long as the disturbed state of the bowels continues, it will be worse than useless to push food. Time must be allowed for the alimentary canal to become partially emptied of its irritating contents before fresh nourishment is introduced. If the child is at all low, it must be supported with small doses of brandy—from ten to twenty drops in a teaspoonful of water or milk and a little sugar, once in two hours. You cannot be too careful in watching cases of infantile diarrhœa, especially in weak children, for it sometimes happens that serious exhaustion comes on quite unexpectedly, and if you do not visit the patient every few hours, a sudden change may occur, and the case be hopeless before you come to its assistance.

I have already drawn your attention to the fact that in these cases of diarrhœa, bacteria often grow and multiply to an enormous extent in the caseine clots. In many cases every part of the intestinal canal is pervaded by millions of these organisms, which grow and multiply in the altered secretions and food which are continually being poured into the stomach. The changes which ought to take place in the food prior to its absorption and conversion into healthy blood are consequently prevented. Children may, under these circumstances, die of inanition, although they have been but too liberally fed during the whole period of the illness. The food they are plied with merely serves to encourage the growth of bacteria, and it actually undergoes changes which interfere with its digestion and absorption. If just at the right time you withhold food, perhaps only for a few hours, everything may right itself; the irritating matters may themselves act a little on the bowels, and thus get pushed onwards by the contraction of the muscular coat of the intestine. Diarrhœa may come on and last for a few hours or so, or even for a day or two, and then the secretions return to their natural state. The child will be out of danger and soon be well again. In treating diarrhœa in children, particularly infants, you must take care that the child is kept warm. One of the principal causes of diarrhœa is cold, and bathing in cold water, and exposure to cold and wet will sometimes bring on diarrhœa even in adults.

You should be aware of the different characters of the stools in different forms of diarrhœa. If they are of the natural color and odor, you may let the diarrhœa go on for a while, for it will probably do no harm, and will most likely stop without medicinal treatment. But if the stools should become much altered—if they should emit a sour smell, and the secretion should have the appearance of rice water, it will probably be necessary to check the discharge. For such evacuations, as well as those which are colorless or almost colorless, consist wholly, or in great part, of secretions poured out from the glands, and from the vessels of the mucous membrane of the lower part of the small and of the large intestine. You will find in such evacuations much altered mucus, with numerous small cells (bioplasts) from the follicles as well as from the surface of the mucous membrane, chiefly of the colon. Not unfrequently you will find a little blood; but there may be more albumen than the quantity of blood will account for. If the increased formation of mucus continue for a considerable period of time, it is often associated with a serious change in the tissues of the mucous membrane itself. After such excessive action has gone on for several days or weeks, there may ensue an excoriated and almost lacerated state of a small portion of the surface of the mucous membrane. A sort of superficial ulcer results, from the surface of which perhaps blood will from time to time escape. By the continual drain of nutrient matter, and general disturbance of the action of the bowel, a low state of health may soon be induced, which, with the local affection, may soon lead to the development of a very serious disease, not uncommon in many tropical climates, but, happily, rarely contracted here. The malady in question is Dysentery, but it cannot be included among "slight ailments."

Not unfrequently, however, in this climate the colon is the seat of great uneasiness, often amounting to actual pain. In many of these cases it is unquestionably the mucous membrane which is affected. The capillaries of a limited area become congested. The congestion not unfrequently passes into ulceration, and we have an approach to that state of things which may, under certain circumstances, be soon followed by dysenteric symptoms. More commonly, if proper precautions be taken, the patient gets better before actual ulceration occurs. If we

13 *

could see the mucous membrane in some of these cases, I have no doubt we should find it, in the immediate situation of the painful spot, swollen, red, and exceedingly sensitive. Every time the muscular coat contracts, the dull pain changes in character and becomes severe. The affection may occur in any part of the colon ; but I think the sigmoid flexure, the cæcum, and one or other end of the transverse colon, are the situations to which the pain is usually referred ; and, as regards frequency, in the order in which I have named them. If small pieces of hardened fæces or the *débris* of food happen to be forced into contact with the spot, sudden attacks of exquisite pain, of a cutting or tearing character, may be experienced.

Not unusually the state of mucous membrane I have described persists for a considerable period of time. This condition may last for weeks, or even months, just as a portion of skin may be deranged by congested vessels, and chronic changes induced in the epithelium, and continue for a long period. Such morbid changes may be stopped by judicious interference, but they may not yield to remedial measures for some time. In the case of the colon, it is of the first importance not to allow anything of an irritating nature to pass along it—to restrain its action as far as possible—and to prevent the formation of wind, and the consequent irregular contraction of the muscular coat.

In some forms of diarrhœa, which are often spoken of as "bilious," you will notice a very peculiar alteration in the character of the stools, which are very dark colored, and not unfrequently may be fairly spoken of as black. Sometimes the color is such as to suggest the idea that bile has passed down the intestine without undergoing the usual changes, and forms the chief constituent of the fæces. In some of these cases it is probable that bile accumulates for a considerable period in the gall bladder, until at last this viscus, having become considerably distended, suddenly expels its contents, which are discharged in such considerable quantity that much passes almost unchanged into the large bowel.

You must be careful not to mistake the color of the motions, which is produced by many preparations of iron for that caused by blood. If a person takes iron his motions will become almost black, owing to the action of the sulphuretted hydrogen of the alimentary canal producing a dark black compound with iron. Salts of bismuth and lead also impart to discharges from the bowel a very peculiar dark color. It is important to distinguish all these changes from those caused by the presence of blood, which is itself much changed in color by the action of the intestinal gases and fluids which act upon it.

The *diet* is of the greatest importance in the management of all forms of diarrhœa. Little liquid should be swallowed while the purgation continues, and everything taken should for the time be tepid or cold, for hot things, and particularly hot liquids, seem to keep up the diarrhœa. Ordinary diet must be withheld for a time. The patient may live upon milk, thickened or not with flour, Indian corn, or lentil flour, arrow-root, sago, tapioca, or other bland, non-irritating starchy matter. Cream, puddings made with eggs, such as boiled batter, may be allowed, but anything containing hard particles that might get embedded in the mucous membrane, or irritate any tender spot that may exist, must be avoided.

Treatment of Diarrhœa.—In all forms of diarrhœa, particularly where there is much abdominal pain, it will greatly contribute to the comfort and relief of the patient if you at once apply warmth to the external surface, and recommend that he be kept in a warm room. He should lie down and rest, and if the attack be severe, he should be in bed. Cold unquestionably tends to keep up diarrhœa, and may in fact cause it. Cold also increases the sufferings of the patient. Hot fomentations to the stomach have been strongly recommended, and certainly afford relief. Various plans may be adopted. One of the simplest is to wring flannels out in very hot water, and have them quickly applied; or two or three thicknesses of dry flannel, held before a good fire until it is quite hot, may be preferred. The wet or dry flannels should be covered with a piece of oiled silk or mackintosh, which will prevent rapid cooling; or a large piece of spongio-piline, made moist with hot water, may be applied. A better plan is to procure, at one of the shops where India-rubber things are sold, a hot-water bottle, made of good strong vulcanized India-rubber. It should be eight or nine inches by fifteen, and covered with woollen material. In cases even of very severe griping pains, great relief will be afforded if the bottle containing hot water be placed closed to the skin of the abdomen while the patient is lying on his side, and kept there for an hour or more. Those who are subject to troublesome attacks of diarrhœa should wear, during winter and summer, a good thick flannel belt made for the purpose.

There are many potent remedies for checking diarrhœa. We have alkalies, the action of which I have already referred to; then there are many astringents, certain metallic salts, acids, and sedatives. Astringents (*astringo*, to bind) are often given in diarrhœa, and unquestionably check it. Amongst these may be mentioned "*Krameria*," "*Kino*," "*Catechu*," "*Logwood*," and several more are in general use. The value of many astringent remedies used in diarrhœa is perhaps, in great measure, due to the Tannin they contain, and this substance itself may be prescribed. It is a powerful astringent, and prevents free transudation of fluid through the walls of the vessels. The precise action of the Tannin is not fully understood. It may act directly upon the tissues themselves, and perhaps alter the permeable or diffusible property of the fluids. At the same time no doubt it acts upon the afferent nerves distributed to the capillaries, and through these causes contraction of the muscular fibres of the small arteries. Thus their calibre is reduced, and the quantity of blood flowing to the capillaries lessened. Logwood, *Hæmatoxylon*, is much used in the treatment of ordinary diarrhœa. You may order the decoc-

tion of Logwood, *Decoctum Hæmatoxyli,* in doses varying according to
the severity of the illness. You may begin with small doses, say from
two drachms to half an ounce of the decoction once in three hours, and
if the diarrhœa continues the dose should be increased to an ounce, and
the remedy given more frequently. Of astringent tinctures, like the Tincture of Catechu, *Tinctura Catechu,* the Tincture of Kino, *Tinctura Kino,*
and the Tincture of Rhatany, *Tinctura Krameriæ,* you may prescribe
from half a drachm or a drachm to three drachms in a mixture, and you
may give this once in three hours, or, if the diarrhœa is severe, once in
two hours. Many practitioners order one of these astringent tinctures
with chalk. Chalk Mixture, *Mistura Cretæ,* and the Aromatic Powder
of Chalk, *Pulvis Cretæ Aromaticus,* are valuable remedies in ordinary
cases of slight diarrhœa. If there is anything irritating the bowels, it
must be removed, or the diarrhœa will continue. As I have already
explained, p. 146, a purgative is necessary to expel the irritating matters before the diarrhœa will cease.

Next, with regard to the use of Opium.—If the diarrhœa has lasted
for a considerable period of time, and the patient is becoming weak and
exhausted, and you have reason to believe that instead of the bowels
being filled with irritating matter, they are empty or nearly empty, the
mucous membrane irritable and sore, with constant and irregular contractions of the muscular coat, giving rise to severe griping and excruciating pain, you will find Opium a most valuable remedy. In such cases
small doses frequently repeated answer best. You may give five or ten
drops of Laudanum in each dose of a mixture for an adult, half as much
in the case of young people, but bear in mind that Opium must not be
given in any form to young children. I prefer to give Opium in severe
cases of diarrhœa in the solid form. A quarter of a grain of solid Opium,
or half as much of the extract, *Extractum Opii,* for a dose. The composition of Dover's powder is known to most of you. Two grains will
contain one-fifth of a grain of Opium. This quantity or more of Dover's
powder, the compound Ipecacuanha powder, *Pulvis Ipecacuanhæ Compositus,* may be given in the form of a pill once in three or four hours
if the diarrhœa persists. Or you may give the patent medicine Chlorodyne, which is so well known—perhaps too well known—to non-professional persons. Chlorodyne is a mixture of many things, but it undoubtedly acts beneficially, and agrees with some persons who cannot
take ordinary preparations of opium. Many other remedies are frequently ordered, but I cannot refer to them in this place.

INTESTINAL WORMS.

I will here make a few remarks upon the important subject of intestinal
worms, for some of these parasites are often the cause of slight ailments,
and at many different periods of life. It is, however, during childhood
that illnesses depending upon the irritation of intestinal worms are most

commonly met with. The ailment may vary from a slight, but almost constant, uneasiness or pain in the stomach, occasioning or accompanied by irritability of temper, to a very serious disturbance of the nervous system, characterized by attacks of convulsions, and even unconsciousness, —in fact, by the epileptic condition, a form of illness which cannot be regarded as slight, and classed under the head of slight ailments, although the affection almost always terminates in recovery.

The intestinal worms most commonly observed in children are called *Thread Worms*, from their resemblance to small pieces of thread.

Oxyuris vermicularis.—The little *Thread Worms* are sometimes found in immense number in the fæces of children, and occasionally they trouble adults. The worms are male and female, the former being the smaller of the two. The female is seldom more than half an inch in length. They inhabit the lower part of the large bowel, and breed in immense numbers in the rectum. The eggs are oval, and are not more than the one five-hundredth of an inch in length in their longest dimensions. They are produced in countless multitudes, and can generally be demonstrated easily enough by microscopical examination of the matter passed by the bowel in cases in which thread worms have been observed.

Children suffering from thread worms are often fidgety, fractious, and excitable. They generally complain of itching about the rectum; and not unfrequently the mucous membrane of the nose and of the lips is in an irritable condition. Sometimes there is diarrhœa and discomfort referred to the lower part of the abdomen.

In order to get rid of these minute pests you may begin with purgatives. A few doses of Castor-oil will often bring away hundreds of worms. Compound Jalap Powder, *Pulvis Jalapæ Compositus*, in doses of from five to twenty grains, according to age. Compound Scammony Powder, *Pulvis Scammonii Compositus*, is still more efficacious, but must be given with caution in the case of weak children in doses of from two to ten grains. But of all the remedies for the destruction of thread worms, bitter infusions are the most potent; and Quassia is, I think, the best. An infusion of Quassia may be made by placing a tablespoonful of *Quassia* wood-chips or shavings in a jug and pouring upon them about a pint of *Cold Water*. In an hour it may be strained. A child may take an ounce or more of the clear bitter infusion twice or thrice times a day. But it is more efficacious to inject the infusion of Quassia into the rectum; and if common salt be added, in the proportion of about a tablespoonful to a pint of the infusion, it will act more efficiently. In bad cases, about a quarter of a pint or more may be injected daily into the bowel with the aid of a little India-rubber ball syringe. If the worms are not very numerous, once or twice will be sufficient. Some cases will resist for a long time all the remedies that you may try; but if you continue to use the injections steadily, the case will at length yield to treatment, though the patient may long have to exercise great care as regards diet, if he would continue free from the troublesome parasites. The tendency manifested by the large bowel of some persons to favor the growth and multiplication of these little Ascarides is very remarkable, and cannot be easily explained.   I feel sure that in some cases which have been completely cured by treatment, a fresh importation of parasites into the intestines has taken place months afterwards.   Other persons, and even members of the same family, eating the same food and living under similar conditions, pass through life without being once troubled by worms.

The large round worm, *Ascaris Lumbricoides*, is occasionally met with. The female is much larger than the male, and sometimes attains the length of twelve inches.   It is of a pale-brownish color, round, about a quarter of an inch or more in thickness, and tapering off at each end to a thin rounded extremity.   The male is only five inches long.   These worms are seldom numerous, and usually not more than from two to four exist in one individual.   They live in the small intestine, but often pass downwards and escape when the bowels act.   Occasionally they make their way into the stomach, and are vomited or pass into the mouth or nose, to the annoyance, and perhaps terror, of the patient.

Hundreds of thousands of eggs are formed and discharged by a single parasite.   The eggs are oval, and about one three-hundred-and-fiftieth of an inch in the longest diameter; and multitudes are sometimes found in the matter passed from the bowel by the patient when subjected to microscopical examination.   They may be seen by an inch or half-inch object-glass.

One of the most potent remedies for the round worm (Ascaris Lumbricoides) is Santonin, the active principle of Santonica, which consists of the unexpanded flowers of some species of *Artemisia*, or Wormwood. The dose of Santonin is two or three grains for a child, and double the quantity may be taken by an adult.   *Santonica* is the unexpanded flower-heads, as imported from Russia, from which the active principle Santonin, *Santoninum*, is obtained.   The dose of the flower-heads is from ten to fifty grains.

The only other entozoon I need mention here is the Tapeworm, of which more than one species is met with in the human organism.   The medicine which is the most efficacious in expelling the Tapeworm is the Oil or Liquid Extract of the Male Fern; but the remedy requires to be given in a particular manner, after the patient has fasted for several hours.   I shall have to consider Tapeworm and its treatment in another part of my course.

VERTIGO, GIDDINESS.

Vertigo, swimming in the head or giddiness, is an indication sometimes of disturbed action of the stomach and liver, and sometimes of deranged circulation and disturbed heart's action.   But this symptom may also be due to affections of parts of the nerve-structure of the brain, or the small arteries which supply it. The exact seat of the lesion may vary; but in animals, injury to the crus cerebri, as well as certain injuries to the cerebellum, are followed by vertigo. For one case, however, of vertigo which is due to serious disease of the brain or its vessels, we shall meet with ten or more which depend upon temporary derangement of the digestive organs.

The giddy feeling after waltzing for too long a time, or turning round many times on one leg, is within the experience of most of us, and is a form of vertigo. You will find in some works on brain affections that vertigo is mentioned as a prominent symptom of serious cerebral disease. If, however, a patient comes to you complaining of vertigo, do not at once shake your head and look grave, even if you have read records of cases in which it undoubtedly was a symptom of some terrible disease of the brain or cerebellum, or was discovered to be due to some tumor or other incurable morbid growth; for if you do give a dismal opinion you may afterwards discover that you have given a foolish one. You ought to know that this, like many other symptoms, may be due to a mere transient disturbance in connection with the circulation, or of the nerves presiding over the calibre of vessels, distributed to a very limited area of brain tissue. You must not forget that giddiness may be brought about by distal derangement, as well as by local temporary or permanent change. Temporary derangement of the stomach or liver, and probably very slight changes affecting both, will, as I have said, account for vertigo as it occurs in many cases which will come under your notice. There is a form of vertigo which is due to mere fancy or imagination. Having experienced the feeling of giddiness on one or two occasions, patients often fancy it is continually coming on. Violent attacks of coughing, especially in the case of weak persons, may occasion severe attacks of vertigo. Patients who have been ailing for some time, though not suffering from any definite malady, and those who have long been troubled with loss of appetite or impaired digestion, are frequently subjects of vertigo, and may often be cured by judicious management, as regards diet and wine or other stimulants, without any medicine. Small quantities of good soup, at intervals of a few hours, and two or three glasses of Burgundy or port wine daily, for a short time, may be ordered in such cases, and will often cure the giddiness and restore the general health in a week or two.

There are some persons who are very frequently troubled with a curious form of vertigo or giddiness, not arising from any organic lesion, or leading to any change which shortens life, or which may even seriously derange the health. In not a few instances vertigo is due to excessive nervousness. I have known highly nervous people of both sexes suffer from the most severe vertigo, preventing them from walking for many days, and for a time liable to come on if the head was only slightly raised from the pillow. Sometimes disturbed co-ordinating power of the muscles of the eye-ball is accompanied by giddiness. Vertigo occurs in many cases of blood-poisoning, and in some forms of fever. It may be brought on by sudden loss of a considerable quantity of blood, as from hemorrhage; and it often occurs in anæmia. In some forms of epilepsy vertigo is a prominent symptom.

The word *vertigo* comes from *vertex* or *vortex*, a whirlwind, which is derived from "*Verto*, I turn." The sensation is sometimes described as a swimming in the head. Objects seem to be moving in a strange and irregular manner. Many cannot look from a great height downwards without feeling giddy. Vertigo may be brought on by taking certain substances. Opium will cause it, also Belladonna; alcohol causes it very commonly. Any one who has seen a person a little tipsy knows how his power of co-ordinating the muscular movements of his body is impaired, and how he rolls about from one side to the other; and in consequence of feeling giddy is unable to walk in a straight line. Tobacco will also give rise to a form of vertigo, especially when it is brought into contact with nerves and nerve-centres, which have not gradually become accustomed to its influence. A slight, temporary failure in the force of the heart's action may cause marked giddiness; and the attacks may recur from time to time, causing much anxiety to the patient and his friends. A few doses of Sal Volatile or brandy frequently relieve this form of vertigo. Only a teaspoonful or less of the stimulant is required, diluted with not more than double the quantity of water.

Peculiar disturbances in vision occur in many cases of vertigo. Things look crooked. Some see only a portion of an object. They can see the upper half without being able to see the lower half of a person, and so on. These disturbances of vision do not necessarily imply anything more severe than temporary functional disturbance, perhaps due to some irregular distribution of blood in the capillary vessels of parts of the central ganglia, consequent upon sudden alterations in calibre of the small arteries, caused by disturbed action of the nerve ganglia which regulate and preside over the action of the coats of these particular vessels. Such symptoms may mean, it is true, something far more serious, but in many cases they certainly depend upon no more grave or important changes than may be determined by taking a little more wine than is good. Swimming in the head is by many considered a form of vertigo. Persons who have been for some time over-anxious, or who have been overtaxing the mind or body, may suffer in this way. In the last case, the unpleasant symptoms will sometimes disappear ten minutes after taking a dose of Sal Volatile or an alcoholic stimulant. If, however, they do not do so, they will probably be relieved by a little attention to diet, by a dose or two of Calomel or Blue Pill. The general health may afterwards be improved by taking a tonic, containing acid and bark, for a week or two.

Aural Vertigo.—Disease and injury to the semicircular canals of the ear may cause a feeling of giddiness and a tendency to fall, as well as vertiginous movements, the direction of which, forwards, backwards, or from side to side, is determined by the particular semicircular canal which is affected. Ménière, as long ago as 1861, directed attention to a class of cases in which noise in one ear,—humming, buzzing, whistling, puffing, —often associated with pallor, headache, faintness, giddiness, nausea, and vomiting occurred in connection with disease of the semicircular canals, or of other parts of the ear. The attacks at first are slight and occasional, but gradually the noises in the head increase in intensity, and are almost constant. At last absolute deafness of the affected ear ensues, and in consequence of the nerve-structures being destroyed, the giddiness and other symptoms cease.

You will, however, meet with the symptoms above enumerated in cases in which there is no reason to suppose that organic disease of the ear or any other organ exists. The attacks, after recurring several times at intervals during many years, will at last cease, leaving the patient perfectly well. Some of these cases seem to belong to the category of sick headache, and the attacks will be relieved by a small dose of Calomel, Blue Pill, or Grey Powder, *Hydrargyrum cum Cretâ*. In such instances it is very probable that there is temporary disturbance of the circulation in the internal ear, as well as in other parts. Moreover, very nervous, fanciful people will sometimes complain of the symptoms of Ménière's disease, but as they quite recover under the influence of tonics, good living, and change of air, it is more likely that the symptoms were due to slight and temporary nerve disturbance, than to definite morbid change affecting nerve or other tissue.

BILIOUSNESS.

It is difficult to adequately explain the various phenomena which constitute what is known as biliousness, although very many persons are well acquainted with the symptoms of the bilious condition, and have frequently experienced them. Whether there is congestion of the liver in all cases, I cannot tell, for I am glad to say that I never saw a *post-mortem* of any one who had died during an attack of biliousness. Whatever may be the essential nature of the malady, it is not fatal. Nay, bilious people are for the most part long-lived. Some physicians who have experience in connection with life insurance business, so far from objecting to take bilious people, are desirous of insuring them. In this opinion I fully concur. There is no doubt that a tendency to biliousness makes people very careful as to their mode of living. They know that if they exceed they will suffer. Bilious persons are often very fidgety about their diet, for if they eat too much a bilious attack usually comes on, and for a time they are completely unfit for ordinary work. Although biliousness is anything but an agreeable malady, nevertheless you may generally recommend bilious patients with confidence for various occupations in which endurance is required. The capacity for going steadily on for a long period of time is in truth often associated with a bilious habit of body. I fancy a very large share of the best work of the world is performed by the bilious. Such a tendency is frequently characterized by much energy and determination to work in spite of the derangement, and although there may be also some irritability of temper or despondency, there is frequently a very remarkable degree of patience, persistence, and resisting power.

Although I cannot give an accurate description of the pathological phenomena of biliousness, I may help you to form an idea of the sort of unpleasant sensations experienced by bilious people, if I describe in his own words, the sufferings of a gentleman who had been bilious all his life, but who nevertheless managed to live to a very advanced age. My friend was a man who might have done great things and left his mark ; but I fear he lost much, and perhaps the world more, in consequence of his not being obliged to work. As in some other cases, a fortune is after all a misfortune. He was, moreover, unwise enough to allow himself to get into that habit of thinking too much about slight physiological derangements which occurred in his own organism, and he gradually got into the bad habit of frequently talking to his friends about his aches and pains. Being rich, he was listened to, and further was spoiled by the sympathy and pity foolishly lavished upon him. As age advanced, the interest of his environment seemed to him to diminish, while the growls and grumblings, excited by sensations within himself, became so loud that at length he determined to seek professional consolation. He consulted the most celebrated physicians, but no one succeeded in curing his biliousness, or in teaching him to bear it patiently. He grievously troubled his family by his reiterated complaints, and by his persistent anxiety about himself. Though on occasions he felt pretty well for a day or two, during many years he failed to make himself contented or happy. Every kind of treatment was tried, but nothing cured the derangement or averted the attacks. Blue Pill afforded some relief, and was the only remedy persisted in from first to last. All his tissues were probably sound, and I doubt whether there was any serious morbid change in any organs after more than ninety years of work. This gentleman was seen by me many times, and wrote down for me a description of his sufferings. Here it is: " Flatulence, distention of the bowels, and painful sensations between the shoulders ; coldness of the feet, twinging pains occasionally under the right shoulder-blade, nausea after eating. Muscular pain about the head and neck—particularly the muscles at the back of the neck." The last is a very common symptom, and a very painful one in many cases of biliousness, and recurs in almost every attack. This old gentleman ate too much, and no wonder he was disturbed at night, and had to complain of " harassing and long-distressing dreams."

He also suffered, as very many old people do, from "irritation of the skin of the body generally, but of his legs principally, and from soreness and eruptions about the mouth, affecting chiefly the upper lip." Such was the long catalogue of recorded symptoms, and the list by no means exhausts all this old gentleman's complaints.

Some who suffer from biliousness differ from my old friend, and seem to alternate between a state of misery and despair and a state of comparative comfort and even hopefulness. You will sometimes find patients bilious and irritable and out of temper, and very indisposed to do what you may wish, unless indeed they have sufficient self-command to overcome their natural bent. Another time you will find the same persons in excellent spirits, and ready to do anything for you, and as agreeable as possible. We may have very contradictory accounts of the same individual; one person tells us that he is a most disagreeable, cantankerous person, while another affirms him to be a most pleasant and excellent man. The conflict of testimony is explained by the circumstance that one informant happened to see him when he was bilious, while the other came in contact with him just after he had recovered from an attack.

It seems curious that we should not be able to fully explain such very prominent and persistent functional derangements as affect important organs in cases of biliousness, more especially as the condition is a common one, and has been often experienced by well-trained scientific and thoughtful members of our profession. But I have never been able to get, from any physicians with whom I have conversed or from any books I have read, what seems to me to be a clear and satisfactory account of the disturbance which occurs in an attack of biliousness, or of the actual changes which affect the action of the peccant organs during the prevalence of the attack. There is, however, no doubt that at the time there is actual disturbance in the liver. When biliousness is experienced, the changes taking place in this organ, as well as in the stomach, differ in important particulars from those which occur under ordinary circumstances.

The liver is not concerned merely in the secretion of that fluid which we know as the bile, but it has to do with many other changes. Among the most remarkable phenomena of the liver are its sugar- and fat-producing powers. It also effects great changes in albuminous matters and peptones, which have just been taken up by the vessels of the intestines and carried to it dissolved in the portal blood.

Concerning any slight derangements which the sugar-forming functions of the liver no doubt undergo from time to time, we know comparatively little; but we do know that these functions may be so disturbed as to result in the establishment of a most serious change in the action of the organ which, when once started, usually persists, and at length, at least in the case of the young, ends in death. In Diabetes, particularly as it occurs in the young, many ounces of sugar are formed during each period of twenty-four hours, and the kidneys are chiefly concerned in the removal of this sugar from the blood, although the tears and other secretions also contain sugar when the diabetic state is established. This formation of sugar, although varying in activity from time to time, and under the influence of remedies, cannot certainly be stopped. It continues in the great majority of well-marked cases, and gradually exhausts the patient, until, after a period varying from a few months to two or three years, death results. On the other hand, I may confidently state that, under certain conditions, which cannot be exactly defined, the liver may be seriously deranged as regards its sugar-forming functions, not only without causing death, but even without apparently deranging the general health or nutrition of the patient. In old age it is not an uncommon thing to find a certain amount, and occasionally an enormous quantity, of sugar in the urine of a person, although its presence was quite unexpected. It would seem that, in old age, the sugar-forming action of the liver may be greatly in excess of what it is in the normal state, and although the sugar pervades the blood and is carried by it to the various tissues and organs of the body, it scarcely seems to disturb their action. At any rate, it may continue uninterruptedly for more than twenty years, and the patient may die at an advanced age of some other malady. Not only so, but any healthy person may for a time form considerable quantities of diabetic sugar, if he will take more than a moderate quantity of cane sugar. A man who took a dose of a quarter of a pound of ordinary sugar passed diabetic sugar in his water for two or three days afterwards; but this temporary diabetic state is not to be induced so easily in every person. The liver is the organ by which the change is effected, and if you think over these facts you will, I think, agree with me in the conclusion that, in many slight derangements of the health, some other functions of the liver, instead of or as well as its bile-forming office, are at fault. The action of the liver-cells, in connection with their influence on the formation and transformation of fatty, albuminous, and amyloid matters, must, therefore, not be lost sight of in our efforts to determine the causation of many slight derangements of the health which seem referable to the liver.

But as regards "biliousness," it seems to me that the yellow tinge of the conjunctiva so commonly observed, the alteration in the color of the skin and its dryness, the disturbed action of the sebaceous glands, the sense of weight in the right side, the derangement of digestion—all point to the fat- and bile-forming operations of the liver-cells as being mainly at fault. This view is confirmed by the fact that medicines which correct the changes just referred to are those which unquestionably act upon the bile-forming process, and as soon as the action begins the patient who suffers from what is known as a bilious attack experiences relief. Some cases of severe biliousness approach so nearly to those cases of temporary jaundice, which I shall presently speak of, that I am almost inclined to regard them as related to that condition. Possibly, it may be correct to consider biliousness a condition which initiates certain forms of jaundice. Biliousness may possibly depend upon an inactive state of the liver-cells, in consequence of which substances remain in the blood which ought to be separated from that fluid and converted into bile. The sluggish state of the circulation, the tendency to the accumulation of the blood in the capillaries and veins, as shown by the distention of the capillaries of the papillæ of the skin and the bleeding which takes place if they are divided, the formation or increase of hæmorrhoids, the turgid state of capillaries near slight scratches or wounds, and the indisposition of the latter to heal, indicate such disturbance of the capillary circulation generally as would result from the accumulation in the blood of substances which ought to be thoroughly eliminated from the circulating fluid.

The Treatment of Biliousness.—The only medicine that relieves many bilious people is a small dose of some mercurial preparation. The old gentleman to whose case I have already referred discovered that blue pill alone gave him ease, and dissipated for a time the unpleasant sensations from which he suffered, and which made him at times perfectly wretched. He took blue pill of his own accord, whether the doctors allowed it or not. For forty years he seldom went four days without the remedy. He tried over and over again to get out of the habit, and many advisers strongly recommended him to give up taking mercurials. He made many attempts, but in a short time his sufferings became so great, that at last he was obliged to return to his favorite remedy. He seldom, however, took more than a grain once in four or five days.

I do not mean to imply that you will cure every case of biliousness if you give mercurials; but certainly the great majority that come under your notice will be benefited. Many cases resist every effort to cure them, but it is the exception to meet with a sufferer who cannot be in some degree relieved by treatment. The bilious habit seems to be due to an unusually sensitive, irritable stomach and liver, which discharge their functions fairly in a moderate degree, but which cannot be made to perform more than this moderate amount of work, without getting much out of order; so that where you have to treat patients suffering from biliousness, you must be careful to give directions concerning diet, which should be very moderate, and lay stress upon the importance of great moderation.

Most of the organs taking part in the digestion and assimilation of the food seem to strike work when a decided bilious attack comes on. If food be taken, the suffering becomes greater. Moderate starvation is what is required in many cases. Bilious people often find advantage from giving their digestive organs partial rest for several days. In this way time is allowed for the return of the organs deranged to their normal state. The fact seems to be that the digestive organs require rest for a time, and if, when an attack comes on, this rest is given, the bilious state passes off, and then the patient feels extremely well, perhaps for a considerable time.

In general, you will find that those who are liable to bilious attacks require very little meat. Free meat-eating will often bring on an attack. Generally, rich foods do not agree. Fatty matters in certain forms and in moderate proportion must be taken, but cooked and half-cooked fatty materials, as in many sauces, soups, fried fish, and meats, are not suitable. Cream or much milk sometimes precipitates an attack. Most forms of alcohol, and any form in quantity, will generally disagree with the patient. Vegetables and many fruits, on the other hand, agree well; vegetable acids seem to help the action of the liver and stomach. From half an ounce to an ounce of lemon juice daily for a time is undoubtedly useful in many instances. Cider in moderation, that is, one or at most two tumblers daily, can be taken by some bilious persons. Citrates, Tartrates, Acetates, may also be given. Light puddings composed of starchy matters of various kinds, such as Rice, Indian corn, Sago, or Tapioca, made with milk and eggs in small quantity, and plenty of bread, may be enumerated among the articles of diet for the bilious. Generally, such persons are of necessity small eaters—their organs rebel before it is possible to damage them by overwork, and so they seldom die of those diseases which cut short the life of so many who enjoy good living, and who possess strong digestive organs. Hence, as I have already remarked, the bilious often live to be old. When an attack comes on, benefit often results from the use of mild purgatives. Effervescing Citrates and Tartrates do good. Liquor Ammoniæ Acetatis and Muriate of Ammonia have been also prescribed with advantage in many cases. I have often recommended grapes, in quantities of half a pound a day, when they can be obtained. Many persons have been relieved by taking from six to ten tumblers of fluid in the course of twenty-four hours, for two or three days at a time. Ordinary soda water, or seltzer, or Apollinaris water may be ordered. The kidneys are in this way made to act very freely, and relief soon follows.

Of the deleterious action of the *east wind* upon the functional action of the liver there can be no doubt; but it is not easy to explain precisely how this results. That the dryness of the air and the constant wind are potent in interfering with the due action of the skin there can be no question; but these effects do not afford an adequate explanation of the facts, since persons shut up in rooms artificially heated, and with the air supplied with watery vapor, nay, people who have kept their beds, are often aware when the wind blows from the east. Northerly and westerly winds may be as cold, and I think as dry, as the east winds, without giving rise to those very unpleasant sensations experienced by the majority of the population who have passed their fourth decade, whenever the wind is in the east. As long as the wind blows from this quarter, people suffer; but a few hours after a change has taken place they feel perfectly well, both in body and mind ; for, as is well known, the temper is often terribly ruffled by a dry east wind.

The *seaside* has the reputation of seriously impeding the action of the liver ; and deservedly so ; for we are assured by many persons that whenever they go to the sea for a week or more, the motions are invariably scanty, and of a very pale yellow or of a gray color. But what is very remarkable is this : that for some time after their return from the sea the hepatic actions of the same persons is unusually free. Although they may consume much less food than when they were away, the motions are more abundant and the fæcal matter properly formed. In these cases there is no doubt that there is increased formation of fæcal matter—that materials which had been accumulating for perhaps a fortnight previously are at length separated from the blood, and the patient in consequence feels greatly relieved and appears to be much improved in health.

Where the bilious state is very severe—and in some cases it is so severe as to incapacitate people from performing any kind of work for the time —you will often afford relief, and in a very short time, if you give a grain or two of Blue Pill or Calomel. Some who suffer from biliousness also experience violent headache at the time ; and this symptom is also relieved by the Blue Pill or Calomel, and frequently in the course of a very few hours after the medicine has been taken. Indeed, some who suffer much, and who are, generally speaking, in anything but a good state of health, may yet be able to get through their work with the help of an occasional dose of a mercurial—from one to three grains of Gray Powder once in five or six days. I am not aware that any deleterious effects are produced by this practice in persons who suffer much from biliousness. Of course it is not desirable for any one to be continually taking mercurials, or any other drugs for that matter ; but it is better to take mercurials now and then than to be utterly incapacitated for one or two days out of every ten or twelve, as is the case with many who suffer from this most unpleasant ailment.

From some experiments performed by Dr. William Rutherford on the dog, it appears that several vegetable substances act as stimulants to the secretion of bile ; and it has been inferred that they act upon man as well as upon the dog. Among the most important of these cholagogues are Iridin, Baptistin, Juglandin, of each of which from two to four grains may be prescribed for a dose, Euonymin in doses of from one grain to two grains, and Phytolaccin, of which the dose is from one-eighth of a grain to a grain. Dr. Rutherford's observations will be found in the "British Medical Journal," February 8th, 1879.

Jaundice is a rather common affection, particularly in summer. It may be due to many different causes, some of which are unimportant and transient, while others are serious and irremediable. The particular form of jaundice to which I am about to refer, may, with propriety, be included under the head of "slight ailments." It is known as *ordinary* jaundice; and I dare say that perhaps thirty or more per cent. of us have suffered from an attack of jaundice, or will do so before the age of twenty-five is passed.

The physiological changes in the system must needs be very much modified if the bile, which is formed in such considerable quantity, instead of being poured into the intestines, is retained in the gall-bladder. In every form of jaundice the bile is formed by the liver, but does not escape by its usual channel. Most commonly the Common Gall-Duct, *Ductus Communis Choledochus*, is plugged up; and the bile, which has been formed by the cells of the liver, and has passed into the gall-ducts, is obstructed in its further course towards the intestine. After accumulating to some extent in the ducts, and in the gall-bladder, it would appear that it gradually makes its way through their coats, and gains entrance to the lymphatics and veins which lie outside them. Hence the bile formed by the liver soon passes into, and circulates with, the blood. Tissues in all parts of the body become stained, and in some cases take a deep yellow color. Textures, both at the surface and in the interior of the body, are thus stained more or less intensely in cases of jaundice.

Not only so, but the excretion of the yellow coloring matter which has been formed originally in the liver, and has been absorbed into the blood, is effected to some extent by the kidneys. Mucus, epithelial cells, casts, and even some crystals passed in the urine are tinged of a bright yellow color, while the urine itself contains a good deal of yellow biliary matter. Sometimes it appears of a dark-green color, owing to the quantity of bile it contains. So quickly in many instances is the bile removed from the blood by the kidneys that the urine is often stained with the characteristic yellow color for some days before the skin acquires the slightest yellow tint. On the other hand, the secretions from the bowels will be found to lose the ordinary color, and after the jaundice has lasted a short time they will be clay-colored or colorless.

Whether the impediment which interferes with the passage of the bile into the intestine, in these cases of temporary jaundice, is due to firm spasmodic contraction of the muscular fibres which surround the lower part of the common gall-duct near its opening in the duodenum, or to the accumulation of mucus and epithelium in the same situation, thus plugging the duct, is not quite certain; but there can be no doubt that there is in all these cases an impediment to the onward flow of the bile, consequent upon some temporary obstruction, which after a period varying from a week to three months or longer gives way without any permanent change or derangement being induced. Patients suffering from temporary jaundice completely recover.

Now I desire to ask your careful attention to the fact that in these cases the jaundice is due not to the accumulation in the blood of substances out of which bile might be formed by the action of the liver-cells, but to the passage into the blood of bile which has been already formed by the action of these hepatic elements, and has passed into the ducts.

As I have already said, the stools appear more or less like clay, or of very light-brown color, in consequence of the biliary matter not having passed into the intestines, where ordinarily it undergoes those complicated changes which take place in its resinous acids and coloring matter, and which end at last in the development of the peculiar chemical compounds which are constantly found in normal fæcal matter.

Even in slight cases of jaundice the bowels are usually somewhat confined. The patient perhaps experiences slight nausea, with indisposition to take food. He gets thin. The nutriment matters he does take do not nourish him properly, and he feels weak and out of health. Some people suffering from jaundice are, however, able to do their work, and students have passed through a difficult examination although they were deeply jaundiced ; but the proceeding is not a wise one.

You see, therefore, that a very large and important organ like the liver may be seriously deranged without the ordinary functions of the other organs of the body being very seriously disturbed. For a time at least we can get on not only without bile flowing into the intestine, but in spite of its distribution to all parts of the body. In these cases, the bile prevented from escaping from the liver is reabsorbed and taken up by the blood, and the coloring matter deposited in many of the tissues. The patient may, however, notwithstanding this great change, be able to perform a certain considerable amount of work, and may be able to use his mind efficiently, although the whole of the blood distributed to his brain is contaminated with a considerable proportion of biliary matter.

But, as I have remarked, you must bear in mind that from time to time cases of jaundice are met with which end, and very quickly too, most disastrously. It is a fact which must not be forgotten, that some of these cases which may run on to a fatal termination in the course of two or three weeks, cannot at their commencement be distinguished from that almost trivial form of jaundice of which I have spoken. Ordinary jaundice may last for a period varying from one week to three months. Probably the average time will be from two to three weeks. When it persists for more than a month, even though there be no grave symptoms, we feel some degree of anxiety lest the case should be due to more than a temporary obstruction of the duct. The longest case of ordinary temporary jaundice which has come under my own notice lasted for upwards of twelve weeks. For the whole of this time the patient, a young man of eighteen, was deeply jaundiced, and no decided improvement began to take place until three months had passed. In cases where the malady is prolonged so considerably beyond the average time, we may suppose that the plug of mucus or modified epithelium in the common duct is firmer than usual. At last, however, the mass, having become softened, slowly escapes, bit by bit, from the orifice of the duct, and gradually the organ returns to its normal state.

That form of jaundice which is very fatal, and which may end quickly in death, is dependent upon serious damage to the secreting and other structures of the liver, and the liver-cells are often completely disintegrated and destroyed. As I said before, I do not know how we can distinguish the terribly serious from the slight ailment when the patient first becomes jaundiced. In the fatal form of jaundice, however, very grave symptoms are developed after the lapse of a few days, and we then become aware of the terrible disease with which we have to deal. But during the first few days of the attack it is, I believe, not possible in many instances to distinguish a case which will end fatally from a case which will terminate in recovery. I allude to this matter because it is really most important not to be over-confident and off-hand in forming a prognosis in this, and indeed in most other forms of, disease. You may perhaps be called to see one of these fatal forms of jaundice, due to what has been called *acute yellow atrophy of the liver*, and, if not aware of the existence of such cases, you might make a very sad mistake in informing the friends confidently that a necessarily fatal disease was only a slight ailment. We ought never to allow ourselves to make light of a malady which may turn out to be very serious indeed. Under such circumstances, we might be deservedly accused of want of care, experience, and knowledge, and regarded as advisers lacking discretion and wisdom, and wanting in power of discerning a most serious disorder, which destroys life in a short time. On the other hand, you must be careful not to needlessly frighten people by detailing all the possibilities of disaster in any given case. Happily, these serious forms of jaundice are not common. In the course of a year we seldom see in the hospital more than one or two of them, and several years may pass without a single case being admitted.

Ordinary temporary jaundice may occur at any period of life, but it is most common between the ages of fifteen and twenty-four; and it is more frequently met with in males than in females. Whether it is that we are apt to exceed in diet more than the other sex at this period of life, or whether the way we live has anything to do with it, I cannot tell; possibly we may be more anxious and nervous about our work and examinations than female students; but it is certain that about adolescence jaundice in men is not at all uncommon.

Jaundice occurring in middle life and old age is not very likely to be of this kind. More probably it will depend upon some more serious change than catarrh of the gall-ducts and the obstruction of the common duct by a plug of mucus. A very common cause of jaundice in middle life is a gall-stone impacted in the duct. Jaundice of this kind is usually associated with great, and not uncommonly sudden, excruciating pain, and its nature can often be at once detected. This form of disease can, however, hardly be included under the head of "slight ailments." You should be aware that jaundice may occur in very young children; and I have known cases in which it existed in intra-uterine life. It is not an uncommon thing for the child at birth to be completely jaundiced, but this usually passes off. It is due to temporary change. I have seen one case in which life was destroyed at or about the eight month of intra-uterine life by jaundice, caused by the impaction of a gall-stone in the common gall-duct. What is the earliest period of development at which the embryo may become affected I cannot say, but it is certain that some months before birth biliary calculi may be formed. Urinary calculi also may be produced even before the development of the kidney in which they are formed is perfected.

Treatment of Temporary Jaundice.—With regard to the treatment of ordinary jaundice there is little to be said. The main point to be borne in mind is that the patient should live on a light diet. Do not let him feed heavily, or he will get worse, and may suffer much. Keep the bowels gently acting by giving small doses of Blue Pill or Gray Powder at intervals of a few days. You may also, or instead, occasionally give a dose of some saline purgative. A drachm or two of Sulphate of Magnesia, *Magnesiæ Sulphas*, with a little Hydrochloric or Sulphuric Acid (p. 141) before breakfast, is of service in this condition, just to promote the action of the bowels. Do not, however, give violent purgatives or attempt to cure the disease off-hand by any course of special treatment. A mustard poultice may be placed over the region of the liver every day, or every other day, for twenty minutes. Another local application which seems to be of use, and which I learned from Dr. Blakiston, is Hydrochloric Acid applied on rags. The strong acid is diluted with twice its bulk of water. A rag is carefully wetted with the lotion, placed over the liver, and then covered with some useless rags or an old towel. This application may be used each alternate day, care being taken that the acid is not allowed to spoil any linen or the clothes of the patient. It produces only a little tingling. The skin should be wiped with a soft, wet sponge when the rag is removed.

I come now to another malady, reference to which may perhaps raise a smile. It is, however, an extremely disagreeable ailment to endure, and it may entirely prevent, or seriously mar, the execution of mental and bodily work.

SICK HEADACHE.

This is one of the most severe of the maladies I have included under the head of slight ailments. The affection is very common, and used to be known as Migraine. Some, who in other respects are perfectly healthy persons, with apparently sound constitutions, and whose tissues generally would seem to be not only healthy, but of an enduring character, suffer from very frequent attacks, and may be for many years hardly ever free from the malady. Nevertheless, sick headache is to be regarded as a very troublesome and inconvenient, rather than as a serious, derangement.

This curious disorder may affect people at every period of life. Some authorities assert with confidence that as we grow older we overcome the tendency to sick headache; but I am sorry to say I know some who have grown old, and many who are growing old, who still suffer. One sees cases of sick headache occasionally in very young children, frequently in young people and adults, and not uncommonly in old age. I know persons of seventy-five and upwards who continue to suffer from well-marked forms of this intractable malady. However, there is no doubt that the tendency of the sick headache is to diminish in severity as age advances; so that many who are martyrs to frequent and severe attacks up to the age of twenty-five or thirty, begin to improve after that period, and towards forty become troubled less frequently, or recover altogether. In others, the attacks become rare, but occur now and then as long as life lasts.

Sick headache is a disease not dependent upon any actual pathological change, as far as can be at present ascertained. It seems to be due to some temporary, but widely-extended, derangement, influencing a number of different tissues and organs, situated at a distance from one another.

I shall endeavor to lay before you the several phenomena of which this malady is composed, and shall try to point out in what respects there is a departure from the normal and healthy action of the several organs and tissues involved. In the first place, as to the headache. This is peculiar, for it is usually confined to one-half or less of the head, *Hemicrania* (ἡμισυς, half, κρανιον, the head). A part of one lateral half of the upper part of the head is the seat of very severe pain, which is occasionally described as of a boring or penetrating character, and may be so circumscribed that the painful spot could be covered by the top of the thumb. Sometimes the pain is situated immediately over one brow, the sensation experienced being like that which would be produced if a sharp and strong instrument was being forced into the head at that particular spot. The pain, varying much in intensity, and somewhat in character, from time to time, may last for a period of from twelve to twenty-four hours, or even longer. It may then shift to the opposite side, and, after lasting there for about twelve hours more, may gradually subside, until the patient becomes perfectly free from pain. In a short time he feels well, and, perhaps, for some days after the attack has subsided considers himself unusually vigorous. From the frequency of the occurrence of cases in which the pain is confined to the region above one or other brow, the condition has been called *Brow Ague.* The term ague is, however, unfortunate, for the affection is far removed from maladies belonging to that class.

Next, as regards nausea and vomiting, which frequently accompany this headache. The stomach derangement in sick headache is often very marked and very distressing; but these symptoms are often preceded by an almost irrepressible tendency to yawn at frequent intervals. There is a sensation apparently situated in the soft palate which almost makes the person yield; but as soon as he has yawned once the desire returns; and this often lasts for some hours, or until vomiting occurs or sleep is induced. There is, as I have said, almost always more or less nausea, and not unfrequently absolute vomiting, the depression accompanying the sickness being sometimes of the most distressing character. It is often as bad as severe sea-sickness. I have known people to vomit fifteen or twenty times in the course of the day, although they were merely suffering from what is called sick headache. In this condition, then, we have temporary, but very decided, and sometimes violent, disturbance of the digestive organs, inability to take food, nausea, and severe vomiting, associated with pain, more or less acute, on one side of, or, it may be, all over, the head. The vomiting is remarkable; for there is not merely straining and contraction of the stomach, followed by the rejection of its contents, but a great deal of secretion is poured into the stomach from the blood or from the glands; and after this has accumulated so as to distend the organ, it is suddenly expelled. It is in this way that many of those who suffer from sick headache get relief. After the removal of the contents of the stomach, which are often of an intensely acid reaction, the distressing nausea and sense of oppression and exhaustion become relieved for a time, but recur if more acid fluid is poured out. What is very remarkable in many of these cases is this: that food may be digested shortly before the vomiting is excited, when an enormous quantity of acid fluid from the stomach is brought up. There can be no doubt that in these cases much acid is formed in the stomach, or secreted by the glands. Indeed, at the very time food is being digested and passed onwards to the duodenum, there is evidence of the formation of other acids beside the ordinary acid of the gastric juice. Oxalic, butyric, acetic, valerianic, are among the organic acids which are developed, owing to some unusual chemical changes taking place in the contents of the stomach. It is the accumulation of this acid mixture which causes the nausea and painful sinking experienced at the pit of the stomach. The nausea remains until the contents of the stomach have been expelled. Vomiting may, of course, be encouraged by the administration of a medicinal emetic, by drinking several tumblers of warm water, or by tickling the back of the fauces. The act of vomiting may be attended with instant relief. I have known cases in which, the moment after the stomach had rejected its contents, the pains ceased, and, for a time at least, the patient is in comparative ease, or feels perfectly well.

In slight sick headache, as well as in more serious head affections, there is evidence of remarkable sympathy and association between the action of the brain and the stomach. The pain that we suffer in sick headache is not due merely to some affection of the cutaneous nerves

15

of the skin of the head and face, as has been held by some, but there is clearly a temporary disturbance in the brain itself, probably in connection with the vessels at least of the surface of the gray matter of the convolutions, for not only does the pain seem to be situated in the brain, but the action of the cerebral matter is unmistakably disturbed. The memory is for the time impaired. Attention cannot be given without conscious and even painful effort. Sustained thought is impossible for the time, and there is a decided longing for mental rest, which, being yielded to, soon results in dozing, or in actual sleep. It might be thought that cerebral disturbance generally, at least when ushered in by functional or organic disease of the digestive organs, would be due to deranged action of the upper part of the alimentary canal only. The most remarkable phenomena undoubtedly point to stomach and duodenal disturbance, and we know that in many diseases of the brain the action of the stomach especially is disturbed—frequent and sudden vomiting being often present. The action of the stomach, as every one has experienced, is much influenced by the brain, and the latter by the stomach. Digestion may seriously derange cerebral action, and may in its turn be modified or completely interfered with by mental or emotional disturbance. This indeed is admitted, but in many forms of sick headache the derangement is certainly more general than the consideration of the subject thus far would have perhaps led you to suppose, and it is doubtful whether the lower, as well as the upper, part, and in some cases exclusively the lower part, of the alimentary canal is not implicated in the attack. I shall presently refer to this point more particularly.

The disturbance of the nervous system in sick headache is so striking and widespread, that some pathologists have been induced to place sick headache among nervous diseases, and to support the conclusion that the derangement not only begins in the nervous system, but that the affection is exclusively nervous. To me, however, it seems more probable, and the conclusion is grounded partly upon personal experience, that the nerve phenomena are second in the order of their occurrence, and that the starting-point of the malady is abnormal functional disturbance in the digestive organs, and, through these, in the blood itself.

That the blood is deranged in cases of sick headache is probable from several circumstances. It has been noticed that any wound or scratch that there may be on the surface of the skin looks angry. The processes of healing and the nourishment of tissues do not proceed as in perfect health. Another reason for concluding that the blood is more or less out of order is that, when the sick headache disappears, very free action of excretory glands sets in. A considerable quantity of urine, often rich in uria and urates, and of high specific gravity, is voided, and this is succeeded by the free secretion of large quantities of pale urine containing a small proportion of solid matter. Gradually the ordinary actions in the several tissues and organs are resumed.

The composition of the blood is also much altered during the attack by the free discharge of certain substances from it into the stomach. The glands, instead of pouring out ordinary gastric juice to digest the food, secrete, and in considerable quantity, a fluid which, instead of quietly digesting the food, irritates the nerves distributed to the mucous membrane, and causes vomiting. The fluid is frequently highly acid, but, as I have remarked, the acidity is due to a number of organic acids which are not to be found in health. Under these circumstances it is useless to introduce food into the stomach, for little or no digestion will take place. The stomach must be allowed to rest for a while, until its contents are rejected, or by degrees driven downwards into the small intestine. It seems, then, probable that certain materials which yield these substances when discharged into the stomach have been accumulating in the blood for some time before the attack of sick headache occurs—that, indeed, the malady depends upon this accumulation in the blood, and that the "attack" corresponds to their discharge into the stomach.

The salivary glands, the little labial and buccal glands, are else affected. Saliva is very sparingly secreted, and the mouth is often in a dry or clammy and uncomfortable state; the mucous membrane dries very quickly; there is often a very unpleasant taste, and instead of the mucous surface being soft and moist, it seems to be besmeared with viscid mucus, and the patient will tell you his mouth is quite out of order. In many cases the action of the salivary glands is certainly suspended for a time, and when the attack is passing off, one of the first points noticed is the pouring of a quantity of saliva into the mouth. With the return of salivary secretion, the unpleasant sensations about the mouth, the dryness, the disagreeable taste, and the clamminess disappear.

The liver is out of order in "sick headache." Its action in many cases seems indeed to be almost suspended for a time. The excrements are sometimes, but not invariably, pale and altered in consistence. The intestine is not stimulated to perform its ordinary contractions, and in many cases flatus collects. Moreover the surface of the liver is sometimes tender to the touch. Not unfrequently there is a feeling of fulness or actual pain in the right side; and often there is distinct yellowness of the skin and the conjunctiva. The action of the alimentary canal is partially suspended, or the intestine scarcely acts at all. Its contents, in many instances, seem to remain almost still for a time during the attack, or are very slowly urged towards the lower bowel. The action of the colon is suspended. No accumulation of fæcal matter goes on during the attack, for fæces are at the time not being formed.

In some cases of sick headache, I think the derangement actually begins in the large intestine. Sometimes there is evidence of moderate, but not excessive, fæcal accumulation, with a passive state of the mucous membrane and its glands, and sluggishness of its muscular coat. The cæcum and ascending colon are very commonly at fault ; and I have often succeeded in feeling the accumulation at this part of the bowel. The patient himself is frequently aware of some discomfort or unpleasant sensation in the right iliac fossa. By palpation you may detect the fulness, and by the tympanitic percussion over this part of the bowel you demonstrate the presence of gas, much of which probably arises from decomposition of materials which ought to have been expelled long before. It does not follow that actual constipation has prevailed, but the bowel has not completely emptied itself. For some time, perhaps for weeks and months, it has not driven down the fæcal matter towards the rectum as fast as it was formed. The lower part of the ileum, as well as the cæcum, is at fault in many instances. Probably Peyer's patches and the solitary glands do not act freely ; and oftentimes their action is further disturbed by the constant presence of faulty secretion, and possibly of the products of fermentation and unusual chemical action in the slowly-moving and almost putrefying mass. The action of the glands themselves is then interfered with ; and the uneasiness and pain which are sometimes experienced may be due to this cause. You must not forget these points, for they are of interest in connection with the causation of many derangements of the health, some of which are by no means slight. I believe that a prolonged, and perhaps almost constantly disturbed, action of this part of the alimentary canal leads to important changes in the blood, and may establish a state of system favorable to the development of important diseases of different kinds. Neither must it be forgotten that when materials remain for some time in contact with the mucous membrane of the large bowel, reabsorption occurs, and thus many noxious matters, which ought to be discharged from the system, find their way in an objectionable form into the blood.

You see, then, in sick headache there is evidence of very widespread, but, at the same time, slight, derangement in many organs and tissues of the body. There is general disturbance of the intestinal canal, alterations in the composition of the blood, and disturbed action of many parts of the nervous system. There are derangements of touch, perverted taste and smell, often disturbance connected with vision, and, not unfrequently, singing in the ears, and other departures from the normal state as regards the action of the organ of hearing. The action of the heart is depressed. The capillary circulation is deranged, there being too little blood in some parts, congestion in others. Digestion is much deranged, and the action of the liver and other secreting organs is seriously impaired for the time. The muscles do not work as they should do. Delicate movements cannot be executed with the usual precision, and sustained muscular effort is difficult or impossible. The body is fatigued. The memory is more or less affected for a time, and in many instances the temper becomes "bilious." To attempt brain-work when you suffer from sick headache would be useless, for the mind will not work to any advantage. Sometimes there is a very distressing faintness, and a feeling of terrible exhaustion ; the heart's action being often very feeble for a time, and sometimes so very weak as to cause alarm. Rest in the recumbent posture for a few hours may be necessary ; but, generally, the heart soon regains its usual power if let alone. Stimulants sometimes increase the stomach disturbance, and prolong the attack ; but if the heart's action is very depressed it may be desirable to administer Ammonia or brandy, in very small quantities, at short intervals, until the organ regains its natural strength, as indicated by the character and intensity of the heart's sounds.

When the attack of sick headache begins to pass off, urine, often loaded with deposits of Urates of Soda, Ammonia, and Lime, and of high specific gravity, is excreted. Then the kidneys begin to act freely ; the bowels also act slightly, and in a few hours more the patient will feel well. It is remarkable that, after all this disturbance in the system, the individual who has suffered should be for a time in better health than usual ; and he may feel exceptionally well and vigorous. Indeed, you will find that many of the victims of this derangement have considerable powers of endurance, which enable them in a great many instances to work on energetically, far into old age. Many who suffer severely, though not fit to work, by great effort may get through their duties, and, perhaps, during a long lifetime may not have been forced to absent themselves for a single day. As far as I know, no harm results from working on through a sick headache, in cases in which this can be done, but, of course, certain kinds of work cannot possibly be executed under the circumstances. Attacks of sick headache may occur once a week and oftener, or the affection may recur not oftener than once in a fortnight, or once a month, or still less frequently. You will sometimes find that the suffering returns almost to the day, after a week or a fortnight, or other interval.

In spite of this almost continual disorder, the general phenomena of the system, essential to the continuance of life, proceed as usual. I think that some of those who suffer, and who take moderate care of themselves, really enjoy certain advantages as regards the prospect of longevity. Their tissues do not seem to grow old as fast as those of many of their more vigorous contemporaries. Periodical sick headaches may, after all, be conservative in their action, and may protect the organism from more serious pathological derangements, thus perhaps enabling persons to live long who might under other circumstances die early. Although the digestive organs may be seriously wrong for a certain time, they get the advantage of resting from time to time for periods varying from twelve to twenty-four hours. If in the affected organism anything happens to be wrong in connection with the alimentary canal, there is the advantage of time being allowed for the derangement to right itself instead of per-sisting until actual morbid change has resulted. There appears to be hyper-sensitiveness in connection with the nerves of the digestive organs

15 *

in many who suffer from sick headache, which, by favoring severe temporary disturbance of a functional character, may prevent damage and permanent structural changes in important tissues. Possibly this may be the reason why many people who suffer from sick headache not only live to be old, but retain their vigor in old age.

Some physicians have thought that an intimate relationship existed between sick headache and the epileptic state, but we meet with so many instances of each condition without the slightest indication of tendency to the other, that I cannot, without some further evidence, accept this opinion as correct. Undoubtedly you will now and then meet with a case which might seem to justify such an inference, but you will also come across cases which, considered alone, might suggest a relationship between epilepsy and many other forms of disease usually considered quite distinct. Indeed, there are few morbid conditions in which nerve derangement exists which might not be adduced as supporting the view of their affinity to the epileptic state. Hysteria, nightmare, waking up suddenly in the night and calling out, nocturnal expulsion of urine, twitchings occurring in the muscles, may all be regarded as belonging to the category of epileptic affections. But if I admitted this view to be probably correct, I should still be disposed to doubt whether any connection between sick headache and any form of the epileptic state had been proved to exist. Some cases that come under our notice would seem to justify the notion that, in certain instances, attacks of sick headache take the place of attacks of gout, and that the two affections are related. But it must be admitted that there are many persons who suffer from sick headache who have no tendency to gout, while many who have gout hardly know what it is to suffer from headache of any kind. Nevertheless, there is reason to think that in both affections the blood is deranged, and possibly by the accumulation in it of nitrogenous materials which ought to be eliminated. Both affections come on at intervals, and often suddenly. Both are relieved by the same general treatment. Both are aggravated by a full meat diet, and mitigated by a diet largely composed of vegetables and fruit. In both there is derangement of the liver, and Calomel and other remedies which act upon that and other excreting organs relieve those who suffer from gout as well as those who suffer from sick headache.

We cannot, I think, accept the generalization that sick headache belongs to the class of neuralgic affections; for those who suffer from severe forms of neuralgia do not seem to be more susceptible of sick headache than other persons; nor, on the other hand, are the victims of sick headache unusually prone to neuralgic pains. I do not see what we gain by calling this, and many diseases in which nerves are affected, " neuroses," or by referring them to " nerve storms," for no one knows what he means by the phrase " nerve storm." Nor has the supposed connection between sick headache and ague, and maladies of that class been proved. There seems to be an alliance between many different diseases, but it is most difficult to do more than point out the connection in general terms. As time goes on, I have no doubt many affections which have received different names, and are now regarded as distinct diseases, will be shown to be much more closely related to one another than we should be led to suppose from the accounts given in our systematic works on medicine. For reasons to which I have already adverted, I should rather place ordinary sick headache under the head of derangements of the digestive organs than include it in the disorders of the nervous system. This question of the nature of the malady has an important practical bearing, for it must influence our views as regards treatment. Now I think I may go so far as to commit myself to the opinion, that if the digestive system and the most important organs of excretion could be made to work properly, and could be kept working properly, the subjects of sick headache would be cured, and, from the time when these results had been obtained, would be free from attacks.

It appears to me probable, for reasons which I have set forth, that some material gradually accumulates in the blood, and by its deleterious action on the nerve-cells of the brain gives rise to the headache, and causes the inability to think, or at any rate renders it impossible to sustain connected thought for many minutes at a time. This inability to think is probably caused by an indirect action leading to dilatation of the capillaries of the pia mater and those in the superficial part of the gray matter of the convolutions. At the same time it is probable that the fluid effused from these vessels, laden with matters which ought to have been eliminated, bathes the nerve-cells, and exerts a deleterious influence upon them. A small dose of Calomel within two hours, or even less time, completely alters the state of things—for the nausea, the headache, the misty confusion of intellect, all disappear. The kidneys soon begin to secrete actively, and in this way the blood is depurated. The stomach and the intestinal canal participate, and then the peccant matter which has accumulated is removed and the healthy function restored.

Treatment of Sick Headache.—I believe we may often succeed, by judicious management, in reducing the number and severity of the attacks of this disorder. You must, in the first place, inquire very minutely into the general habits of the patient, and, of course, advise him to correct any irregularities he may have committed as regards quantity and quality of food, and the times of taking it. To lay down a strict dietary is, however, useless, nay, it might be mischievous, and more harm than good result. Many doctors make themselves ridiculous, and their patients miserable, by the absurd importance they attach to severe restrictions as regards particular articles of diet. The victim of sick headache will not gain anything by feeding as if he was in prison, and exercising as if he were under sentence of penal servitude, or undergoing the "cure" at some strict German bathing establishment. You may cut off his beer,

wine, and all things containing sugar; you may order him to take so
many pieces of dry toast at breakfast, without a particle of butter, and
only allow him skim milk and lime-water to drink.   You may limit him
to a biscuit for lunch, and allow a small chop, with bread pudding, made
without any sugar, for dinner, and a cup of water arrow-root for supper,
or no supper at all.   You may make him walk so many measured miles,
rise at a certain hour, and retire at a time when most people consider
the hour for a little quiet reading or other harmless enjoyment has
arrived, and all to no purpose; nay, instead of getting better, he may
tell you that he is worse, and feels less happy and contented than before,
and less able to bear his suffering.   Your advice, as regards living, should
be considerate, but not too strict; for, in the first place, we do not know
enough about the real nature of the malady to justify us in accurately and
arbitrarily laying down the law of living; and, secondly, experience has
incontestably proved that persons who suffer from sick headache get on
better, upon the whole, if they live fairly well in the intervals, and starve
for the short period during which they have to suffer.   As regards wine,
it will be generally found that light wines, such as hock, suit the sufferers,
if they require stimulants at all; but many who suffer from the malady
do not require any form of alcohol whatever.

There are many cases of sick headache that have resisted every attempt
to cure them; indeed, it must be confessed that, up to this time, no
certain method of "cure" has been discovered.   While the headache
lasts, and the action of the stomach and liver, and, indeed, of the secreting organs generally, is suspended, even the most digestible substances
do harm, and I know of no medicine that invariably affords relief to the
patient.

Some of those who suffer from this unpleasant affection can tell, some
days before the derangement begins, that they are about to have an
attack.   There is a disagreeable taste in the mouth, with a degree of
dryness, particularly at the tip of the tongue; a feeling of distention or
fulness over the stomach; sluggishness or inaction of the bowels; lassitude, and an indisposition to take active exercise; slight or considerable
depression of spirits, and an inclination to sleep.   The appetite may still
be good; but there is often some degree of discomfort after taking food,
and very frequently a feeling of regret that anything in the shape of food
had been taken at the time.   Now, if the patient, by whom the import
of these premonitory symptoms is understood, takes two or three grains,
or even one grain, of Gray Powder, with a little Colocynth, and, perhaps,
a saline draught the following morning, he may completely escape the
impending attack.   He may feel more or less out of sorts for a day or
two, but he does not get the severe headache, and, perhaps, also escapes
the sickness, though very likely he experiences a slight degree of nausea.
This surely indicates that matters which had accumulated in the blood
have been removed by the purgative, and have thus been prevented from

exerting a deleterious influence, culminating in the headache, and causing other symptoms.

But what should be done in these cases? What methods of treatment afford the best chance of relieving the patient who actually suffers? If you cannot always cure the patient you may do something to prolong the interval between the attacks, and to mitigate the severity of symptoms when they occur. If the sick headache is not severe, persuade the patient to think as little about it as possible. Recommend him to go about his ordinary work, and tell him to try by his manner to prevent people from discovering that he is ill; for too much sympathy and kind inquiry concentrates his attention upon the malady, and makes him feel worse. If anything appears to annoy him, he should keep quiet, and restrain himself from expressing any decided opinion until he is well; otherwise he may get the character of being a very ill-tempered or cantankerous person, when, in truth, he is nothing of the sort. It is his headache, not himself, that does the wrong.

I. TREATMENT DURING AN ATTACK OF SICK HEADACHE.

Rest.—During a severe attack of sick headache, the patient, if this be possible, must have complete rest, so that the organs which are deranged may be allowed to gradually right themselves. The mind and the nervous system need repose as well as the stomach, liver, and other organs. When the suffering is very great, and particularly in cases in which there is that distressing feeling of nausea, and frequent or occasional attacks of actual vomiting, the patient must lie down. But one meets with many instances in which he is able to continue his usual avocation, in spite of the headache; and I am not aware that any one has discovered that his sufferings were actually greater, or lasted longer, than when he adopted another plan, and gave way as soon as the headache came on, and lay down in a darkened room until the attack passed off. In bad cases, however, and especially if the patients are weak, and in other respects out of health, absolute rest in the recumbent posture must be recommended from the commencement of each attack.

Starving in Sick Headache.—The patient who is suffering from an attack ought to starve for the time, and thus rest the stomach until the attack passes off. It is very remarkable that many who suffer from this troublesome disorder are able to discharge even active duties without taking any food at all for perhaps twenty-four hours or longer, although in ordinary health the same person would get completely faint if, fasting, he attempted to do the same amount of work. A person may get up with a sick headache and be quite unable to eat any breakfast, and yet he may perform the ordinary duties of the day, and perhaps continue working up to nine or ten o'clock at night without having taken a particle of food, and yet without suffering. The same man in his ordinary health might not be able to postpone breakfast for an hour without feeling faint and exhausted. This peculiar state in which abstinence from food does not occasion exhaustion may last for forty-eight hours, during which period not an ounce of solid matter may be taken, and yet it does not follow that the nutrition of the body will be in any way impaired, or the health damaged for any length of time. The patient will not lose in weight, because the organs soon resume their natural functions. When the appetite returns, and the victim is able to eat again, plenty of nutrient material will be poured into the system and rapidly appropriated. Abstention from food for twenty-four hours is usually long enough to allow the organs which are deranged to right themselves. But in any case during an attack of sick headache, it is not of the slightest use to attempt to force the patient to eat. Even bread and butter is apt to disagree. The starchy matter of the bread instead of being digested is apt to undergo other changes, and butter and other fats suffer decomposition, various organic acids being formed, which, after a time, irritate the stomach, and cause it to reject its contents. Even meat is not digested, but if the patient feel exhausted, a little cold beef-tea may be absorbed, or beef-tea which has been artificially half digested with the acid of pepsine, p. 110. If patients object to starve from the fear that they will get very weak, you may tell them to try a little mutton broth or beef-tea, which should be entirely free from fat, and should be sipped. Of course, as far as any real advantage is concerned, they might just as well take nothing, for the little that is introduced under these circumstances cannot in any way help nutrition, although it may, on the other hand, somewhat interfere with the return of the stomach to its normal state. The fact is, that temporary abstinence from food, as above suggested, can do no harm whatever, and this course is necessary if the patient desires to gain his normal state of health in the shortest time possible, and with the least degree of suffering.

Warmth.—Exposure to cold often precipitates an attack of sick headache if one is about to come on. Indeed, many sufferers attribute the illness to the direct influence of cold. I have thought on some occasions that instead of catching an ordinary cold from undue exposure, I had contracted the greater, if less lasting suffering,—sick headache. Sick headache is certainly relieved by warmth. A warm bath sometimes removes the headache, and almost always gives relief for the time. In slight attacks of sick headache complete relief may be obtained by putting the feet into hot water, or even by simply well warming them before a good fire. An ordinary hot-water bottle, or, better, a vulcanized India-rubber bottle filled with hot water and applied to the stomach, sometimes appears to be of use, and is at any rate very pleasant under the circumstances.

Counter-Irritation.—There is no doubt whatever that considerable temporary relief is afforded during an attack of sick headache by the employment of counter-irritants. A mustard plaster (half mustard and half linseed) to the back of the neck or to the pit of the stomach will relieve the pain, or half of one of Rigollot's mustard leaves, a piece of writing-paper intervening between the mustard and the skin, may be applied in one or both situations; but one of the best applications to be used in these cases is described on p. 97. In recommending the external application of strong Hydrochloric Acid, you must, however, always be very careful to give explicit directions, or you will get into great disgrace in consequence of the destruction of bed-clothes and the serious damage to wearing apparel.

Acids.—It is curious that in many cases in which acids are produced in undue proportion by decomposition of various materials in the stomach, there should be a natural desire for things having an acid taste. Many persons certainly experience a distinct longing for acid drinks, which undoubtedly afford relief in some cases. Lemon or Lime juice and water is very grateful to some, and seems to allay the distressing nausea often present.

Tea-Drinking in Sick Headache.—Some persons sustain themselves during an attack of sick headache by drinking several cups of tolerably strong tea in the course of the day. The tea seems to keep them up, to mitigate the severity of the headache, and to relieve the nausea. Tea is condemned in the most unqualified manner by many members of the profession; but I cannot help thinking that the public forms a more cor rect estimate concerning the value of this celebrated infusion. I doubt whether it would be possible to persuade old women or old men, or even young men, as a class, to give up tea. The majority of people do not believe that tea does half the harm attributed to it; and with this opinion I am inclined to agree. If, however, you were ailing, and were to consult many of the most distinguished members of the profession on the matter, you would almost certainly be enjoined to give up tea, whether the malady was dyspepsia, constipation, or sick headache; and, indeed, for many slight ailments, the most important curative measure would seem to be to abstain from tea. Some practitioners express this opinion with amazing confidence and absolutism. Milk and water or wine and water are suggested as substitutes—substitutes for tea! Your medical adviser fairly argues that something or other must be wrong, and infers that you take something that you ought not to take; that this something must be at the root of the evil; and then concludes, but not, in my opinion, with good reason, that the particular peccant matter is nothing less than *tea*. Now, it is almost hopeless to attempt to alter the views of those whose minds are "made up" upon such a matter as this; and, as regards the deleterious effects of tea, not a few medical minds will be found in this happy state. No one is to be allowed to say a good word for tea. Tea is held to be the almost universal cause of dyspepsia, and there is an end of the matter. But, in spite of its condemnation, tea is at this time more largely drunk than ever. Probably more than two hundred million pounds of tea per annum are consumed in the United Kingdom alone; and, if its influence is as bad as some assert it to be, it is wonderful how few people discover its deleterious qualities. Seldom, I believe, does tea do the harm that has been attributed to it. In many cases of sick headache, four or five cups of good tea, at intervals during the day, will unquestionably mitigate the severity of a bad attack, and, perhaps, enable the sufferer to pursue his ordinary avocations in a way that he could not otherwise carry out. Strong coffee seems to suit some persons who cannot take tea.

Vomiting sometimes goes on for four and twenty hours, and sometimes for a longer period. The patient may be much exhausted, and the stomach become weak and very tender. Three or four days often pass before the patient regains his normal state of health, and is again able to digest food.

2. TREATMENT IN THE INTERVALS BETWEEN THE ATTACKS.

Now, as to the treatment in the intervals between the attacks. After having tried many different systems of diet, with the view of preventing attacks of sick headache, as I have already mentioned, I have come to the conclusion that, upon the whole, the best plan is to live pretty well, and not to be too fidgety as regards food. In one or two days after the attack has passed off, the stomach begins to digest, and, in most cases, it will readily digest the ordinary things taken in health. I do not think that a restrictive diet, of any kind, is of much advantage; and if the plan adopted lowers the general health, there is no doubt that the attacks of sick headache will not only come on more frequently, but they will be more severe. I should say to those who suffer from this troublesome ailment, "Live fairly well while you can, and when the sick headache comes on, entirely abstain from food for a time. As soon as the attack has passed off, live as usual, and think as little as possible of the malady." A great many persons are certainly *too* careful, as regards diet, in sick headache as well as in many other slight ailments. I fear, too, it must be confessed that many doctors encourage this, and give minute directions, as to food, which are as unpractical as they are meaningless and useless. A parcel of very absolute rules is laid down for patients' guidance, many of which rest upon no principles whatever, and are but needless arbitrary enactments. If they were called upon to give their reasons for the rules they have made, they would find themselves in a very serious difficulty. Many of the very precise directions that have been given to people suffering from slight ailments are really quite ridiculous. Even if some patients are a little silly, it is certainly not our duty to treat them as if they were utterly devoid of sense. Give reasonable and necessary directions as to diet by all means, and see that patients do not exceed in any way, but do not write minute directions concerning the precise thickness of the bread and the exact quantity of butter, and do not give written orders as to whether the toast is to be taken hot or cold, buttered or without butter. Such trumpery minutiæ will be regarded as feeble affectations by all sensible patients.

If people, who are merely dyspeptic or bilious or inclined to headache, are allowed to be too particular as to what they may or may not eat, they get very fidgety, and, perhaps, at last loathe almost all food. In consequence they lose in weight, simply because they do not get food enough to sustain them. Thus such persons often get into a low hypochondriacal condition, and some real, and perhaps serious, illness may come on.

Many who suffer from sick headache discover, if they will only try the experiment, that they can eat pretty much as other people do in the intervals between the attacks; and, if they can manage to eat fairly well, they will find that, instead of suffering from a greater number of attacks, they escape with fewer. Most who suffer from sick headache require, and can take, but very little stimulant. Many are better without any stimulants whatever. Beer will often precipitate an attack, and wine generally disagrees. A teaspoonful of sherry, taken between meals, is sufficient to bring on an attack in one predisposed to the ailment. There are, however, exceptions to this; for I know some who find that a little sherry or beer helps them in the intervals between the attacks, and does not seem to bring one on unless it happens to be imminent.

All sufferers from sick headache should do all they can to avoid worry. Peace of mind and freedom from anxiety are of course to be desired for every one, but those prone to the malady we are considering should be doubly careful, and should avoid undertaking responsibilities which make them anxious. So also they should exercise as much self-control as possible, and endeavor not to give way to a feeling of restlessness and fussiness, which only increases the severity of the attacks which they have to suffer.

Many saline medicines, which increase secretion, seem to be useful to those who suffer from sick headache. Small doses of Nitrate of Potash, *Potassæ Nitras,* Bicarbonate of Potash, *Potassæ Bicarbonas,* the so-called effervescing Citrate of Magnesia, or *Liquor Ammoniæ Acetatis,* or *Liquor Potassæ,* may be ordered to be taken in a largely diluted state early in the morning before the breakfast, and the last thing at night. Or you may give half a tumbler of *Vichy Water,* or *Lithia Water,* or *German Seltzer Water* at the same time of the day, for a few days at a time, in the intervals between the attacks of sick headache.

Some bitter preparations also seem to be of use. You may give Infusion of Orange, *Infusum Aurantii,* or Infusion of Quassia, *Infusum Quassiæ,* or Quinine; or, as I have suggested before, you may try the effect of tea or coffee in somewhat larger quantity than they are usually taken.

A good deal has been said lately about Guarana. It is prescribed in powder, in doses of from ten to thirty grains twice or three times a day.

16

Its active principle has also been extracted, and may be prescribed in doses of from one to three or four grains. I am indebted to Messrs. Savory and Moore for a specimen of Guaranine. It looks something like quinine, but is more flocculent. The taste, though bitter, is very unlike the taste of that substance. There is also a Liquid Extract of Guarana, *Extractum Guaranæ liquidum*, the dose of which is from twenty to thirty minims. I am sorry to say that, although benefit seems to have been derived by some, many have tried this remedy without gaining the hoped-for advantage from its use.

General treatment in the intervals of comparative good health must not be forgotten. Tonics of various kinds are often useful. You may give Quinine in one- or two-grain doses twice daily, about eleven and four o'clock, or Quinine Wine, or Tincture of Quinine. Various other bitter tonics and the mineral acids may be prescribed in many cases with advantage. The above remedies must, however, be withheld as soon as the headache begins and while it lasts.

If the patient suffers from constipated bowels, you must give mild purgatives. If the various excreting glands do not sufficiently freely perform their work, you must prescribe those remedies which act upon the liver, kidneys, or other organs at fault. Whether Calomel should be given now and then is a point upon which there is much difference of opinion. Some patients undoubtedly derive great benefit from small doses of this drug. From one to two or three grains, taken at intervals of three or four days, is, as I have before remarked, treatment which really deserves in certain cases to be called curative. There are, however, a few persons who cannot take Calomel. If you give even half a grain, the salivary glands will begin to act within three or four hours, and soon secrete violently. The saliva flows from the mouth, the tongue and cheeks swell, the teeth become loose, and the patient is in too much suffering to take food, and too ill to digest it properly if he could take it. You must be aware of this extraordinary susceptibility to the action of Mercury, and do not order it if the patient or friends assure you that it has this effect. Sometimes Calomel seems to weaken patients terribly. Small doses purge them too much, and harm, instead of good, results. On the other hand, I can assure you that the confident unqualified condemnation of mercurials that has lately been so fashionable rests on no foundation of fact. It is one of those fads or fancies which, being acted upon, are very interfering with our usefulness to the sick. It is, of course, easy to bring forward numerous instances where persons have been known to take Mercury almost daily for thirty or forty years, not only without suffering, but, from their own account, with great benefit. Indeed, some will tell you that they cannot get on without an occasional small dose. Many Mercury-takers have lived to be very old. I could give examples of life being prolonged beyond eighty-four years, although one or two grains of Blue Pill had been taken every fourth or fifth day for forty years. I have been told by people that they had been distinctly warned by their medical adviser upon no account to take Calomel, on the ground that if they did take the drug, it would almost kill them, or would at least provoke some serious and lasting injury to tissues and organs, and damage the constitution. Such assertions are merely arbitrary utterances. It is a fact, as I have told you before, that Calomel enters into the composition of many powders which have a great reputation for exerting a soothing effect upon irritable children, and which are given even to young infants for the sake of improving the temper. It is wrong for practitioners to lay down the law against the use of such a remedy as Mercury. The public are sufficiently capricious to make it difficult to advise them for the best, and it is very injudicious on the part of a skilled practitioner to encourage fancies and prejudices. Calomel, by helping the action of the stomach and liver, restores digestion, and even an infant soon regains its good humor. Adults experience a pleasant sensation if digestion goes on quietly and effectually; while, on the other hand, if the digestive process is interfered with, the most amiable persons will find it difficult to keep themselves in that desirable state. If they do not feel out of temper, they probably experience despondency, and feel melancholy and out of heart.

So far, the reputed substitutes for mercurials which I have tried have not succeeded as I could wish; but I have not yet had an opportunity of giving in a sufficient number of cases of sick headache and other maladies where the liver is at fault, the new remedies recommended by Professor Rutherford.

3. OF THE MANAGEMENT OF SICK HEADACHE WHEN THE PATIENT CONTINUES TO WORK.

The following plan has been found to answer, in several instances, in mitigating the severity of the attack while the patient continued his usual avocation. The victim may become conscious of the attack as soon as he wakes in the morning, and, instead of attempting to eat any breakfast, he should take only a cup of rather strong tea. In the commencement there is a feeling of weakness and lassitude, often accompanied by giddiness; but the patient can, nevertheless, walk about, and so far from feeling exhausted, as he certainly would do if, under ordinary circumstances, he was deprived of the first and, with some, most important, meal in the day, he will, very probably, not feel the slightest demand for food. In an hour or two he may take another cup of tea; and the dose may be repeated at intervals through the day. A little milk and sugar may be allowed; but, probably, the simple infusion of a good tea, taken warm, would be best.

In this way the patient may get through his work, with difficulty, no doubt, and, perhaps, he may feel somewhat miserable; but the time passes more quickly than if he were lying down and contemplating his pain. Towards evening, in many cases, the discomfort becomes less, a sensation of emptiness, not difficult to bear, is experienced, and this is gradually followed by an actual desire for food. But the most striking change which sets in about this time, and which is an invariable indication of a favorable turn in the progress of the malady, is the free secretion of urine, after the action of the kidneys has been nearly suspended for four-and-twenty or forty-eight hours, or more. At first, a small quantity of very acid urine, of high specific gravity, makes its appearance in the bladder; but this is soon followed by a very free secretion of pale urine, of low density, and great relief of all the distressing symptoms is at once experienced. The stomach will now bear a little light food. The large bowel begins to resume its function, and next morning the patient will probably wake up feeling nearly well. If, however, the headache still troubles him when he rises, it usually passes quite away during the day.

It is true that in many cases the attack is often more severe, and its duration longer, than I have indicated; but the general plan of treatment suggested should be the same—complete abstinence from solid food, the administration of tea, coffee, or even plain water, at intervals of two or three hours, until the headache nearly ceases and the nausea disappears. Some people like warm water flavored with lemon-juice; and you may add, with advantage, Supertartrate, or Nitrate, or Citrate of Potash, or some other salt known to act as a diuretic.

It would appear that during the attack of headache most organs of the body, and notably the secreting organs, strike work. It is useless to try to violently and immediately excite them to action, for you would do harm by such attempts. You must wait for a few hours; and as soon as you see the slightest tendency of a return to activity, I believe you may be of use in saving time and hastening the return to convalescence. A free flow of urine, I am sure, is advantageous, and lemon-juice, nitre, with plenty of water, will often effect this object. Purgatives do harm if given too soon; and I have not been satisfied as to the advantage derived from many other remedies that have been warmly recommended during the attack. Neither warm baths nor cold baths seem to be of use; and with the exception of tea or water flavored with lemon-juice, with, perhaps, some simple saline diuretic, the less introduced into the stomach during the twenty-four or thirty hours of suffering the better. In conclusion, let me impress upon you the inference that sick headache is not an unmixed evil. The condition has its advantageous side, for he who is subject to the malady generally finds no difficulty in keeping temperate, and the delicacies of the table are to him scarcely a temptation. Thus he is less likely to suffer from early failure and degeneration of important organs than many apparently healthy persons who may overwork them and subject them to undue strain.

Drowsiness.—Patients sometimes come to consult us in consequence of a persistent sleepy state. They will tell you that they feel as if they could sleep all day as well as all night. If they sit on a chair for a few minutes, they drop off to sleep; if they take up a book or a paper, it soon falls from their hands in consequence of an irresistible drowsiness. If they go out for a walk, they soon begin to experience a strong inclination to lie down and yield themselves up to sleep. Patients who suffer in this way sometimes come for help to their medical adviser. They may feel pretty well, and in good health, with the exception of this irrepressible drowsy feeling, and they ask you what they can do to get rid of a tendency so very troublesome and inconvenient.

In many cases this drowsy state seems to depend upon some imperfect action of the digestive organs. Sometimes it may be traced to overfeeding. Sometimes to taking too large a meal in the middle of the day. Sometimes beer or a too liberal allowance of wine seems to be the cause of it. If you give mild purgatives and mineral acids before meals, and saline medicines which act upon the intestinal canal, you will often succeed in curing the patient. When the liver is in fault, as is not unfrequently the case, you will find the advantage of giving a small dose of Calomel, Blue Pill, or Gray Powder (from one to two grains will be sufficient) every third or fourth night for three or four courses.

Cold bathing also is often useful. As soon as the patient rises in the morning he may have a cold shower-bath. There is no need of a large quantity of water. A shower-bath of two or three pints will be sufficient. If the drowsiness is very troublesome, two moderate shower-baths a day may be tried—one at about eleven, the other at four o'clock—cold or tepid, according to the time of year. In some cases, in addition to the cold bathing, a mild purgative every night for a week will be found useful.

Wakefulness and Restlessness.—The very opposite condition to drowsiness afflicts some patients. They come to you complaining that they cannot sit still or rest quietly for a time. They experience a strong desire to be continually walking about. They cannot stay for long in one place, and do not feel satisfied unless they get constant change of scene. You inquire if there is any cause for this restlessness, and, as a rule, the invalid assures you that, although everything is going on in its usual way, he cannot feel satisfied, quiescent, or composed. Sometimes vague frights harass the patient. When he goes to bed at night, instead of dropping off to sleep in a natural way, he lies tossing about. The pillow seems uncomfortable, and soon gets too warm for the head. A very miserable night is passed, and the patient only gets a little sleep towards morning, and perhaps wakes up feeling tired, exhausted, and unrefreshed. The mental disturbance in these cases depends upon some temporary derangement which cannot be accurately defined. If upon inquiry you learn that the restless state has existed for a considerable time, you must induce the patient to thoroughly change his mode of life. If he is in business, recommend him to get away and take a holiday for

16 *

a time. Send him to some place where he will get complete change of scene for a month or more. The diet must at the same time be carefully regulated, and in all probability the patient will return home well, and able to go on with his daily round of duty just as steadily as he did before the illness commenced.

Persons who suffer from wakefulness are often ordered to take Chloral, and after finding out the efficacy of the remedy, some very imprudently continue its use without consulting their medical adviser. In a short time they discover that they cannot sleep at all without the drug, and at last they become complete slaves to its use. It has happened that from want of due care an overdose has been taken, and death has resulted. It is important to caution all persons for whom you prescribe Chloral, never to take this drug unless it is specially ordered for them. More dangerous even than Chloral-taking is the hypodermic injection of narcotics, and it seems to me that this method ought never to be employed in cases of occasional wakefulness, and I think that in all cases the rule should be observed of never leaving the syringe and morphia solution in the patient's custody, nor should any one be allowed to perform the operation for you. In those cases only in which, owing to chronic incurable disease, accompanied by constant severe pain, the unfortunate patient can get no sleep or peace without the aid of morphia, and only very exceptionally, should this rule be relaxed, and non-professional persons permitted to inject the narcotic.

Patients oftentimes complain of feeling tired and exhausted as well as restless, and sometimes they will tell you that they cannot walk half a mile in consequence of being muscularly weak. You must carefully inquire into the state of the various functions of the body, and suggest what you can to rectify the action of any which are improperly discharged. (See p. 113.) Generally, you will do well to send such patients for a moderate tour in a pleasant part of the country, where they can see a good deal without walking very far. You must particularly caution them against over-fatigue. Many persons suffering from this or other conditions requiring change, are advised to take a walking tour in Switzerland or the Tyrol. So they go with all despatch, and having arrived at their destination, begin their pedestrian cure. Not having been accustomed to much exertion for many years, they set to work and, perhaps, walk twenty miles or more a day. Instead of feeling better, and gaining strength, they soon feel terribly tired and exhausted, and return home in every respect worse than when they set out. Such an expedition, under the circumstances, is a mistake. You must strongly impress upon such patients that they are not to walk more than a mile at first, and if they are tired, they are to sit down, or, better, lie down on a sofa, and read a novel, or otherwise amuse themselves. They should, as we say, moon about, or potter about in the open air several hours daily, without taking any active exercise. In this way, most sufferers will soon begin to improve, and when this is the case, they may by degrees extend their daily walk until they are restored to health.

Nervousness.—There is another condition, which is usually called "nervousness." In this state there can be no doubt that the mind is, in some degree, temporarily affected. There may be undue emotional excitement. The least thing may arouse fear or dread; but instead of the nervous, excited state impelling the patient to be more active in his work, he finds it almost impossible for him to discharge his ordinary duties. A large proportion of the population seems never to have experienced anything approaching to nervousness, but some people suffer from it in a terrible degree. I have been told by patients that for some time they had been conscious of an indescribable anxiety, for which they could not account, and from which, by no reasoning with themselves, could they get relief. They know and acknowledge that there is no reason for anxiety; but, nevertheless, a sort of ill-defined dread seems to hang over them. They fear that something or other is about to happen; and this most painful state of mental disturbance sometimes lasts for a considerable time, causing the patient great suffering. With this state is frequently associated considerable depression of spirits. The subject of it feels as if everything was going wrong with him. He may be getting on just as well, and making quite as much, or even more, money than usual, but nevertheless feels discontented and depressed, as if something terrible had happened. People who suffer in this way sometimes tell you that they are certainly going to the workhouse, and all this sort of thing, although they know themselves to be prospering. If a patient in this state of health should happen to lose a few shillings, he will feel quite convinced that everything is going to the dogs, and nothing will persuade him to give up the despairing views of life which have somehow arisen in his mind.

People who suffer from extreme nervousness, combined with a restless, unsettled state of mind, occasionally do very curious things. A man may wake up suddenly in the middle of the night and with the conviction he smells fire. He gets out of bed, strikes a light, goes over the house, finds nothing the matter, and goes to bed again. In another hour or two, perhaps, he wakes up a second time, and goes through the same proceedings as before. Many people whose nervous system is a little overwrought, wake up at night, and jump out of bed, and, perhaps, light a candle before they are quite aware of what they are doing. A further development of the same tendency may lead to sleep-walking, of which condition again there are many different degrees. Children of highly nervous temperament are likely to suffer from attacks of chorea. These and many more severe disturbances of the nervous system seem to depend upon a highly sensitive or excitable state of certain parts of the central nerve organs, rather than upon any abnormal or morbid change. They are, however, often associated with a special type of organism; and

frequently it will be found that cardiac disease, affecting either the mitral
or aortic orifice, or both, also exists, or is developed before the period
of adolescence.

But sometimes an unusually restless and excitable state of the nervous
system temporarily troubles people, and may come on at almost any
period of life. The patient in such a state should be advised to visit
friends, or take a holiday abroad. You should urge him to leave for a
time his ordinary avocations, and very likely in a few weeks he will
recover from his nervousness. Upon careful inquiry, you will find that
many who suffer in this way have been long in the habit of taking too
little sleep. There is hardly anything in which individuals more widely
differ from one another than in the time required for sleep. Some can
do with six or seven hours, but it is quite certain that many require nine
hours. Nervous people, as a rule, are benefited by a long night's rest
now and then, and require an average of eight or nine hours.

Of late years, very much has been written on the subject of nervousness,
and attempts have been made to show that we are much more "nervous"
than our fathers were. It seems to me that the evidence adduced in favor
of the statement is, to say the least, very far-fetched. The so-called
brain-workers are supposed to be great sufferers. It is said that people
are more sensitive to heat and cold, and require to live in rooms more
highly heated than was the case even a few years ago. It must, however,
be borne in mind that a far greater number of the existing population
are able to have the advantage of warm rooms in cold weather than formerly, and, in consequence, the majority enjoy better health, and live
to be older. That large incomes engender a good deal of fussiness, and
little aches and pains which are made too much of, is, I dare say, true ;
and if this is "nervousness," an increase no doubt exists, and such
"nervousness" will increase as prosperity increases. But I cannot help
thinking that if our fathers had been as prosperous as we are, as large a
percentage would have suffered from "nervousness." However this may
be, it is quite certain that if our modern habits and systems are productive
of increased nervousness, they are at the same time conducive to health
and longevity. There is no doubt whatever that the general health of
the population has improved, and is improving, that the average duration
of life is on the increase, and if the sum of human happiness is not much
greater every succeeding decade, it ought to be so ; and the fault lies in
the circumstances that individual evil inclinations are capable of counter-
acting the natural influence of highly advantageous external circumstances.
Upon the whole, I doubt very much whether there is anything to justify
many of the statements made about the increase of nervous disorders.
Whenever money is made rapidly, luxury and folly will increase ; but
the silly rich, after all, constitute but a very small part of the population—so small a part that, in the life of a country like England, their
existence is hardly noted, except by themselves and the few whose inter-

est leads them to minister to their requirements and to pander to their caprices.

Dr. G. M. Beard, of New York, has lately called attention to the increase of nervousness in the United States, but I think his remarks can only apply to a very small fraction of the population of some of the large cities. This author seems to think very much of pork as a food, and to have formed a low estimate of those whose stomachs are not strong enough to digest it. The dethronement of pork, says Dr. Beard, is having a disastrous effect upon the American people—"Pork, like the Indian, flies before civilization." Really it seems very hard that people who cannot digest pork should be put down as unduly nervous, over-sensitive, and the like, and be accused of undergoing deterioration and decay. I have no doubt that the American nation will survive and increase in numbers and in vigor, "the dethronement of pork" notwithstanding.

As regards the effects of overworking the brain in the case of the young, while it may be admitted that, now and then, instances of mental strain are met with, such cases are exceedingly rare, even in these days, as compared with the number of persons, young and old, who are suffering from the very opposite condition—from too little mental exertion. I should say that, as a fact, far more *disease is caused by too little brain work than too much.*

Neuralgia.—I will now offer a few remarks concerning a very important condition which is well worthy of attentive study, but of which I can now treat only very briefly and imperfectly. Every one of you must have heard something about *Neuralgia* and *Neuralgic pains*, though no one has yet been able to give an adequate explanation of their causation in many cases. Sometimes these pains are no doubt due to a temporary change induced in the nerve itself, which may possibly be beyond the means of investigation. Perhaps the capillaries distributed to the nerve-fibres constituting the trunk of a large nerve may be unusually distended with blood. Possibly the circular muscular fibres of the little arteries ramifying amongst the bundles of nerve-fibres may be temporarily relaxed through nerve influence; and thus the capillaries distributed to the particular nerve or particular part of the nerve may become much dilated, and thus pressing upon the adjacent nerve-tubules, very severe pain may be occasioned.

That the trunk of the nerve is the seat of attack in certain ordinary forms of neuralgia is certain, and pain like that of neuralgia may often be produced by pressing or stretching or squeezing a nerve-fibre. If a sensitive nerve-fibre be pressed upon by a tumor or growth of any kind, or be stretched over a tumor, great pain generally results, and it may continue perhaps for months if the circumstances causing the alteration in the nerve persist. In certain cases, on the other hand, the precise seat of the affection is undoubtedly in the peripheral distribution of the nerve where it breaks up into expansions, plexuses, or networks of extremely delicate fibres.

Neuralgic pains, then, are generally associated with branches known to consist principally of sensitive nerve-fibres. Perhaps the fifth nerve is the greatest offender in these cases. You may have neuralgic pain closely resembling that of toothache, and affecting the very same nerve-fibres, the tooth itself being free from disease. The pain may be so acute as to lead both the patient and his adviser to conclude that some morbid change is going on in the pulp of the tooth. The dentist is consulted, and, unless he is thoroughly up to his work, the tooth may be injudiciously extracted, and upon examination found to be in perfect health. The patient, however, goes away with the conviction that, although he is minus a sound tooth, he has at any rate experienced the last twinge of pain. But, alas! before many hours have passed the suffering returns as bad as ever. Torture as severe in all respects as that from which he had previously suffered is again experienced, though perhaps to the sufferer the pain may seem to be situated in an adjacent tooth. The patient might have one tooth extracted after another without the neuralgic pain being cured. Extraction is not the proper expedient in these cases.

In some instances it is probable that the attack depends upon some change taking place in the circulation, and that in consequence partly of the pressure exerted by the distended capillary vessels, and partly in consequence of changes produced in consequence of exudation amongst the ultimate ramifications of the nerve-fibres, or around their bioplasm, pain results, and may persist for some time until the conditions become slowly altered. In a few very intractable forms of toothache, or rather of neuralgic pain apparently originating in the tooth-pulp, it is probable that the nerve-centre is the seat of disturbance due to vascular congestion, brought about by reflex action.

In cases in which the pain depends merely upon some temporary disturbance in the branch of the fifth nerve which supplies the tooth, or in the tooth papilla itself, the probability is that it will yield to very simple treatment.

Treatment of Neuralgia.—Sometimes a good sharp purgative will cure the patient at once, but more frequently it is necessary to follow up the purgative with tonics, and especially preparations of bark, or Quinine itself, a mild purgative being also given every few days. In this way you very often cure obstinate neuralgic pains. You must, however, bear in mind that it sometimes happens that if Quinine is given by itself it may under some conditions of the system increase the pain, even for some time; while if you give a purgative in the first instance, or combine purgative medicine, such as Sulphate of Soda or Sulphate of Magnesia, with it, the Quinine will often act perfectly well and cure the patient. When the pain is intense, and is decidedly a neuralgic pain, coming on at about the same time of the day, and lasting about the same length of time, you must order a considerable dose of Quinine at once—five or ten grains,—and then from three to five grains twice or three times a day. Some people can take as much as ten grains of Quinine twice or three times a day for several days with great relief to various nerve ailments. Quinine may be given in the form of pills, or you may place the bitter powder on the tongue, or it may be diffused through water, or dissolved in water containing a few drops of free Hydrochloric, Sulphuric, Nitric, or Phosphoric Acid. The usual way of giving Quinine is the last. We order a six-ounce mixture as follows: Aromatic Sulphuric Acid, three drachms; Quinine, thirty-six grains; Syrup of Lemon, half an ounce or more, and water to six ounces. The dose will be half an ounce, or one tablespoonful, with an equal quantity of water, three times a day, between meals, for a fortnight.

The old *Muriate of Ammonia, Chloride of Ammonium, Ammonii Chloridum*, is a very valuable remedy in certain cases of neuralgia which are not relieved by Quinine. Some consider it as a specific, and say that it seldom fails. The remedy should be given in good doses, and it is often useless to order less than twenty grains or half a drachm. It is not pleasant to take, as it has a peculiar salt taste which is disagreeable to most palates. However, those who have suffered much from neuralgia are usually ready to try anything that affords them prospect of relief.

Salicine is sometimes of use, and may be given in doses of from five to eight grains every three or four hours for one or two days. *Salicylate of Soda* has been largely prescribed in the treatment of severe forms of rheumatism, and has been given for neuralgia. It is not much used in slight forms of either disease, but occasionally it does good. In many cases of acute rheumatism it acts admirably in lowering the quick pulse and high temperature. It must be given with care, and the patient taking it must be well looked after, as sometimes it lowers the pulse and depresses the heart's action to a greater degree than is desirable.

Iron. Arsenic.—Many preparations of iron may be ordered in cases of neuralgia, particularly if there is reason to think that the state of the blood is at fault. *Arsenic* in small doses, and given with due care, may be prescribed if the pain is very severe. It is well not to continue arsenic for more than a month at a time. You may order from three to five minims of Fowler's solution of arsenic, *Liquor Arsenicalis*, with a little syrup of ginger and an ounce of water, three times daily, soon after food has been taken.

Opium.—There are several forms in which opium may be given. A small dose of Dover's powder, *Pulvis Ipecacuanhæ Compositus* (from two to five grains), at bedtime, followed in the morning by a mild saline purgative, if persisted in for a few days or a week, will relieve and sometimes cure certain forms of neuralgic pain.

Hypodermic Injection.—You may, too, inject a solution of Morphia under the skin if the pains are very severe. The sixth of a grain, or less, of this drug is sufficient for subcutaneous injection. The operation is performed with the aid of a little injecting syringe made for the purpose, one of many forms of which I show you. In this way, for the time being, you may relieve the most exquisite nerve pain ; but too often it happens that, as soon as the effects of the Morphia have worn off, the pain returns. You must know that people are nowadays too apt to get into the way of prescribing sedatives for themselves after they have found relief, and thus they may do themselves great harm. You must, therefore, always exercise caution in prescribing and recommending this class of remedies, and be careful to tell patients they ought never to prescribe them for themselves. More particularly as regards hypodermic injection it is my duty to impress upon you the importance of not allowing the patient, under any circumstances, to get into the way of operating upon himself. There is really great danger in this, for the process is very simple and easily performed ; and as the relief is great, patients are very apt to assist themselves without waiting for the doctor. Of those who take this injudicious course, not a few get into the habit of narcotizing themselves on the slightest excuse. Whenever they suffer slight pain they at once resort to hypodermic injection. As soon as the effects begin to wear off, the pain recurs, and the dose is repeated. A vicious habit is soon acquired, and it is difficult indeed to prevent many of those foolish persons from going to extremes and making themselves slaves of the remedy. Very painful cases of the kind come under our notice from time to time, and every now and then death results from an overdose. Patients who have contracted this habit of self-injection not uncommonly lose all control over themselves, and introduce narcotics hypodermically, just as other weak-minded individuals become a prey to drink or indulge in other vices. We shall before long have societies for the entire suppression of hypodermic injection, if this treatment becomes much more fashionable than it is.

Dr. Sansom's Disks.—Of late years some excellent little disks of gelatine have been prepared, each of which contains a given quantity of the drug we may desire to inject. All that is necessary is to dissolve the gelatine disk in a few drops of warm water at the time when it is required. The solution may then be taken up by the syringe and injected into the subcutaneous areolar tissue of the patient. I believe my friend, Dr. Sansom, was the first to suggest the employment of these disks, which are also used when it is required to apply atropine and other remedies to the conjunctiva.

Chloral-Hydrate and *Croton Chloral-Hydrate.*—Chloral is of great use in procuring sleep in many cases of severe neuralgia, especially when the patient has been kept awake night after night ; but you must give it with the greatest caution, and only order one, or at most two, doses on the prescription. Take care also to write full directions how and when the aught is to be taken. The dose of Chloral is from ten to twenty grains, with a little syrup, and Peppermint or other water. The most convenient form is the syrup of Chloral-Hydrate, one drachm of which contains ten grains of the drug. Peppermint or Ginger covers the taste of the Chloral better than anything else. In cases of old catarrh and emphysema it should not be given. I have seen it do harm in several instances in which the heart was weak and the right ventricle dilated. *Croton-Chloral* or *Butyl Chloral-Hydrate*, which was much used a few years ago, when it was first discovered, has not been heard of so much lately. It is prescribed in doses of one or two grains, to be taken every two or three hours. In the "Lancet," for January 31, 1874, Dr. Burney Yeo reported some cases in which the remedy had been of great service in relieving very severe neuralgic pain; and in the same journal, for December 2, 1876, you will find some cases recorded by Dr. Skerritt, of Bristol, in which the remedy relieved bilious headache, facial neuralgia, and giddiness. Five grains were given twice a day.

Rheumatic Pains.—I must now say a few words about another kind of pain which is very common. It is, perhaps, not so severe as bad forms of neuralgic pain, but it nevertheless occasions much suffering, and in some cases is so severe and so constant as to prevent the patient from following his avocations. I allude to the so-called *Rheumatic Pains*, which affect various tissues and occur in many different parts of the body. The character of the pain differs somewhat in different cases, sometimes occurring as sharp, evanescent twinges, which either flit about, as it were, from place to place, or seem to be obstinately fixed in certain joints, the severity of the suffering altering only in degree. A good many old men and old women, living in damp, cold, country places, will tell you they have been martyrs to rheumatism for more than half their lives.

When the blood is in a state favorable to the development of those changes which result in rheumatic pains, you may be exposed to cold, damp air for a short time, towards sundown, conscious of a slight chilly feeling, and in two or three hours you feel very decided aching of the muscles of the forearm, or upper arm, or of the leg, back, or other part of the body. Perhaps some of the tendinous structures about the wrist or ankles are the seat of fixed, continuous pain, which becomes worse on exertion, and makes it a matter of great difficulty to lift anything, or to perform the ordinary movements. Very commonly the muscles at the back of the neck, from their insertion in the occipital bone downwards, are so painful that you cannot turn or bend the head. Partly from the pain and discomfort experienced, partly from the effect of the altered blood on sensitive nerves of the body generally, you feel quite ill and must lie down. Now you soon find out that external warmth gives great relief. Sit before a good fire, wrap yourself up in a railway rug, take a warm bath, or hot-air bath, or a Turkish bath, and the pains will soon disappear. If you go to bed and freely perspire, you will feel better within an hour. But, perhaps, after a few hours more you have evidence that the pain has not gone, showing that the changes which caused the pain in the first instance have been followed by phenomena which determine a more lasting departure from the normal state.

Rheumatic pains are often preceded by, or are associated with, flatulence, heart-burn, and other symptoms, indicative of deranged digestion. Some suppose that the peccant matter, which causes the pain, is actually secreted by the stomach, while others consider that it results from the occurrence of unusual chemical changes occurring in the recently absorbed constituents of the food. In favor of this latter view may be adduced the fact that the subjects of rheumatism are almost invariably made worse by beer, while rheumatics who can be persuaded to give up this popular beverage, almost invariably improve. The rheumatism, however, returns whenever the beer is resumed.

Rheumatic pains differ from neuralgic pains, inasmuch as they commonly arise in muscles and fibrous tissues, while neuralgic pain is generally seated in a nerve-trunk or its ramifications. The dental nerve and its branches, or the superior maxillary, or frontal, or certain cutaneous branches in various parts of the body, are more frequently affected than other nerves. Rheumatic pains, on the other hand, seem to be situated deeper, more in the substance of tissues, and to emanate from the ultimate ramifications of the nerves, distributed to tendons or fasciæ, or to the muscles themselves.

Lumbago is a form, and a very unpleasant one, of muscular or fibro-muscular rheumatism. Sometimes it is very obstinate and very difficult to cure. The patient is obliged to rest in bed ; and it may be a fortnight or more before he is able to bend his back without great suffering.

Rheumatic pain seems in many cases to arise near the insertion of a muscle. The point of attachment of the deltoid to the humerus is a frequent spot for the development of rheumatic pain, which may be so severe as to interfere with the raising of the arm, and to render the putting on of a coat without assistance a most difficult proceeding. Sometimes the pain persists in this situation for several weeks.

The intercostal muscles are not unfrequently the seat of very severe rheumatic pain which is sometimes mistaken for pleurisy. The muscles of the side and of the hip are also frequently affected. Rheumatic pain in some of the fibres of the diaphragm and of the abdominal muscles has unfortunately led the practitioner to express the opinion that a patient was suffering from peritonitis, and some days perhaps will have elapsed before this terrible and erroneous diagnosis has been controverted.

The nerve-fibres distributed to the muscular fibre cells (organic muscle) may be the seat of organic pain as well as those distributed to voluntary muscle. It is to be remarked with reference to the latter, that those parts of the muscle situated nearest to the tendon are most frequently the seat of the pain. Here, of course, the circulation through the vessel is slowest, and there would be the greater chance of any exudation poured out from the blood producing a deleterious influence upon the finer branches of any nerve-fibres with which they may come into contact.

In various forms of rheumatism, then, we infer that certain of the fibrous tissues are the seat of pathological change. Exudation is probably poured out from the blood as the circulating fluid slowly traverses the sparsely scattered capillaries of the tissues. The nerve-fibres close to the capillaries (see p. 230) suffer. The exudation coagulates, and part of it is at length converted into fibrous tissue, so that the affected textures become thickened, and the movements of the joints and of the tendons and muscles in their neighborhood seriously impaired. In many old cases of chronic rheumatism the patient becomes seriously crippled, and the movements of some joints are greatly impeded if not altogether stopped. It would almost seem as if in bad cases of rheumatism the fibrous tissues were the seat of a sort of slow inflammation ; and that the exudation poured out in the interstices of the bundles of the fibrous tissue gradually increased in amount as the disease advanced, and that the resulting fibrous tissue underwent condensation and contraction, greatly interfering with the action of the tissues in question. The movements of the large joints at last cease altogether; this change being partly due to the pathological phenomena I have described, and in part to the circumstance that the pain accompanying every effort to move has gradually discouraged the patient from making any attempts. The limbs become quite stiff, and the patient is dependent upon others, even for every mouthful of food he swallows. We often see extreme cases of the kind in work-houses in the country. If you visit some of these institutions, you will almost certainly discover several persons who, for many years, have been complete cripples from rheumatism, and are bedridden and incapable of moving any one joint in the body.

The inquiry as to the actual state of things at the seat of pain during the early stages of the disease in ordinary rheumatic affection, is an interesting one, but I am sorry to say I cannot tell you what are the essential differences between a slightly rheumatic and a perfectly healthy tissue. The facts of the case justify the conclusion that certain materials, probably soluble, are formed in undue quantity in the blood—that the solution transudes through the walls of the capillaries in situations where the vessels are few and the circulation is slow, that the contact of the fluid with the fine ramifications of the nerves close to the capillaries causes pain, that in consequence of the formation of more fluid of the same character in the blood, that which has been already poured out cannot be absorbed. The accumulation thus brought about accounts for the persistent character of the pain. Whether the pain is caused by the direct influence of the effused fluid on the fine nerve-fibres, or upon the bioplasm or living matter connected with them, is a question which is open to discussion. There can be no doubt that stretching of the terminal ramifications of nerve-fibres or pressure upon them will give rise to pain, and it is not unreasonable to infer that fluid differing in its composition from that which bathes them in health would also cause pain and disturbance of nerve action. The mere stretching and pressure to which the nerves are subjected are not, it may be fairly objected, an adequate explanation in many cases, as for instance, in those where there is persistent rheumatic pain not associated with any tension or swelling of the tissues. The views above suggested, however, receive support from the fact that in many cases after very free secretion has gone on for some time from skin, kidneys, and bowels, the reabsorption of any exuded fluid does take place and the rheumatic pain ceases.

With regard to the muscles there is almost invariably imperfect action, and some muscles during an attack pass into a state of complete inaction. The muscular tissue which has been many times affected by the rheumatic state, gradually wastes, and the muscle itself after becoming very weak soon exhibits structural degeneration. Near the tendon the contractile tissue undergoes condensation, and slowly degenerates into fibrous tissue, while in the fleshy parts adjacent, fatty degeneration often occurs. Shrinking, wasting, thickening, and contraction proceed until muscle after muscle deteriorates, when the limbs fail to execute their ordinary movements. I need hardly say more concerning the very serious results consequent upon the long continuance or frequent recurrence of the rheumatic state. Every one must see the importance of doing all he can to check the pathological changes, or failing this, to cause them to take place as slowly as possible, and to retard the development of that dreadful state of helplessness and incapacity which are too often the consequence of rheumatism.

MEASURES TO BE ADOPTED FOR THE TREATMENT OF RHEUMATISM.

General Hints concerning the Prevention and Relief of Chronic Rheumatic Affections.—All who suffer from rheumatic pains should be made to understand that by acting in a certain way they may greatly diminish the tendency to rheumatism if they cannot completely check it, while by acting in a different manner they may greatly encourage the progress of the morbid change. All rheumatics should be instructed concerning the great importance of promoting the free action of the secreting organs generally. Their medical adviser should particularly direct their attention to the great importance of frequent and free action of the skin, kidneys, and bowels, in order that the materials which tend to accumulate in the blood, and which are concerned in the causation of the rheumatic state, may be removed as fast as they are formed, and expelled from the system.

In our climate a tendency to slight rheumatism is so common that I should say at least half the population suffered more or less. It is noticed, too, at every period of life. The so-called *nervous, neuralgic,* and *muscular pains* are very often of a rheumatic nature. These may get well of themselves, or be relieved or removed by a purgative, by a few doses of Bicarbonate of Soda or Potash, or by one of those effervescing salines now so commonly sold, or by a few ordinary warm baths, or, in the case of the young, by active exercise followed by free perspiration. A somewhat more decidedly developed rheumatic condition often brings patients to us for advice; and here and there, I am sorry to say, we find this to be but the state precursory to a severe attack. In the great majority of cases, however, the morbid condition yields, in a few days or a week or two, to remedial measures based on the principles already brought under your notice.

The first thing to bear in mind in the treatment, I might say of every form of rheumatism, is that free action of the skin should be encouraged. Warm baths of various kinds, and in many parts of the world, have been held in great repute for their curative properties. The Turkish bath is often of great use to those who are troubled with rheumatic pains. It is, however, a rather long business, and the patient who adopts it must have two hours or more at his disposal. I know people who take a Turkish bath twice every week with advantage, and consider that they could not get on without it.

Those who cannot, or will not, adopt the advice given them to take Turkish baths may, perhaps, not object to an ordinary warm bath, twice or three times a week, staying in the water from twenty minutes to half an hour, or until they perspire freely. I think the action of the ordinary warm bath in rheumatism is improved if the water be made alkaline. This may be done by dissolving in it a quarter of a pound of washing-soda. The vapor bath is also of great use, and so is the hot-air bath. Very simple arrangements for vapor or hot air may now be obtained.

By free perspiration, the removal from the blood of a large quantity of water holding various substances in solution is effected. Thus thirst is excited. The patient drinks freely of aërated or other water. In this way those noxious materials which would otherwise accumulate in the tissues are gradually removed, and the patients, perhaps, escape much suffering.

Shampooing is also of great use in slight cases of muscular and fibrous rheumatism. By judiciously pressing and squeezing the muscles, and by rubbing the skin, the removal of fluids from the interstices of many tissues is promoted.

You know it is very important for the free action of the muscles that the fluid which bathes the contractile tissue, and which undergoes alteration during the action of the muscle, should be frequently changed. If some portions of the fluid remain in contact with individual fibres, the materials resulting from the decomposition taking place during the action of those fibres will accumulate and, necessarily, interfere with their free

17 *

action, probably also affecting the action of the nerves, and thus occasioning rheumatic pains. You will find that, generally, muscular pains may be relieved by exciting the action of the skin, the bowels, and the kidneys. Alkaline remedies have this effect, and are invariably useful to those who suffer, perhaps because in this condition there is an invariable tendency to the development in the system of organic acids, particularly lactic.

Alkalies may be given in all forms of rheumatism. You may order *Bicarbonate of Potash*, or *Liquor Potassæ*, or *Bicarbonate of Soda*. These are very old remedies, and concerning their influence in relieving rheumatic pains there cannot be the slightest doubt. In many slight cases of pain, twenty or thirty grains of Bicarbonate of Potash, dissolved in two ounces of water, will be found to relieve in three or four hours. Sal Volatile helps its action, and also stimulates the heart a little, and thus the blood is driven more quickly through the capillary vessels, and absorption promoted. You may order the alkali to be taken about half an hour after meals, for a week or a fortnight at a time. But you must take care not to let a patient go on taking *Liquor Potassæ* or *Bicarbonate of Potash* from one year's end to another, or you will probably be consulted on account of the appearance of phosphates in the urine, with, perhaps, irritable bladder. Retention of urine may follow, and considerable quantities of pus may be formed. Sometimes the patient becomes very low and weak ; and I am not sure that serious changes in the blood, and even purulent inflammation of joints, have not resulted from the too long continued use of alkalies. *Potash* and *Soda* are very valuable remedies, if given with judgment, and if people are not allowed to go on taking them as long as they like. You must not forget to explain to patients how long you wish them to continue taking any medicine you prescribe, or you will sometimes be astonished, if not alarmed, to find that a somewhat obedient patient, for whom you have prescribed a pill, has been daily taking it for years.

If a patient suffering from rheumatism finds that alkalies disagree with him and disturb his digestion, you may try salts of vegetable acids, particularly the Citrates and Tartrates, for these become converted into alkalies in the system, and the urine may even be rendered alkaline by them as well as by the ordinary alkalies. Lemon and orange juice, and many fruits, also act beneficially in some cases.

Among diuretics, the ordinary Nitrate of Potash or Common Nitre, dose from five to ten grains, in water, three or four times a day ; the Acetate of Potash, in doses of from ten to fifty grains, in two ounces of water, three or four times daily ; the Bitartrate of Potash (*Potassæ Tartras Acida*), in doses of twenty to sixty grains or more, in two or three ounces of water, three or four times in the twenty-four hours (sometimes also acts as a purgative), and the Citrate of Potash, in the same doses as the Acetate, are the most generally useful.

Guiacum.—In former days, Guiacum was much in favor in the treatment of chronic rheumatism, and I have found benefit result from its use.
You may prescribe the resin, *Guiaci Resina*, in doses of ten grains made
into pills, or finely powdered and mixed with milk, three or four times
a day, or the *Mistura Guiaci*, an ounce of which may be ordered twice
or three times daily. Perhaps the least unpleasant form in which to take
Guiacum is as the Ammoniated Tincture, *Tinctura Guiaci Ammoniata*,
in a mixture with some bitter tincture or infusion. Mucilage and a few
drops of *Spiritus Chloroformi*, with water ; or peppermint, mint, or other
water, may be used to cover the taste.

Iodide of Potassium.—You will often find that severe lumbago pain,
fixed pains in the muscles and fibrous tissues in many parts of the body,
and severe chronic aching about various joints, which have troubled
people for months, will be relieved by a few doses of Iodide of Potassium
(*Potassii Iodidum*). You may begin with three grains, three or four times
a day, and gradually increase the dose to five, six, eight or ten grains.
The Iodide should be dissolved in a considerable quantity of water, and
should be taken about an hour or more after meals. You may also give
with it half a drachm of *Liquor Cinchonæ* (Battley's), and a few drops
of *Tincture of Ginger*. Although I cannot justify the practice, on scientific grounds, I often give with the Iodide, Nitrate of Potash (five grains).
The Iodide probably acts upon the painful textures, partly by promoting
the absorption of exudation, but I think chiefly by taking the place of
Chloride of Sodium, driving this out, and thus promoting free circulation
of fluids and saline matters through the interstices of the textures. Don't
accept the conclusion, implicitly received by many, that the beneficial
action of Iodide of Potassium is evidence of the syphilitic origin of the
malady. This is one of the new delusions. Some authorities attribute
half the ills we suffer from to syphilis, and even think that a syphilitic
taint accounts for the majority of ailments they cannot otherwise explain
or account for. If neither you nor your father nor your grandfather had
syphilis, the origin of disease is to be discovered further back in your
ancestral line, if, indeed, it is admitted possible by syphilitic authorities
that three generations can exist without having acquired the disease.
Some authorities seem to think that no one exists who is entirely free
from syphilitic taint. Both Iodide of Potassium and Bichloride of Mer-
cury (from the $\frac{1}{32}$ to the $\frac{1}{16}$ of a grain for a dose) are extremely valuable
remedies in very many affections which are not in any way due to syphilis.

Bromide of Potassium, *Potassii Bromidum*, is useful in cases in which
the rheumatic pain is, in part, neuralgic in character. It may be given
alone, or with the Iodide, in doses of from ten to thirty grains. Salicine
and Salicylic Acid and Salicylate of Soda (*see* p. 191) are useful in some
cases of chronic rheumatism, and quinine is frequently of advantage.

I have observed, and in many instances, that after the persistence of
slight but evidently rheumatic pains for many days, perhaps for two

or three weeks, the patient, without resorting to any special treatment whatever, experiences unusually free action of the skin at night. Even in midwinter, as soon as he gets warm in bed, he sweats profusely, and for the whole night,—finding his nightshirt quite moist and his skin thoroughly soft and soddened in the morning,—although no change had been made in his bedclothes nor in his diet, and he had not taken any medicine whatever. The free sweating had not only come on of itself, but, perhaps, persisted night after night for some time. So remarkable and unusual is the free action of the skin that oftentimes a patient is alarmed, and seeks advice with the object of stopping the cure. On inquiry, it is found not only that the rheumatic pains have been much less severe since the free sweating at night came on, but that the patient feels in much better health. He is in better spirits—lighter, as he says—and stronger and more active. His mind clearer. His bowels act unusually well, and his water is excreted freely, and is perfectly clear and destitute of the accustomed sediment. The tongue is clean and the appetite is good. But notwithstanding his conviction that he is in better health than usual, he fears the very free sweating may weaken him, or in some way do harm, and therefore seeks advice. Now, so far from interfering with the free perspiration, you may assure your patient that a natural cure is being effected, and that it is desirable not to stop it. After a week or two the perspiration will diminish, and the patient will feel well, and will not be troubled with rheumatic pains for some time to come. Such facts are of the greatest interest, and are well deserving of your careful contemplation. We may learn from them even more than we can learn from many serious cases of disease. And though, if we act rightly, we may object to interfere, our attention is forcibly directed to certain phenomena, from the consideration of which the principle of treatment to be pursued, in the case of those who are not so fortunate as to suffer a spontaneous cure, may be deduced.

Moderate, but habitual, natural action of the skin, liver, and other emunctories, probably prevents altogether the development of the rheumatic state. Free action for a time cures the rheumatic condition, if present, and this free action may be brought about by changes within the body. In the absence of this action, however, we endeavor by artificial means to excite it. And if the rheumatism is really severe, we should resort to the best means we possess to bring about these curative influences as soon as possible.

Questions like the following will doubtless occur to some, but I regret to say that I cannot adequately answer them : "Why in some organisms only this spontaneous cure is observed? Why some never suffer from rheumatism, and so need no cure? Why some suffer terribly in spite of all measures adopted for their relief, and why some die in consequence of the extreme degree and inveterate character of the rheumatic phenomena?" Some would refer the difference to nerve action only, and there can be no doubt concerning the amazing variation in rapidity and intensity of nerve action in different individuals. Some people seem to be "all nerve." Others appear to get on, and very well, with extremely slow and apparently blunted nerve action. Between these two extremes many degrees of difference are to be noticed. If the nerve mechanism presiding over the physiological changes in the system is well developed and highly active, derangement will be corrected ere there has been time for its existence to have been made evident to the consciousness of the individual; but when nerves and centres are dull, and small and sparse in proportion to the extent of area they have to govern, response is slow, and physiological derangement may even pass into pathological change, and result in structural alteration of a most serious and irreparable character without the patient being aware that he is even out of health. Nay, we see the most grave morbid changes running a long course, damaging in the most decided manner, it may be, many important tissues and more than one organ, and at a comparatively early period of life, although the patient has not experienced even discomfort. On the other hand, sensitive, constantly ailing people often lead long, complaining lives, and die in old age, without a single organ having passed into a state of actual disease. In such instances as the last, the patient is endowed with highly active nerve organs. In the first, very decided pathological change fails to exert any influence upon slowly acting and blunted nerve organs. In the one, broad and obvious lesions progress until action is greatly deranged or death results; in the other, illness is prevented or is self-cured before it progresses to any extent. Very decided and well-timed interference at an early period, and the utmost care all through, would alone save patients of the first class from serious disease, and perhaps death; while no treatment, or only treatment of the simplest character, would be needed by the more sensitive nervous person. Slight ailments in some organisms cause much ado, while in others grave pathological actions of great intensity may occur, and serious structural morbid changes run their course for a considerable time without being discovered, and without giving rise to any symptoms sufficiently distinct to attract the attention of the patient.

The Diet in Rheumatism must be nutritious, but care should be taken that the patient does not exceed. All rheumatics should be careful not to partake too freely of meat and allied substances. Farinaceous substances and fatty matters do no harm, but while many ripe fruits agree well, and some—oranges, lemons, cooked apples, prunes, and some others—are useful, sugar in large quantity is certainly not desirable. Milk is excellent, and rheumatics may take it in quantity. Various puddings, such as batter, sago, tapioca, etc., made with milk and an egg, may be recommended. Acid wines, like the commoner forms of claret, often do harm, and indeed may occasion rheumatic pains. Beer is especially hurtful, and should invariably be withheld. In treating cases of rheumatism you must impress upon patients very strongly that beer, as well as claret and some acid wines, seriously interferes with the improvement which otherwise would probably result from the remedies you prescribe. If stimulants are required at all, you may allow in the twenty-four hours two or three tablespoonfuls of brandy with seltzer or other mineral water, or the same quantity of whiskey with lemon juice and water.

Importance of Warmth and Warm Clothing.—Cold, damp, ill-ventilated rooms are especially hurtful, and exposure to sudden changes of temperature often gives rise to very severe and acute attacks of rheumatism. Those who are prone to rheumatism may feel annoyed if they perspire much, and are too often unwise enough to try to check the tendency to perspiration by wearing very light clothing, and thus not uncommonly they precipitate an attack. Not only should all persons who have even a slight tendency to rheumatism wear woollen next the skin during the day, but at night they should either have a flannel night-dress or a flannel jacket over their cotton garment. If the shoulders and arms be exposed at night with insufficient covering, very obstinate rheumatic pain, which may last a considerable time, is sometimes the consequence.

A departure from the healthy state of the blood may originate either in the circulating fluid itself, or may be determined by changes in the tissues and organs which it nourishes. The change in the blood may, in its turn, react upon and influence the action of some, and, indeed, almost all the tissues and organs in the body. When this is the case, the phenomena are said to be "general," to distinguish them from phenomena of the same general nature which are restricted in area, and are spoken of as "local." We may speak of *general tissue changes, general fever, general inflammation*, as contrasted with changes of phenomena similar in their nature, but which are local, and affect only a very small portion of the body. Among the most important and most common general changes are those departures from healthy action known as *fevers* and *general inflammations*. So common is febrile and inflammatory disturbance that it is doubtful whether a single example could be adduced of a mammalian organism which had reached maturity without having suffered more or less from some such pathological changes. Few of us pass a month without experiencing, in our own bodies, some degree of febrile or inflammatory disturbance, and many are seldom entirely free for many weeks at a time from phenomena of the kind.

Of Catching Cold.—Before bringing under your notice the actual phenomena which characterize all fevers and inflammations, I propose to direct attention to the consideration of that most common of all febrile disorders, and the best known of all slight ailments—*an ordinary cold*—in the course of which a certain degree of febrile and inflammatory action invariably occurs.

Most people have "caught cold" probably many times in the course of their lives, and though they may have suffered on some occasions severely, there is no reason to suppose that any tissue in the body has been damaged in the slightest degree, or that any structural disease has resulted in consequence. Whenever you are unfortunate enough to take cold, you should make the most of the opportunity, and carefully study the changes as they go on in your own organism.

When the cold is coming on, you may perhaps shiver a little, or you may experience a creeping sensation, apparently in the skin of different parts of the body. Although you may feel quite chilly, if you place a clinical thermometer in your arm-pit, you will be surprised to discover that it indicates a rise of three or four degrees above the normal in the temperature of your body, and the very striking and important fact will be impressed upon you that, although you feel extremely chilly and inclined to shiver, and desire warm clothing, or to sit by the fire, with a good blanket over you, the temperature of the body is decidedly higher than it ought to be, and in fact may have risen from a little under 98° Fahrenheit, the point at which it stands in health, to 100°, 101°, or 102°. You need not be very much disturbed or frightened if you should find that it marks 103°. You will also notice that, as soon as you get into a free perspiration, all the uncomfortable sensations which you have experienced during perhaps several hours, will disappear. If, as soon as you feel warm, and especially if you have perspired a little, you again use the thermometer, you will find that the temperature has fallen a degree or two. After you have perspired very freely, it will fall lower still, and probably stand at the normal.

I shall endeavor to show not only that a cold is a form of fever, but that in many colds there is evidence of a certain, and in some a considerable, degree of inflammatory action. The mucous membrane of the nasal passages, of the larynx, trachea, and bronchial tubes, of the pharynx, and many of the small glands connected with these surfaces, are red and "inflamed." The capillary circulation in them is impeded, and if a minute examination be made we shall find evidence of undue growth of the bioplasm of the epithelium and adjacent structures.

Many of the symptoms which usher in an ordinary cold precisely resemble those which occur when some special form of fever or, it may be, severe inflammation is about to attack the patient. In the last case the shivering and other phenomena may be more severe, but the difference is one of degree; in fact, a cold must be included among the *Febrile Diseases.*

But let us for a moment go further back in our inquiry as to the nature of the malady, and try to discover the change which, so to say, constitutes the first departure from the normal state in the case of a common cold or other simple form of febrile attack. The event in question usually precedes by hours, and it may be days, the manifestation of any symptoms. The actual process of taking cold is never *immediately* followed by any phenomena which disturb the health or which indicate to the patient himself that he has passed, or is about to pass, from the healthy into an abnormal state. This fact alone—the existence of an interval between the commencement of the operation of the disturbing cause and the development of distinct derangement in the physiological actions of the body—seems sufficient to show that the symptoms are not due to nervous disturbance alone, and conclusively points to the conclusion that the change excited is of such a nature that it does not result in immediate consequences.

The condition of the organism which favors " taking cold " is not one of perfect health. The circulation at the time is feeble, and the blood itself not in a perfectly healthy state. Instead of passing quickly through the cutaneous capillaries, the circulation is retarded in the surface-vessels, partly on account, as above suggested, of feeble heart's action, but mainly, I think, owing to the muscular fibres of the smallest arteries being relaxed, and the consequent dilatation of the tube of the vessel. The blood, very slowly traversing the cutaneous capillaries, being far too long a time exposed to the cooling influences perhaps of a draught of cold air, becomes the seat of chemical changes which differ from those ordinarily taking place in the blood constituents. The particular chemical compounds formed under these circumstances are not readily excreted. Remaining in the blood, they accumulate, and minute bioplasts grow and multiply. At length an influence upon the nerves is exerted, and then ensues the chilliness and other symptoms due to the derangement of the action of many tissues and organs of the body which mark the invasion of the illness. After a time the materials in question begin to be eliminated, and the patient gets well.

If we promote the action of the excreting organs, we follow the " suggestions of nature " and expedite recovery. Now some may think all this a rather fanciful explanation ; but if we consider what happens in slight rheumatism, we shall, I think, be convinced that the conclusions arrived at are supported by facts. When the rheumatic state comes on, the patient experiences pain in the muscles and fibrous tissues in many parts of the body distant from one another, which pains are relieved in a very short time if free action of the skin, kidneys, and bowels is established. There is no doubt whatever that certain alkaline, diuretic, and purgative medicines excite the desired action, and thus the morbid condition is relieved or cured. The increased flow of urine, caused by giving diuretics, is followed by thirst, to quench which the patient resorts to cooling drinks. Thus the tissues get well washed out, and the peccant materials which, by their action on the nerves, cause the pain, are by degrees highly diluted and dissolved away, or in the blood are converted into materials which are readily removed from the body by different emunctories. We have thus accounted for the formation of morbid materials in the body, and have explained how these derange many physiological actions and occasion pathological phenomena. Further, it has been shown how these noxious substances are removed, and by what means their removal, or, in other words, the recovery of the patient, may be assisted and hastened.

Preliminary Changes and Attendant Phenomena.—As regards the accession of a cold, or other febrile or inflammatory attack, the first indications of derangement in the ordinary physiological processes are much the same; but the intensity of the changes varies greatly in different fevers and inflammations. For some little time before you "catch cold," you are conscious of not being in the ordinary state of health. Without feeling very weak or low, you are inclined to lie down; and, perhaps, if you followed your own inclination, you would go to bed, and in this way try to obtain relief from the discomfort and sense of oppression and general uneasiness. In a short time some degree of soreness about the nose is usually experienced, and this is often associated with dryness of the nasal cavity and of the throat. The tongue feels more or less dry and uncomfortable. Little or no saliva is secreted; the skin, too, often feels hot and dry. When the skin is perfectly healthy, it is smooth and supple, but when a cold, or any general fever or inflammation, is coming on, a change usually takes place. It becomes more or less harsh, and even rough, small particles of the outer layer of the cuticle being partially detached. The surface, in consequence, feels dry and rough, and when rubbed, bran-like particles, consisting of the scales of old cuticle, are removed.

Very frequently the patient experiences slight uneasiness about the head, perhaps not amounting to actual headache, but a little pain, it may be, over the brow, or heaviness there or at the back of the head, or in the back of the neck, or in all these situations. The pain in the neck is probably caused by some derangement affecting the nerves distributed to those muscles by the action of which the head is raised and drawn backwards. This pain just below the occiput often lasts for several days and is very troublesome, the slightest movement of the head being difficult in consequence of the pain which is excited.

When a cold or fever is imminent, you usually feel weak and disinclined to take exercise. If it is necessary to walk, you have, as it were, to force yourself to do so. There is little appetite, and perhaps no desire to eat an ordinary meal. Rather than solid food, you feel inclined to take a cup of warm soup or strong beef-tea, or ordinary tea or coffee, or gruel, or hot wine and water. There is very generally indeed a demand for fluid when a cold is coming on. You feel dry and thirsty, and almost instinctively seek for water, iced water, or lemonade. It is unquestionably advantageous to take fluids when these sensations, which usher in a cold in the head or other febrile attack, are experienced. For although, as Dr. J. C. B. Williams long ago showed, by resisting the longing for fluid, and bearing with the thirst for two or three days,

18

the catarrhal symptoms may be lessened, at least for a time, the discomfort and distress are often so great that the patient prefers the inconvenience incidental to the cold to the suffering which results from carrying out this dry system of treatment for its relief or cure, and it is doubtful whether the duration of the illness is by this plan in any way shortened. I have thought that in some cases the cold has been cut short by taking plenty of fluid, and thereby exciting free action of the skin and kidneys. The premonitory symptoms of a cold are unquestionably often much relieved by a basin of hot soup, or even warm tea or coffee. As you are probably aware, the treatment everywhere most popular is a glass of hot wine or spirits and water. You will hear in every part of the country of cases of various terrible forms of disease which have been at once stopped or cut short by a stiff glass of hot brandy, whiskey, or gin and water. Although the secretion from the mucous membrane may be diminished by withholding fluid for a time, it is also quite certain that general relief of the discomfort and unpleasant symptoms may be obtained from the very opposite system, that of drinking freely of fluids which excite the action of the skin and kidneys, and thus wash out of the system various deleterious matters which have accumulated in the blood.

The Body-heat of Man and Warm-blooded Animals Fixed and Definite.—The temperature of man and the higher animals in a state of health is fixed within a very limited range, and, as I mentioned in one of my early lectures, it is worthy of note that this fixed and definite temperature of the blood in the case of warm-blooded animals is maintained at the uniform standard, although the temperature of the medium in which the animal lives may vary greatly from time to time. The temperature of our body is the same in summer and winter, or at the most varies little more than a degree of Fahrenheit's scale. A man in the polar regions will have the same internal temperature as one living at the equator. In the cold climate there is very little sensible perspiration. In the hot one perspiration never ceases, and the cuticle is always wet and soddened. By constant changes in the rate at which heat is evolved in and carried off from the body, the internal temperature of the blood is kept very nearly uniform. It is remarkable that the limit of variation in health is so slight, for we may regard it as proved that the blood cannot vary to a greater extent than is represented by two degrees of Fahrenheit, without a departure from the normal state of health.

Whether the air be cold or hot, whether a person take violent exercise or lie quietly in a warm bed, whether food be taken frequently or withheld for many hours, the temperature will not exhibit more than a very slight temporary disturbance, and whenever a change does occur, the temperature will very soon return to the normal point.

Rise of the Body-heat in all Fevers and Inflammations.—In every form of fever and in every kind of inflammation the temperature of the body or of the affected part, and therefore the blood, rises. You must not forget that, although, as I have said, the patient may feel excessively chilly, nay, though he be seized with decided rigors, so that he is excessively pallid, the face being pinched and destitute of color, or actually livid and cold to the touch, his limbs trembling and his teeth chattering, the temperature of his blood will be higher than in the ordinary condition of health. So far from the blood being entirely or only affected, it is more probable that in many cases the rise in temperature begins in the tissues outside the vessels. The blood-corpuscles, as they pass through the capillaries, take heat from one place and distribute it to other parts, so that a considerable rise in one spot may be soon reduced, and the heat diffused over a wide area, and thus cause a slight rise in the temperature of the body generally. Even in the flea-bite, if it were possible to place an instrument among the distended capillaries and tissues of the affected part, the temperature, I venture to say, would be found higher than in the tissues just beyond the affected area. In extensive inflammations, as was shown by Mr. Simon, the temperature of the blood which leaves the inflamed part is always decidedly higher than when it passes into it.

There is not a fever known to us in which the temperature does not rise above the normal; neither is there any inflammation which is not characterized by phenomena which occasion the development of an increased degree of heat in the inflamed part. This generalization is to be extended to all the higher animals. Every creature capable of suffering inflammation or the feverish condition exhibits, during the attack, elevation of temperature. There is, in fact, a very intimate connection between the increased development of heat and the states *Fever* and *Inflammation*, and we may go so far as to affirm that the existence of either of these pathological processes without a rise in the temperature is not possible. In both fever and inflammation it would seem that the circumstances which determine the maintenance of the equable body-heat of health are deranged, either generally, as in the fever, or locally, as in the inflammation. Heat is developed faster than it can be carried off, or the processes by which it is carried off are for the time interfered with, or both circumstances are concerned in determining the rapid rise of temperature which is often observed in various fevers and inflammations of marked intensity.

Is there Increased Oxidation in Fever and Inflammation?—This question is one of much importance in reference to the consideration of the real nature of the febrile condition. It would be answered directly and most positively in the affirmative by most pathologists, but, as we shall see, the facts known by no means justify an off-hand and confident answer. The secretion from the kidneys of a person suffering from feverishness is usually concentrated and of high specific gravity. You will frequently find it loaded with urates, and often there will be *Excess* *of Urea.* Deposits of uric acid are common. The *Excess of Urea* is shown in a very simple way. To about half a teaspoonful of the urine in a test-tube you add an equal bulk of strong nitric acid, and plunge the lower part of the tube at once into cold water, shaking it from time to time. In the course of a few minutes crystals of Nitrate of Urea will begin to form, and if the specific gravity of the urine is 1.030 or higher, it may become almost solid from the quantity of crystals formed.

The circulation of the blood and the action of the various organs in the body are greatly disturbed, and there is departure from the normal state in many respects, both as regards the chemical processes going on in the blood, and the presence and accumulation in quantity in the circulating fluid of substances which ought to be removed from it in a very dilute state as fast as they are formed and passed into it. Instead of this, many of the excrementitious matters are in such a high degree of concentration that they readily separate from the fluid in which they are dissolved, and in the case of the urine some are deposited soon after the secretion has been passed and has become cool.

These and many other phenomena, which are undoubtedly due to exceptional chemical change, are often set down to excessive oxidation, although a careful consideration of the facts would lead us to entertain the opposite conclusion, that oxidation was deficient instead of being in excess.

In many books you are told that body-heat is invariably the result of the combination of carbon and other elements with oxygen—that the increase of temperature in all fevers is due to increased oxidation. There is, however, evidence of a most striking kind that in various morbid conditions in which the temperature of the body considerably exceeds the normal standard the process of oxidation is much interfered with. If, for instance, a man has one lung solid from the air-cells being plugged up with lymph poured out from the blood, as occurs in pneumonia, is it not unreasonable to maintain that oxidation is going on to a greater extent, or is more complete, than in health? In this case are not the air-cells filled with solid matter, which renders the entrance of air less constant and its renewal quite impossible? And yet we are assured that the elevation of temperature in pneumonia, and in all other febrile and inflammatory states, is due to increased oxidation, and to that alone. Again, the body of a person who has died from a terribly severe attack of acute rheumatism can hardly be considered to be in a state favorable to free oxidation. Nevertheless the temperature, which at the time of death may be as high as 107° or 108°, often rises three or four degrees of Fahrenheit during the first hour or two after death. How, then, can we reasonably attribute this rise of temperature to increased oxidation? Consider not only that the rise continues for some time after the lungs have ceased to act at all, and the heart can no longer propel a drop of blood along the vessels, but that for many hours, or even days, before death the conditions of the system had been most unfavorable to the introduction of air and its free distribution to distant parts, as also to its absorption by the tissues and fluids. We can show that in all probability the high temperature is due to the increased growth of bioplasm, not to increased oxidation.

The generalization that the elevation of temperature in fever and inflammation is due to increased oxidation is, I think, a grave mistake. It is more probable that the phenomenon is occasioned by changes in the bioplasm or living matter of the blood and tissues of a nature far removed from the process of oxidation. I shall have again to refer to this very interesting subject, and hope to consider it more in detail.

Method of Ascertaining the Temperature of the Body.—The actual temperature, as indicated by the thermometer, is found to vary slightly, according to the part of the body which is selected for observation. If, for example, you place the thermometer under the tongue, you will find, as you would anticipate, that it will mark a degree or so higher than if the same instrument is placed in the arm-pit. In medical observations on the body-heat we restrict ourselves to observations in two places, the mouth underneath the tongue and the arm-pit. But if you try the mouth, in the case of children, you will not unfrequently have the bulb of your instrument bitten off. Such an accident is serious, for good clinical thermometers cost from twelve to sixteen shillings each. It is, therefore, upon the whole, better to take the temperature in the arm-pit only. In order that you may be able to compare the records of different cases, you must take care to work in precisely the same way, and to place the thermometer in the arm-pit for at least two minutes, if the bulb is a very small one, and for double that time if it is not of the smallest size. You will have little difficulty in using the small thermometer, even in the case of the most irritable and violent children ; for you can always put it in the arm-pit and keep the child's arm nearly still for the length of time required.

Thermometers for medical observation, *clinical thermometers* as they are called, may be obtained of all the instrument makers. Those with the smallest bulbs respond very quickly, and the index comes to a stand in two minutes, or even in less time ; but the degrees are small and more difficult to read off than those of larger instruments, which require to be inserted in the arm-pit for four or more minutes before you can feel sure that the mercury has come to a standstill. Of late a great improvement has been made in the construction of the very small thermometers. The bore is so fine that observers whose eyesight is not the most perfect often find it difficult to see the index. By grinding the glass away somewhat at the sides and making the front of a greater convexity, the effect of an elongated lens is produced, and the almost invisible mercurial thread is made to appear as a broad band of mercury, which can be seen without the slightest difficulty.

18 *   O

Further Consideration of the Essential Phenomena of Fever and Inflammation—Rigors and Cold Stage—Hot Stage—Sweating Stage.— When a severe form of fever or inflammation is about to attack a patient, instead of mere chilliness and a sensation of creeping or tingling of the surface skin, an actual rigor is experienced. This is often so intense that the patient trembles in every limb, his teeth chatter, and he feels dreadfully ill. The very bed on which he lies may be perceptibly shaken, so violent and so general is the nerve and muscular disturbance.

Among severe inflammations, a sharp attack of inflammation of the lungs, *Pneumonia*, and among fevers, small-pox, *Variola*, and scarlet fever, *Scarlatina*, are ushered in thus. If you were called to the patient as soon as he was taken ill, you would see his limbs trembling violently, his face pale and anxious, the patient himself would be considerably depressed, suffering from nausea, and probably every now and then violent retching would add to his distress. If you put your hand on his pulse, you find it quick, feeble, and small; and if you place the thermometer in his axilla, you will find the temperature higher than normal, perhaps by four or five degrees.

It would seem that the blood is diverted from the general surface of the body, and is driven in greater proportion to internal parts— to the lungs, to the intestines, to the liver, and to other internal organs. These preliminary symptoms, with the shivering which is developed in a remarkable degree, represent what is known as the "cold stage" of an ' intermittent fever." *Ague* is a very remarkable form of feverish attack, inasmuch as the several special stages which are to be traced with more or less distinctness in all fevers and inflammations are very manifest, and are well defined and sharply marked off from one another. In the cold stage, blood not only leaves the surface, but temporarily parts with much of its water, which then occupies the interstices of the tissues. After a time it again enters the blood or passes off by the intestines, in which case it may be altogether removed from the body, as in Diarrhœa, or in Cholera, in which disease the blood becomes of a thick and tarry consistence, and stagnates in many of the vessels, scarcely moving at all in some of the capillaries which are distributed to very important organs of the body.

The shivering and other symptoms which constitute the first indications of derangement in febrile diseases are referable to conditions favoring the formation of deleterious matters in the blood itself. In some cases these are due to changes originating in the organism, in others to the introduction of a poison from without.

The phenomena which mark the accession of a common cold correspond to the cold stage of the ague-fit. I think it probable that the so-called collapse stage of cholera is also analogous to the first stage of the ague-fit, and consider that it represents, only in the most severe form, the general phenomena which usher in every form of febrile and inflammatory attack. It is in a sudden and very severe attack of this most terrible disease, Cholera, that we see the cold stage of a fever in its highest conceivable degree of development; for, in fact, the collapse is so severe and so widely diffused, so manifestly deranging the action of every tissue and organ in the body, that in too many instances death results in a very short time. But Cholera, like other febrile affections, has not only its cold stage. If the patient lives, the terrible state of collapse at length gives place to great heat and dryness of skin, and this *hot stage* in turn is followed by a *crisis* or critical change, when the kidneys and skin again resume action. The blood regains its color and begins to freely flow along its accustomed channels, and the various glands and tissues gradually recover from the shock they have suffered and return to their normal state. The patient, in fact, soon becomes convalescent.

The feverish condition which in cholera follows the stage of collapse, after a varying interval of time, is called Secondary Fever. Happily, few of you have seen either a case of ordinary cholera or the secondary fever, which was not so common, but not a few of your teachers have seen and done their utmost to save many a case. In most epidemics the disease was very fatal during the cold stage, and where very much water had been already drained off from the blood into the intestinal canal the patient died in collapse. In some of the cases which recovered the secondary fever was so slight that it attracted little or no attention; but occasionally I have seen it very marked indeed, and have lost patients from secondary fever who, some days before, had passed through severe collapse and were considered to be recovering. I believe that this febrile stage of cholera corresponds very closely to the prolonged feverish condition characteristic of *typhus* or *typhoid*, for example, and to the so-called hot or *febrile stage* of an intermittent. In an ordinary cold the feverish state usually lasts but a very short time, perhaps not longer than from ten to twenty-four hours. In *typhoid fever*, however, it may last for six weeks or more, and in acute rheumatism it may extend over two months. During the whole of this long period the temperature of the patient's blood may not once, even for a single hour, fall to the normal standard, though in many cases it falls and rises several times in the course of the attack, passing three or four degrees above the normal, and then perhaps going down to that point, again rising, and so on. In an ordinary cold or catarrh the chilly stage is usually followed, in the course of five or six hours, by free perspiration, which immediately affords great relief, and in many instances seems to cure the patient at once.

In fevers and extensive inflammations the nervous system generally is affected. In some forms the action of the brain is very much disturbed. Soon after the preliminary phenomena of the common cold have occurred, the pulse increases in frequency, and there is, possibly, severe headache, the whole of the head, perhaps, feeling full, almost to bursting, as if it had been forcibly distended with more than it could properly contain. The action of the mind is affected. No one when he is attacked can perform much intellectual work. His memory suffers, and to think at all is a painful effort. He probably feels more inclined to lie down and do nothing. If he goes to bed, instead of falling asleep he tosses about from one side to the other in an uncomfortable way; perhaps he dreams of all kinds of horrible things, and wakes up suddenly, finding the mouth, fauces, and tongue dry and uncomfortable. There is still more or less feeling of fulness and distention about the head. The patient again tries to go to sleep, only to be disturbed by more unpleasant dreams and to wake again, perhaps frightened, in a short time. Oftentimes there is chilliness, or a creeping sensation is experienced over the general surface, the muscles seem fatigued, and there is a general feeling of lassitude. These phenomena indicate a wide-spread disturbance of the nervous system, cerebral, spinal, and ganglionic, caused probably by the action upon the nerves and nerve-centres of certain materials which ought to have been eliminated, but which have unduly accumulated in the blood.

Such are some of the broad phenomena which almost every one has experienced who has taken a bad cold or has suffered from any form of fever. In severe and specific fevers and general inflammations all these nerve phenomena are more strikingly developed, and trouble the patient for a longer period of time. In any well-developed fever, for instance, the patients may pass many sleepless nights. They may be troubled with headache for a fortnight or three weeks, or even longer, and may be restless and wakeful during the whole of the time.

The chilly sensation, like the *cold stage* of an ague-fit, is succeeded, after a varying period of time, by a very different state of things. The blood returns in volumes to the surface of the body. The little arteries dilate, the capillaries are distended, the color returns and is intensified, and the skin becomes hot to the feel, but it remains dry. There is often headache, and the patient will perhaps tell you that his head feels ready to burst. This is the *hot stage*, which is soon followed by the last or *sweating stage*. The skin is bathed with perspiration, which continues it may be for several hours, so that the cuticle becomes completely soddened and softened. In this way a quantity of water with certain organic matters dissolved in it, and often amounting to several pounds in weight, is very quickly removed from the blood.

The action of the skin and other excreting organs of the body, which had been partially suspended during the accession of the attack, and in many cases for some days before, is a general fact of great importance, and marks the temporary abatement or actual cessation of all febrile and inflammatory disorders. If these phenomena can be caused to come on somewhat earlier than in the natural course of events, the duration of the febrile or inflammatory attack is to that extent reduced. As soon as the sweating comes on the patient may feel relieved, but until it has occurred he may experience much discomfort. Till then you may have felt very anxious about the case. We are unfortunately unable to ascertain at the commencement of the attack how bad the patient is likely to be; we never know to what extent the grave symptoms of the malady may continue to increase, or for how long a time the patient will continue to get worse. Until sweating and free secretion have occurred we can seldom judge as to the probability of recovery or the duration of the time of illness.

Of Free Secretion which Leads to Recovery.—Recovery is associated with the gradual removal from the organism of substances which probably have been accumulating for some time in the blood and nutrient fluids. These substances are slowly removed by the agency of the kidneys, skin, bowels, and other emunctories. When the skin acts pretty freely, you become thirsty and imbibe a quantity of fluid, which is again quickly removed by the kidneys. The bowels act freely, although perhaps for some time before the illness and during part of the attack they had been confined, or had only acted imperfectly, especially when febrile action was most intense. The glands of the mucous membrane of the intestinal canal, like other glands, do not act as freely in the early period of a cold as they do in the healthy state. When, however, the patient returns to the normal condition these glands act freely, and the tendency to constipation and defective action passes off.

Moreover, as the feverishness abates there will be increased action of several glands as compared with their activity in the ordinary state of health. Not only do the kidneys and the cutaneous glands act in an unusual way for some time after recovery, but the glands of the mucous membrane of the nose and those of the mucous membrane of the air-tubes also continue to secrete freely for some time. Many of us while in perfect health might leave our pocket-handkerchiefs behind without experiencing inconvenience, but when suffering from a cold it is well not to be neglectful. A quantity of secretion is poured out from the mucous membrane of the nose, and in many cases also from that of the windpipe and bronchial tubes.

The secretion is modified mucus. In the healthy state the mucus which is formed is extremely small in amount. This mucus is principally produced in minute glands connected with the mucous membrane and which open upon its free surface. The same glands, when the fever of an ordinary cold is passing off, secrete an undue quantity of mucus. Exaggerated action proceeds in connection with all the mucous surfaces, and persists for a certain period of time, varying from twelve or twenty-four hours to many days. The patient then usually gets better, and everything slowly returns to its normal rate of action.

Now this very free secretion, in certain cases, is a matter of serious importance. There are certain forms of inflammation of the mucous

membrane of the air-tubes, including the nasal passages, in which there
may be an undue secretion of altered mucus, amounting to six or eight
ounces in the twenty-four hours. In some sad cases, happily not very
common, an excessive quantity of secretion is so quickly poured out
that it accumulates in the smaller air-tubes, and death may be caused
by suffocation in the course of a few hours.

The mucous membrane of some persons' air-tubes is constantly in so
sensitive and irritable a state, that whenever the weather is either cold
or damp they suffer more or less. Such patients ought to spend their
winter in a warmer climate, where they can be out in the open air almost
daily; for if they remain in London they generally have to be shut up
in warm rooms for a great part of the winter, a course very detrimental
to the general health, and likely to render the mucous membrane still
more irritable and sensitive to adverse atmospheric changes as life advances.

Coryza is the scientific name for a cold associated with the secretion
and removal of a considerable quantity of fluid secretion and viscid
mucus from the secreting follicles and surface of that part of the mucous
membrane which lines the nasal passages and adjoining cavities. *Catarrh*,
Gravedo, are also terms applied to a cold in the head. The word Coryza,
κορύζα, is supposed to be derived from κόρος or κάρα, the head, and ζέω, to
boil. I am not, however, sure whether this derivation is perfectly accurate. The condition was, perhaps, so called because some people, suffering from a very bad cold, say that they feel as if the blood in the head
was in a boiling state.

**Of the Principles upon which the Treatment of a Cold should be
Conducted.**—As regards treatment, I suppose many would say "let a
cold alone;" "it will get well of itself;" "do nothing." I am quite
ready to admit that an ordinary cold will get well without any active
treatment. Nevertheless, a bad cold is a very unpleasant affection in
many ways, and it is desirable to mitigate its intensity and shorten the
attack, if we can do so. Besides, as I shall have to explain, many
serious maladies in their early stage may be easily mistaken for an ordinary cold, and in many cases real advantage does result from the early
adoption of judicious treatment. We will, therefore, endeavor to decide
as to the principles according to which the treatment of a cold and allied
derangements should be conducted.

The phenomena characteristic of an ordinary cold, as I have just remarked, are present during the period of accession of many forms of
fever, and sometimes in a greatly intensified state. You ought, therefore, to know whether, and by what means, these symptoms may be
modified, or the changes which usher in convalescence encouraged, so
that the latter be made to occur somewhat earlier than they would do if
the malady ran its ordinary course. Obviously, the thing to try to do in
the treatment of maladies of the class we are considering is to bring on

the period of perspiration as early as possible and to excite the action of the various glands of the body.

The blood has been diverted from the surface to the internal organs of the body, and we want, if we can, to determine its flow towards the skin, in order that much of its water and some of its organic constituents may be removed by the glands and discharged in the form of perspiration. External warmth will relieve the feeling experienced when a cold is coming on, and I think that sometimes the malady, and possibly some severe acute affections, may be cut short in this way. The patient is told to get into a warm bed or to take a warm bath. But the application of cold externally has been as strongly recommended as warmth, for the very same purpose in the same cases; and you might be led to suppose that here, as in some other instances, opposite and conflicting practices had been advised and adopted for the relief of the very same malady. But this is not really so; for whether you wrap a patient in a sheet dipped in warm water or in cold water, it makes very little difference, except that a cold sheet is somewhat more disagreeable to the patient than a warm one. Cold, wet packing will bring about just the same action as warm packing or a warm bath. For the chilly feeling produced by the first contact of the cold wet sheet is soon followed by reaction, and is replaced by a gentle glow, succeeded by free perspiration.

Diuretics.—But besides trying to excite perspiration, you may endeavor to cause various eliminating organs to act freely. You should give unirritating diuretic remedies, such as *Liquor Ammoniæ Acetatis*, *Citrate of Ammonia*, *Citrate of Potash*, *Nitrate of Potash*, and *Chlorate of Potash*. These all act, more or less, upon the kidneys, and increase the flow of urine; some of them act upon the skin, and in other ways promote the removal from the blood of noxious substances which have accumulated in it. They and many other remedies are thus of use in the treatment of an ordinary cold and allied ailments. I often suggest the following prescription:—Spirit of Mindererus (*Liquor Ammoniæ Acetatis*), two ounces; Spirit of Chloroform (*Spiritus Chloroformi*), from one to two drachms; Nitrate of Potash (*Potassæ Nitras*), sixty grains; or Chlorate of Potash (*Potassæ Chloras*), from one to two hundred grains; Syrup of Orange, of Squill, or of Tolu, half an ounce, and water to six ounces. The dose is half an ounce, or a tablespoonful, with as much water, once in two hours, or less frequently, for three or four days.

Purgatives.—And, lastly, the elimination of noxious matters which have accumulated in the blood may be further promoted by exciting to a moderate extent the action of the intestinal canal. In a cold the bowels are generally more or less confined, and in many cases there has been but imperfect action, perhaps, for some time previous to the attack. I therefore recommend you to make full inquiry upon this point, and, if necessary, order for the patient some mild laxative that will act upon the bowels and favor excretion. Thus you may, perhaps, shorten by a

day or two the period of the duration of the cold.   In the highly feverish condition which often comes on soon after a surgical operation, relief may be afforded in the course of a few hours by the administration
of purgatives, sudorifics, and diuretics.   One or two grains of *Calomel*
will be found to act admirably in many of the most serious of these
cases.   The temperature falls soon after the dose has been taken, and
the patient often experiences great relief long before the medicine begins to act on the bowels.

The fact of improvement so immediately following the use of remedies which increase the action of the skin, kidneys, and bowels, favors
the conclusion that the fever is due to the accumulation of certain materials in the blood, the elimination of which is followed by relief, and,
as we say, the resolution of the fever.   It is important to consider these
matters, the more so just now, because there is too great a tendency to
altogether discard the use of many medicines which are of great value in
the treatment of disease.

**Of the Recognition and Management of Affections which Begin like
an Ordinary Cold.**—Some cases which at the outset seem to be nothing
more than an ordinary cold or catarrh, do not prove to be of this nature, but issue in some form of serious acute disease.   Those terrible
fevers which occur in all the large cities of Europe, and which carry
off so many thousands every year, may come on just as an ordinary
cold does.   During the period of accession the symptoms are much the
same, and both the patient and his doctor may for some days think
there is not much the matter.   The patient feels so strongly convinced
that he is suffering only from an ordinary cold that he goes about just
as usual.   When, however, he gets worse from day to day and feels
decidedly weaker, he begins to be alarmed.   At length he is obliged to
take to his bed, his temperature is found to be and to remain above the
normal, perhaps rising to 102° and 103°.   By this time the practitioner
is able to determine the nature of the case.   Instead of the attack being,
as the patient himself supposed, an ordinary cold, it turns out to be a
specific fever, of a kind which not unfrequently destroys life.   It may
be that under the most favorable circumstances, and with the best nursing and medical treatment, the rate of mortality will not be less than
one out of every seven or eight attacked by the disease.   It is a fact that
many serious attacks of fever begin just like an ordinary cold.   Now
if you happen to be called in just when the fever is coming on, and
you thoughtlessly remarkt that " this is only an ordinary cold ; I need not
do anything," think of the dilemma in which you may be placed.   When
the severe nature of the disease becomes apparent, you will be, as it were,
convicted of having made a very serious mistake.   Very likely neither
the patient nor his friends will have any further confidence in you, and
you may be pronounced to be an ignorant person, who knows very little
about his profession.   You may in consequence get out of heart and feel

altogether dissatisfied with yourself. As a fact, it may have been impossible for any one to make a diagnosis at a very early period of the attack; but the right course would have been to have waited until the premonitory symptoms passed off, or until some definite characteristics of a special malady had manifested themselves. You should always carefully inquire into all the facts of any given case, listen attentively to what the patient has to say concerning the symptoms which disturb him, and do all you can to relieve them, postponing any decided expression of opinion as to the precise nature of the disease until your next visit, when you may perhaps be able to speak with decision.

Even if the disease should be only a common cold, you will, nevertheless, find in practice that many persons who experience suffering, discomfort, or even mere inconvenience, strongly desire to be relieved of their troubles, and as quickly as possible. Of the sick who send for you, a considerable proportion will certainly expect that you will *do something for them.* Though if you were in the same condition yourself you might be inclined to leave the case to nature and not take any medicine nor desire to follow any course more unusual than indulging in a little more rest than when in good health, your patient will expect you to prescribe something that will relieve him or help him to get well. And unquestionably you may help persons suffering from a severe cold if you give sudorifics, diuretics, and a gentle purgative.

Especially in the case of children is it necessary to be very cautious in committing yourself to a positive opinion at an early period of a febrile attack. You may mistake a serious case for a slight one, or the reverse. You will be astonished at the very serious aspect sometimes presented by many a case of mere stomach disturbance. A child who has partaken of unripe fruit may be very ill indeed a few hours afterwards, with a temperature of 104°, flushed face, quick pulse and respiration, with a suffering, anxious look. An inexperienced practitioner would perhaps tell the friends that some severe fever or other acute disease was certainly about to establish itself, when, perhaps, a few hours afterwards the bowels act, the temperature falls to the normal, and when he next visits his patient he finds him well, and the friends laughing about his gloomy prognostications.

In children suffering from slight ailments, I have observed the temperature rise from the normal to 104°, or even higher, and descend to the normal, within twenty-four hours, so rapidly may considerable changes in the temperature of the blood of children occur. Such cases, I need scarcely say, require simple treatment. A purgative dose of castor-oil is sometimes needed, and the patient is well again as soon as it operates. The child, as often happens, is very thirsty, and you may allow it to drink water. Plenty of *toast and water* may be given, or plain water, if the patient likes it better, provided it has been well boiled. Water or milk and water will help the skin and kidneys and bowels to act freely,

19

and in consequence the feverishness will subside and the patient regain the usual state of health. Sometimes, however, a feverish attack instead of subsiding continues for several days. The child may be ill for a week or two, and require careful management, although no definite fever is developed. Neither scarlet fever, nor typhus fever, nor any other specific disease may be manifested; but a general feverish state may be established, and may continue for several days, and then gradually subside, leaving the patient thin and weak and out of health.

It must be admitted that in former days many doctors gave too much physic and were somewhat too fussy. In these days, however, I fear there is a tendency, or more than a tendency, to err in an opposite direction. Some practitioners, having convinced themselves, seem to be most anxious to convince the public and the profession that the chief duty of a medical adviser is to study, note, and carefully watch the progress of a malady—to observe, if he is qualified to do so, the minute changes taking place in the tissues of the sick man, in order that he may discover facts which will increase our knowledge of the nature of the pathological processes, and possibly lead to the enunciation of new principles of treatment for the benefit of sufferers in the next and succeeding generations. But this view of medical aspiration is not always appreciated by the patient, especially if the doctor's visits are not purely of an honorary character, and even then it will be found that there are some few patients so peculiar in their notions as to object to their bodies being used for observation, or their sufferings studied and noted as interesting pathological phenomena, which may be further elucidated as the case proceeds. You must really bear in mind that patients want to be relieved as well as watched, and unless you can be of some use to them—unless you can advise and help them, they may regard you as a nuisance, instead of discovering in you a consolation. But, further, we really ought to do all we can not only to remove bodily aches and pains, but also to relieve our patients' minds. You will not reduce the mental anxiety of a sick man if you tell him you can do nothing to relieve his pain, nothing to expedite his recovery, nothing to avert impending morbid change or to mitigate the severity of the disease. I find that some doctors, if they get ill, even though the illness is obviously not a serious one, become very anxious, and of all sick people they are oftentimes the most difficult to manage. They usually think themselves worse than they are, and are almost invariably desirous that something practical should be done. I have sometimes ventured to discuss with a medical friend the actual nature and import of the symptoms from which he was suffering, but I generally find that my friend is sadly disappointed if I do not propose to "do something" for him or suggest some operation to relieve him. If I suggest to a medical patient that the malady will probably get well of itself, he will, perhaps, feel disappointed, if not hurt; but if I propose that he should take a few doses of the Liquor Ammoniæ Acetatis,

Nitrate or Chlorate of Potash, and Sal Volatile, a practitioner of even a philosophical turn of mind will feel quite happy, and will take the medicine ordered with regularity, and bear his ailments with cheerfulness.

I advise you to bear in mind the principle upon which the treatment of a cold or an ordinary febrile attack is to be conducted, and I recommend you to be careful not to commit yourselves too hastily to a positive opinion as to the exact nature of a febrile attack which has only lately come on. It is important not to make too light of it, on the one hand, or on the other to cause needless alarm by suggesting to anxious friends that what is probably only a most trifling and unimportant temporary derangement may turn out to be a grave disorder.

OF THE ACTUAL CHANGES IN THE AFFECTED TISSUES IN FEVER AND INFLAMMATION.

I now desire to consider more particularly the actual phenomena of Fevers and Inflammations, and the general nature of the minute changes upon which they depend.

I have said before that in all fevers and inflammations there is an elevation of temperature. Whether the rise begins in the blood or in the tissues outside the capillaries, is a question concerning which some difference of opinion may be entertained. In some cases it is certain that the tissue elements exhibit the earliest departure from the normal state, and in all probability it is there that the rise in temperature begins. But the blood is soon affected, for in all cases the blood in the adjacent capillaries becomes hotter, and it is by the movements of the blood that the distribution of heat is effected. On the other hand there is no doubt that some fevers and inflammations begin, so to say, in the blood.

In every form of marked inflammation and fever the vessels of the affected part contain more blood than they do in the normal state. Particularly the capillary vessels and the small veins are distended. If you watch the phenomena of local inflammation in one of the lower animals, as for example that form which may be excited in the web of the frog's foot by the application to one spot of a small portion of mustard for a few minutes, and carefully observe the alteration in the circulation thereby induced, you will gain much important information concerning the nature of the process. You will notice in the first place that the vessels have become much dilated, while the movement of the blood along them gets slower and slower. At last the circulation completely stops. If at this stage of pathological change the mustard be removed and the web be kept perfectly moist, it will be found that the movement of the blood will begin again, and that much of it will find its way on to the small veins. In fact the disturbance will soon cease. The normal state of the circulation will be restored, and without any damage whatever to vessels, nerves, or other tissues having taken place.

In fever there can be no doubt that the same sort of change occurs in the capillaries, but the degree of change is so slight that it is not in all cases to be demonstrated. You may look upon a cold as a slight fever, while a chilblain may be adduced as an example of a slight inflammation.

Some authorities consider that febrile disorders should be classed among nerve disorders, and the arguments advanced in favor of this view also apply to the case of inflammations. But would it not be unreasonable to include flea-bites, and boils, and abscesses in the class of nervous diseases? In point of fact, nerves and nerve-centres are invariably affected in all fevers and inflammations, however slight. Indeed, no changes whatever which involve alterations in the diameter of the small arteries can take place in the body without nerves being concerned, and the essential phenomena both of fever and inflammation are intimately connected with disturbed arterial and capillary action. Still these conditions cannot properly be regarded as nerve diseases. The pathological action does not begin in nerve structures, and the nerves and nerve-centres, so far from being the points of departure of the morbid change, are only affected in consequence of preliminary changes in other textures.

The phenomena of some fevers and general inflammations are due to changes which have taken place in the blood, and there is, as I have remarked, undoubted evidence of the blood being, as it were, the starting-point of all the phenomena. The disease begins in the blood. A poison, or *materies morbi*, may infect the blood in the first instance, and through the blood various tissues and organs may suffer. It is very probable, I think, that the afferent nerve-fibres distributed to the capillary vessels are disturbed either by the action upon them of the altered fluid which transudes through the vascular walls, or, in certain cases, by the growth and multiplication around them of minute particles of morbid bioplasm (disease germs) which also traverse the thin walls of the capillaries, thus leaving the blood in countless numbers and passing into the interstices of the surrounding textures. In Scarlet Fever (*Scarlatina*) the "rash" depends upon the capillaries of the surface of the skin being dilated to such an extent that the redness of the affected parts is as intense as that of the skin of the lips in the ordinary state. The bright red color of the skin of the lips is due, as you are probably aware, to the number and considerable diameter of the capillaries of the skin of the part, and to the circumstance that these vessels are covered by a thin layer of epithelium only. In scarlet fever the redness is due to a dilatation of the vessels, somewhat like that which occurs in those of the skin of the cheek when we blush. In the fever, however, the blush lasts for a much longer time. The period of vascular congestion of the cutaneous capillaries is, in most febrile diseases, fixed and definite; but it varies considerably in duration, as well as in the course which it takes in different kinds of fever. In eruptive fevers, then, and in some general inflammations, the "eruption" or "rash" results from dilatation of the capillary vessels, which lasts for a certain time. The mechanism instrumental in bringing about the result and the precise changes taking place in the vessels are considered on page 231. I do not say that the redness of the skin is due to increased supply of blood, for probably a less proportion of blood goes to the part than in the normal state. In a given time less blood passes along the vessels, but they are distended, and more blood remains in them; their walls being stretched are much thinner and more permeable than in the normal state. The blood is not actually stagnant, but it circulates very slowly.

Slight exposure of a part of the body to cold may cause a severe febrile attack. In considering how cold operates, I think we shall find the following explanation in accordance with the broad facts of the case: The heart's action being at the time feeble, blood will be flowing but slowly through the capillaries of the skin. The blood will, therefore, for a much longer time than usual, be exposed to the detrimental influence of cold. No wonder that under such circumstances chemical changes of an unusual kind are induced. Substances are formed which injuriously affect the tissues and interfere with the proper performance of many of the normal phenomena of secretion and nutrition. The noxious materials dissolved in the fluid, transuding with it through the walls of the capillaries, would come in contact with the delicate nerve-fibres and mar their action. As long as such matters remain in the blood there must be in many ways a departure from the healthy state; but as soon as these compounds have been eliminated, the organism will be restored to its normal condition. For these reasons the free action of organs concerned in excretion is, as I have already stated, of the first importance, and is associated with the subsidence of the fever and the discomfort which accompanies the attack.

There are several affections which may be correctly termed either *fevers* or *inflammations*. If in many cases you looked at the local phenomena only, you would use the term *inflammation*, while to the general symptoms consequent upon the local change and varying with it in intensity, you would apply the term *fever*. Not only is inflammation the cause of fever, but fever in many cases leads to inflammation. In truth, there is no inflammation without a degree of fever, and there is no fever in which the phenomena essential to inflammation are entirely absent. That which is common to both, to all fevers and to all inflammations, is the increased growth of bioplasm, consequent upon increased facilities of access, or of the greater abundance or greater permeating property of the nutrient fluid. This increased growth of the living matter is invariably associated with a rise in the temperature of the tissue or organ in which it takes place, above the normal standard. *Erysipelas* may be fairly called an inflammation, though in many respects it exhibits all the characteristics of a fever. In the slightest local inflammation, however limited its area may be, a flea-bite for example, the phenomena are essen-

19 *

tially the same as in a fever, only they are circumscribed to a particular spot. If you consider the actual changes which occur in both pathological states, you will find that they approach so nearly in their essential features as to justify me in advancing the generalization that *Inflammation is a local fever and Fever is a general inflammation.*

If we consider the actual phenomena of fever and inflammation, as
they are revealed by careful microscopical examination of complex
tissues involved, we shall find that we have :—1. *Temporary enlargement
or dilatation of the capillary vessels, which soon become filled with blood.*
2. *If this state of the vessels lasts for a time, exudation of fluid occurs and
minute particles of bioplasm pass through the capillary walls, and grow
and multiply in the new situation.*   3. *The bioplasts of the vessels, nerve-
fibres, and other tissues, being supplied with more nutrient matter than in
the ordinary state, grow larger and tend to divide and subdivide.*

The particles of *bioplasm*, or *living matter*, in all the tissues and fluids
affected are invariably enlarged in all *fevers* and *inflammations*.   I believe it to be impossible for fever or inflammation to occur without this
enlargement of the bioplasts or particles of living matter, without the
temporary increase of the living matter of the part of the body affected.
The living particles always experience increased nutrition under the conditions present when fever or inflammation exists, and this phenomenon,
this increase of the bioplasm, is invariably associated with a rise in the
temperature of the part.   Rise in body-heat in fever and inflammation
is constant, and I must ask you to note the important fact that it is associated with *slow and impeded capillary circulation, with the exudation of
fluid and minute particles of living matter from the blood, and with the
increased nutrition and growth of bioplasm.*   So far from depending
upon *increased oxidation*, inflammation and fever often coincide with
impaired respiratory function, and the introduction into the blood of
far less oxygen than in health, and with the formation and removal of
less than the ordinary proportion of carbonic acid.

Slight fevers and inflammations do not necessarily result in permanent
tissue changes.   Many leave no traces behind them.   There may be no
degeneration of any tissue in the body, no structural change, no evidence
left of the attack.   After a fever or inflammation the organism may be
left precisely as it was before the attack occurred.   Nay, one or more
attacks of feverishness during early life seem to be the rule.   Almost
every child suffers.   Indeed, amongst young vertebrate animals, dogs
for instance, attacks of feverishness occur in almost every individual, and
the disease is often fatal.   In many cases, however, the feverishness after
a few days passes off, leaving no structural change or damage.

Of a Flea-bite.—If we thoroughly understood the phenomena which
result from the "bite" of a common flea, we should know very much
more about the exact nature of the changes which occur in such serious
inflammations as erysipelas than we do at present.   Possibly, also, such

information might enable us to suggest means by which an attack might be prevented, or at least the inflammation kept from spreading until a considerable extent of the surface of the body was involved in the disease.

You may remember that in one of my early lectures I described how, by the minute but exquisitely sharp lancet of an insect, the formed material of a cell of cuticle might be easily injured, and in such a manner that a part of the bioplasm in its interior would be exposed to the contact of the fluid which moistens the tissue. I showed that, under the circumstances, the access of the surrounding nutrient material to the bioplasm in the interior of the cell must be greatly facilitated. It is obvious that much more nutrient matter would reach the bioplasm in a given time when the so-called cell-wall was thus damaged than when it was intact. In the normal condition of the cell, every particle of nutrient fluid must slowly permeate the thick layer of formed material which constitutes the outer part of the cell, the so-called cell-wall, before it can reach the bioplasm and be assimilated by it. When the formed material has been torn, nutrient fluid will pass at once to the bioplasm and come into immediate contact with it. As the ordinary formed material or "cell-wall" consists of several layers of firm cuticular matter, not very permeable, the ordinary passage of soluble nutrient substances through it must necessarily be a slow process. But when the formed material is injured so that the bioplasm is exposed, the access is free and the pabulum is at once appropriated. The result is the rapid increase of the bioplasm or living matter. Outgrowths or diverticula soon make their appearance at different parts of the circumference of the mass. Some of these are from time to time detached, and being freely supplied with pabulum they grow, and multitudes of separate masses of bioplasm quickly result. These are *pus-corpuscles*, many of which may in this way be formed from the bioplasm of an epithelium cell in a short time.

Pus may result in the course of a few hours by the growth and subdivision of any form of bioplasm, if it be supplied with an unusual amount of pabulum. The appropriate pabulum coming into contact with the bioplasm, the latter *must* take it up and *grow*. If the excess of pabulum were not taken up by the bioplasm and converted into the quickly growing living matter, *pus*, it would become decomposed, and the products resulting from decomposition would infallibly cause the death of every particle of bioplasm in the neighborhood. "Mortification" of a portion of the affected tissue would result. The bioplasm of any tissue, then, as well as that of which white blood-corpuscles and lymph-corpuscles are composed, may give rise to a form of bioplasm, pus, a kind of living matter having general powers and properties, irrespective of the particular form of normal bioplasm from which the "pus" may have been derived. The formation of pus from the bioplasm of an epithelial cell may be studied in the epithelium of the skin, as well as in that of the air-tubes, the bladder, and other mucous surfaces. If living pus be examined, active *vital movements* will be observed in almost every corpuscle; and I beg you to study these wonderful movements for yourselves and ponder over them, for they are worthy of your thoughts. *See* p. 248; *also* "Disease Germs" or "The Microscope in Medicine," 4th edition.

We are just now, however, chiefly concerned with the changes which occur in the skin *beneath the epithelial layer* in an ordinary flea-bite. These involve the vessels and nerve-fibres, and are of the highest interest. The lancet of the flea, I need scarcely tell you, goes deeper than the deepest layer of the cuticle, for it penetrates the vessels and occasions changes in the capillaries as well as in other tissues of the skin. This is of importance, inasmuch as an excellent illustration of the remarkable phenomena which occur in inflammation of a complex tissue is afforded. Here we have a comparatively circumscribed inflammation admirably adapted for the investigation of the actual phenomena which constitute the inflammatory process as it occurs in a compound tissue, like the true skin. In consequence of the wound inflicted upon the capillary vessels, there is of course slight escape of blood into the adjacent tissues. This hæmorrhage gives rise to a very small deep red punctum or spot, which does not disappear on pressure, called a *petechia* (from the Italian *Petechio*, a flea-bite). The important fact to which I now wish to direct your attention is not the petechia caused by the escape of a minute quantity of blood, but the less intensely red area around it, which does disappear when the finger is pressed upon it, so that the blood may be for a moment driven out of the distended capillaries. A short time after the lancet of the flea has penetrated the cuticle and subjacent tissues, there appears this bright red blush around the point which indicates the position of the wound. The area forming the round red spot, with the appearance of which most of us are familiar, is, I suppose, of the same diameter in all cases where the lancet of the flea is of the same size, the wound of the same depth, and the irritating poison discharged the same in amount.

In the case of an ordinary flea-bite, then, the injury is not confined to the particular portion of tissue transfixed and injured by the lancet, but the disturbance extends some distance around. Those who have not studied flea-bites should do so, and I need hardly assure you that you have abundant opportunities in the wards of the hospital for the observation of flea-bites in every state of change—from the most recently inflicted injury to the case in which the redness is disappearing and the bright red tint is giving place to the ordinary color of the adjacent skin.

If in a recent bite you carefully notice the redness, you will observe that the red blush ceases at a definite line; the red tint does not *gradually* shade off into the hue of the surrounding skin, but the red limiting line is abrupt, and, if the skin happens to be pale, what is seen is a little circular patch about the one-eighth of an inch or more in diameter. This area is of a bright red color, almost as red as the cheek, and if you look closely you may often see a dark spot in the centre, which, as I have said, is the perforation made by the lancet of the animal, rendered evident by the passage into it of a little blood.   Now there is no doubt that the redness depends upon the distention of the capillaries by blood.   These little vessels obviously contain much more blood than they do in their usual state.   As regards the precise manner in which this redness is produced there is, however, room for some difference of opinion, and we have, indeed, yet much to learn in connection with this interesting phenomenon.   There can be no doubt that the capillaries of the red area contain twice or three times as much blood as the adjacent capillaries of the skin.   Now you are probably aware that when we blush, the cutaneous capillaries of the cheeks are suddenly distended, and their diameter, of course, is considerably increased.   If it were not so, the difference in the quantity of blood would not be sufficient to produce the intensity of color which is so remarkable.

You see, then, that an instrument which is much less than the smallest needle, having passed directly through the skin, has quickly led to dilatation of the capillary vessels for a certain distance, perhaps the one-sixteenth of an inch or more, around the line of perforation ; but none of the vessels beyond the circumscribed line are dilated, though they freely communicate with the dilated vessels.   Does this action depend upon some influence exerted upon certain fine nerve-fibres lying in the course of the wound, or is it due to any direct influence upon the vessels themselves?   This last suggestion may be dismissed at once, because by no direct influence upon vessels of which we have knowledge can such a phenomenon be produced.   There is no doubt, whatever, that the change in the diameter of the vessels is occasioned by injury to the nerves, and it is probable that the congestion of the capillaries depends, not upon injury done to nerves by the passage of the lancet of the flea, but upon the influence exerted on the nerves in consequence of the escape of a small quantity of irritating poisonous material, which is extruded at the same time, and poisons and irritates the nerves in the course of the wound and those at a short distance around the line of penetration, and thus causes change in the nerve-centre.

Alterations of Calibre of the Small Arteries.—The redness of the flea-bite is due to dilatation of the capillaries ; but what is very remarkable and of great interest is this, that the little arteries which communicate with and supply the capillaries with blood must be dilated to a *certain definite* extent.   Of this you may convince yourselves by trying the following little experiment.   Press the finger firmly upon the skin corresponding to the flea-bite and skin around it, so as to drive the blood from the distended vessels into the neighboring capillaries.   The whole of the skin subjected to pressure of course becomes perfectly pale, the area corresponding to the flea-bite being as pale as the skin around, from the capillaries of which the blood has been temporarily driven.   Now a

few seconds after the finger has been removed, the blood streams back
into the vessels of the area of the skin rendered white by the pressure, so
as to restore the exact tint which existed before.   The flea-bite will resume the precise degree of redness it had before pressure was applied,
being neither paler nor darker.   The pressure has caused only a temporary change.   Although the blood had been completely squeezed out of
the capillary vessels, the moment it is allowed to return it fills these vessels and distends them to precisely the same degree of dilatation as
before.

By this simple experiment we conclusively prove not only that the
capillary vessels are dilated, but dilated to a definite extent, so that
every capillary will resume the same diameter, and is capable of retain-
ing this, at any rate, for some hours, though the blood may be thoroughly
squeezed out and allowed to run back as often as you please.   How is
this brought about ?   By what mechanism is it effected and how can the
phenomenon be accounted for ?   The change is complex and not to be
explained in a few words ;   but as it illustrates some very important physiological and pathological principles the matter is well worthy of attentive consideration.   In the first place, we must take note of the conditions which determine and regulate the flow of blood at a certain rate
through the capillary vessels, and these are somewhat complex.

The capillaries are elastic tubes, which have no power, as far as is
known, of active contraction.   They can be distended, and they will
recoil or contract so as to be very much less than their ordinary diameter, indeed, they may be so reduced as to appear like mere lines, their
cavity being for the time obliterated, and not a blood-corpuscle passing
through them.   Nevertheless the capillary has no active power of contraction or dilatation.   Its thin walls are eminently elastic, and yield if
blood or other fluid is forced into the tube by pressure.   If they are
allowed to react, the fluid will be gradually expelled and the cavity of
the tube almost obliterated, the capillary vessel looking like a fine cylin-
drical cord.   If the little arteries are distended and enlarged, more blood
will be permitted to pass into the capillaries, and these tubes will be
distended and their walls stretched.   If the diameter of the arteries
becomes reduced, the capillaries will shrink.   These phenomena are
repeated whenever the pressure by which the blood is forced into the
vessels is reduced or increased.

*The Degree of Contraction of the Minute Arteries determined and
maintained by Nerve Action.*—And now as to the vessels which pour
their blood into the capillaries.   The smaller arteries, we know, are
capable of undergoing very great alterations in calibre, the alterations
being of an *active* character.   By *active* I mean that the diameter of a
small artery can be maintained for a time at a certain uniform standard,
the canal being completely obliterated, or increased to twice the area of
its usual section, or half the area, as the case may be, and this irrespec-

tive of any temporary changes produced by mechanical pressure applied from time to time.

The smaller arteries are encircled by numerous muscular fibres, placed as close as possible to one another, often arranged in very many layers. This muscular tissue constitutes the greater part of the thickness of the arterial walls. An idea may be formed of the arrangement of the muscular fibre-cells of a small artery, and of the manner in which, by contracting, the tube of the vessel may be constricted, and of the mode of distribution of the nerve-fibres, if the accompanying figure, p. 229, be carefully examined. When the encircling muscular fibres contract, the tube of the artery is, of course, diminished. When the muscular fibres undergo relaxation, the tube of the vessel will be enlarged.

The calibre of the artery is entirely dependent upon varying degrees of contraction or relaxation in the contractile fibres, and the change takes place in all little arteries from time to time. This is not a passive change, like the mere dilatation and recoil of the elastic capillary vessels, but a change due to varying degrees of contraction or relaxation of the muscular fibres which encircle the tube, and which may be retained at a precise point without the least variation in extent or vigor for a considerable time. The contraction of the muscular fibres may even remain constant in spite of an alteration in the pressure by which the blood is driven into the tubes.

Next, we must inquire by what means a definite degree of contraction and relaxation of the muscular fibres of the little arteries is determined. It has been conclusively proved, partly by the results of experiment and partly by reasoning based upon the fact of the arrangement and distribution of nerves to muscular fibres, which has been demonstrated by microscopical investigation, that the wonderful changes in question are brought about through the instrumentality of nerves and nerve-centres only. For every set of minute arterial vessels there is a nerve-centre, and by alteration in the condition of this nerve-centre the calibre of the little arteries, or, in other words, the degree of contraction of the muscular fibres of their coats, will be determined. Each nerve-centre is connected with other centres by intercommunicating fibres, so that a very few arteries only may have their calibre altered, or the change may occur in hundreds and thousands of vessels, distributed to a large extent of tissue at the same moment.

Everything I am telling you is based on observation and experiment, and I shall be able to show you in microscopical preparations the actual nerve-fibres concerned. We can easily demonstrate the muscular fibres of the minute arteries of the body of man and vertebrate animals generally. We know, too, that there are nerves abundantly distributed to these arteries, and that the nerves are connected with ganglia.

Of the Ganglia governing and regulating the Calibre of the small Arteries.—In many instances I have followed fine nerve-fibres distributed to the muscular fibres of a minute artery for a long distance, and have traced them to their origin in an individual nerve-cell in the nerve-centre.

The nerve-centres connected with these and other nerve-fibres concerned in governing and regulating the flow of blood through the arteries and capillaries are extremely numerous. The arrangement of the centres or ganglia and of the entering and emerging nerve-fibres can be most easily studied in the coats of the intestine of any small animal; but for investigating the structure of the nerve-cells themselves, the little green tree-frog (*Hyla viridis*) should be selected. If you examine the mesentery near the intestine of this animal and the areolar tissue in the back part of the abdominal cavity, you will find the ganglia as numerous as is indicated in this drawing. If you take a portion of the mucous membrane of the small intestine of man, or of one of the higher animals, say not more than a quarter of an inch square, and prepare it carefully, you may find from half a dozen to a dozen or more ganglia. Each ganglion will contain from two or three to two or three hundred cells, and every individual cell will have at least two fibres issuing from it.[*] By this investigation you will be able to gain a correct notion of the general nature and structure of the nervous apparatus which exerts an influence upon every part of the vascular system, and particularly of the finest ramifications of the nerves distributed to the walls of the small arteries, veins, and capillaries, and, in certain cases, to the tissues which intervene between the capillaries.

Ganglia and intercommunicating bundles of nerve-fibres exist in every part of the intestinal canal of man and the higher animals. Although no nerve ganglia exist very near the ultimate distribution of the nerves to the small arteries of the skin of the body and to the tissues of the limbs, we know that these nerves are all connected with nerve-centres exhibiting the same general structure and arrangement as those found in connection with the mucous membrane of the intestines and other viscera of the abdomen and thorax. All belong to the so-called Sympathetic system. Nerve-centres or ganglia are placed in certain special parts of the trunk, and from these bundles of nerve-fibres are derived which are distributed to the vessels of the head and extremities. The minute arteries by which blood is distributed to the muscles of the limbs, to the large nerves, to the brain and spinal cord and their membranes are as fully supplied with nerves, and are as much under the influence of nerve ganglia of the sympathetic system, as are the arteries of the lungs or the heart, or those of the liver, kidney, or other secreting organs.

I propose now to describe more fully the mechanism by which the varying calibre of the small arteries is determined. You will form a correct idea of the degree to which little arteries may contract if you take note of what is represented in this drawing (not introduced in this

---

FIG. I.

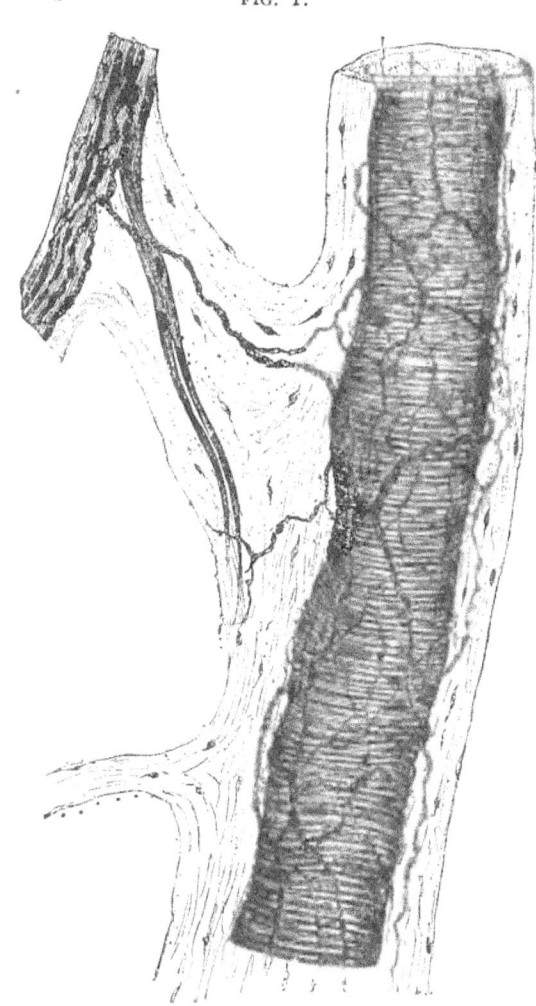

A small artery from the bladder of the hyla or green tree-frog, showing the distribution of fine nerve-fibres to the muscular fibre cells of the vessel. The nerve-fibre can be followed from the nerve trunk *a* to the vessel. In the connective tissue to the left are seen two muscular fibre cells with nerve-fibres distributed to them. These belong to the tissue to which the artery was distributed, and are not connected with the vessel. $\times$ 215. About the middle of the figure the tube is somewhat constricted, in consequence of slight contraction of the muscular fibre cells in this part of the artery.

$\frac{1}{1000}$ of an inch —— $\times$ 215.

work) of the arteries of the Pia mater of the common sheep, which were injected, immediately after the death of the animal, with Prussian Blue fluid. (For the composition of this fluid and the method of injecting, see "The Microscope in Medicine," or "How to Work with the Microscope.") The walls of the vessels, with their muscular fibre-cells, are well shown. The little arteries at the time of death have contracted, so as to produce great irregularity in the calibre of the arteries. You see in one place the muscular fibres of a considerable length of the vessel have vigorously contracted, so as to obliterate the canal. Very few blood-corpuscles could have passed through this part of the vessel at the time of the contraction of its muscular fibres. This firmly contracted portion of the little artery is immediately continuous with another part of the vessel where the coats are relaxed, and the diameter of the tube here would be perhaps twenty times that of its continuation in the contracted portion of the vessel. Many different portions of small arteries in various degrees of contraction are represented in different parts of the drawing. (A very slight degree of contraction is seen in the little artery figured on page 229.)

We must yet go somewhat more into detail before we can expect to find an adequate explanation of the changes which take place in the coats of the small arteries during life, by which variations in their calibre are determined, and which are intimately connected with the causation of the phenomena of the flea-bite. It must be borne in mind that the arteries are not the only small vessels which are supplied with nerve-fibres. It has long been known that to the coats of the small veins nerve-fibres are abundantly distributed, but the general arrangement of the finest fibres has not been fully investigated. They exist in great number, and, indeed, in much greater number than would be expected, considering the paucity of the muscular fibres of the veins and the thinness of the coats of these vessels. From the great number of the nerve-fibres one would incline to the notion that some were concerned in transmitting impressions to the nerve-centre. If all are motor fibres, their number in proportion to the amount of muscular tissue is far greater than elsewhere. But besides the distribution of nerves to small arteries and veins, I must beg you to pay attention to the arrangement of the nerve-fibres which belong to the capillary vessels.

Of the Nerves of Capillary Vessels.—You will not find it stated in any of your text-books, even at this time, that nerve-fibres are distributed to capillaries. Not only is this the fact, but upon many capillaries a considerable number of fine nerve-fibres may be seen to ramify. As long ago as 1860 I succeeded in demonstrating this new set of nerve-fibres, distributed to the capillary vessels, which had not been previously described. Numerous observations upon the capillary vessels of various vertebrate classes have convinced me that the capillaries of vertebrate animals generally are freely supplied with nerves; or, to speak more

accurately, that just outside, or at a short distance from the outer surface of the walls of the capillaries, very fine nerve-fibres exist, which
in many cases form a lax network or plexus of extremely delicate nerve-
fibres on the outer surface of the vessel.

The fact is not of anatomical interest only, but the distribution of
the nerve-fibres in question has an important bearing upon questions
concerning the action of the minute vessels during life. Upon carefully
examining capillaries in many tissues of the frog, according to the plan
I have described in "Microscope in Medicine" and "How to Work
with the Microscope," you will meet with little difficulty in demonstrating the nerve-fibres to capillary vessels. I could show you more than

FIG. 2.

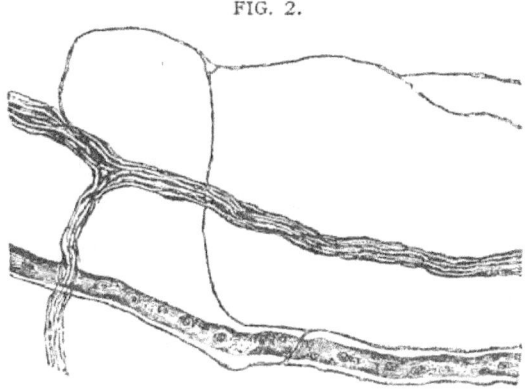

From an interval between the fibres of the mylohyoid muscles of the hyla, *a*. Trunk of fine dark-
bordered nerve-fibres with fine fibres coming from them, one of which may be traced to the capillary
b, while others are distributed to the muscular fibres, which are not represented in the drawing. The
arrangement of the nerves supplying the capillary vessel is well seen. From a specimen mounted in
glycerine and more than ten years old. × 215.

twenty preparations from the frog in which branches of nerve-fibres to
the capillary vessels are seen, without the slightest doubt. The fact cannot be explained away. There is no question whatever about the delicate fibres in question being nerves, because in many instances I have
been able to trace the fibres from their distribution outside the capillaries to their connection with the ganglion cell, without one break in
the continuity of the matter of which they consist. But many will not
believe that a structure which may be demonstrated in a cold-blooded
vertebrate animal like the frog necessarily exists in the higher vertebrata
and in man. I have, however, succeeded in demonstrating nerves to
capillary vessels in several mammalian animals and birds, and have been
able to permanently preserve several of the specimens. One of the best
animals for the investigation is the white mouse, because there is very
little connective tissue in this animal to obscure the extremely delicate
nerve-fibres. Upon the whole, however, I prefer the bat's wing; and of
the arrangement of the nerves upon the capillaries and in other tissues

connected with the thin membrane of this wonderful organ I have preserved several specimens. I have represented a very clear specimen in
the accompanying figures 3, 4. It has been magnified only 215 ; but to
see the points clearly a magnifying power of 700 is required.

Of Demonstrating the Nerves distributed to Capillaries.—In order to
see the delicate nerve-fibres and the capillary vessels, it is necessary to
obtain a structure in which the capillaries themselves can be seen without much dissection or the necessity of section cutting ; for if you have
to dissect the tissue, you will tear the capillaries, and then you will not
be able to follow the nerve-fibres for any great distance. In the bat's
wing, and also in the bladder of the frog, you have a natural dissection
almost ready for observation. (Arrangement shown in several enlarged
copies of drawings.)

Of the arrangement of nerve-fibres in a tissue, a considerable extent
of which is altogether destitute of capillary vessels, one can hardly point
to a better illustration than is afforded by the cornea of a small animal,
particularly the hyla or little green tree-frog. The nerve-fibres in this
transparent fibrous tissue are exceedingly numerous, forming extensive
networks of wonderfully delicate nerve-fibres, with which, at short intervals, small masses of bioplasm are connected. From these the fibres
grow, and the net-work of nerve-fibres increases in extent as the cornea
expands in dimensions. A thin section, which includes the anterior
surface of the cornea (placed uppermost so as to be just beneath the
thin glass cover) is most favorable for observation. High powers ought
to be used (from 300 to 1,200 diameters). In such a specimen you can
trace all that is represented in my drawings. The nerves divide and
subdivide at short intervals, and extensive networks of excessively fine
fibres are formed, which lie on different planes, and are to be found in
every part of the corneal tissue, though the networks are more numerous
near the anterior surface than in other parts. These nerve-fibres might
be regarded as extensions of those belonging to capillary vessels. At
the margin of the cornea some are undoubtedly continuous with the
latter, but many of the nerve-fibres of the corneal tissue may be followed to bundles of nerve-fibres at the margin of the cornea.

**Of the Mechanism by which the Capillary Circulation of Man and
Animals is regulated.**—My chief object in troubling you with this somewhat detailed anatomical description is that I may be able to explain the
probable action of these fine nerve-fibres distributed to the capillary vessels, and give some account of the very important office they discharge
during life. It is true that much of this discussion strictly belongs to
the province of physiology, but inasmuch as the inquiry has a most important bearing in connection with the determination of the nature of
the phenomena occurring in the simplest pathological changes, in a flea-
bite for example, I shall make no apology for referring to it here. Without the facts above referred to, and deprived of the inferences deduced

CAPILLARY VESSELS AND NERVE-FIBRES FROM THE BAT'S WING.

FIG. 3.

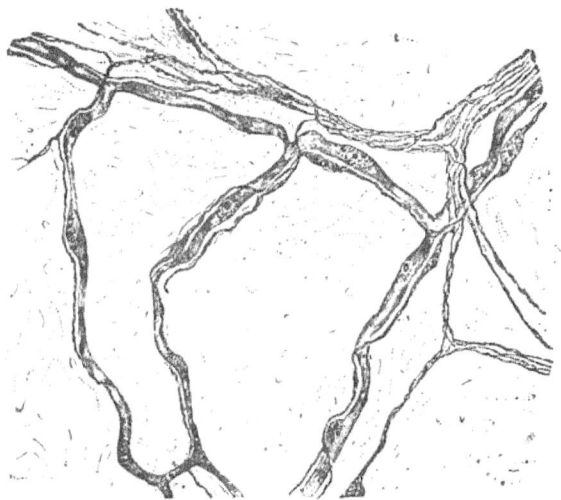

Capillaries and very fine nerve-fibres distributed to the bat's wing. In many parts of the specimen the nerve-fibre could be followed from a bundle of fine nerve-fibres to the capillaries. Two instances of this are shown in the drawing.

$\frac{1}{1000}$ of an inch —— × 215.

FIG. 4.

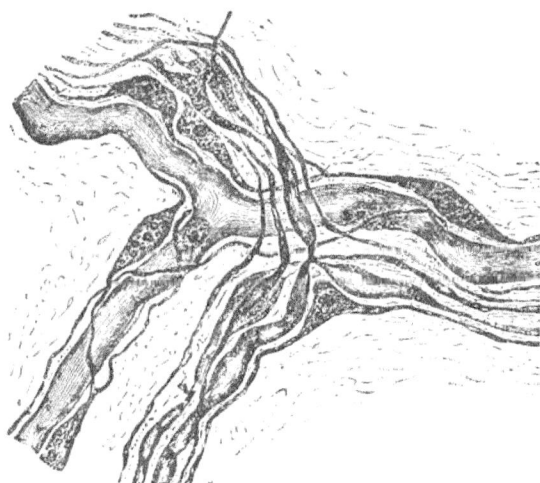

A small part of Fig. 3 highly magnified. The distribution of the nerve-fibres to the capillary and their relation to its walls are well seen. The mode of branching and division of some of the finest nerve-fibres are also well shown in the lower part of the drawing. × 700.

20*

from these observations, I should be unable to explain to you the phenomena of inflammation or fever as these pathological changes occur in
man and warm-blooded animals.   In order to make my meaning clear,
I must refer to this diagram, which is, as it were, made up from observations actually carried out on several different specimens.

FIG. 5.

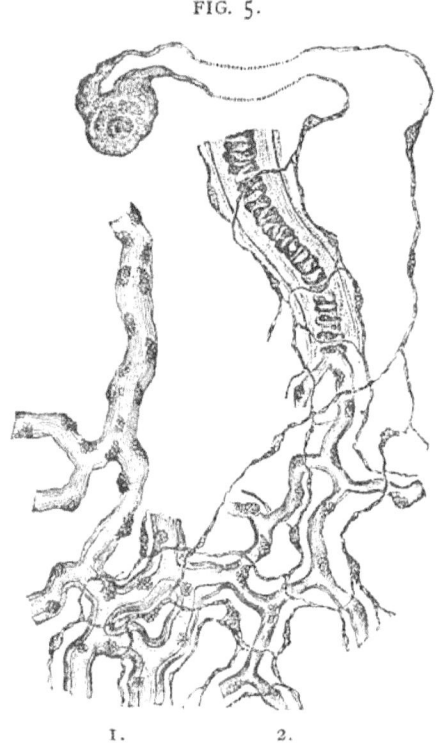

1.   2.

Diagram to show self-regulating mechanism connected with the minute arteries and capillaries.
a, artery with muscular fibre-cells; the dark lines show its diameter when dilated. *b*, small vein.
c, capillary net-work. Over No. 1 the capillaries are dilated and over No. 2 they are contracted. *d* is
a ganglion cell with at least two sets of nerve-fibres connected with it, one of which, *e*, divides and
subdivides, giving off nerve-fibres, which are distributed to the artery *a*, while the other, *f*, is continuous with the plexus of nerve-fibres ramifying close to the capillary vessels. Nerve-fibres are also
distributed to the small vein, *b*, but these are not represented in the drawing. The bioplasm of the
vessels and nerve-fibres is shown.

The vessel to the left, *b*, is intended to represent a small vein, while
that marked *a* is a small artery, and the net-work of small tubes below,
which are continuous with both vessels, are the capillaries, outside which
you see here and there delicate fibres, *nerve-fibres*.   These are really
distributed to the capillary vessels in very much the same manner as is
represented here.   The nerve-fibres distributed to the capillary vessels
join to form a fine nerve-trunk, and are by continuous fibres connected
with a cell, *d*, of the nerve-centre.   *e* is the nerve-fibre distributed to

the artery, and *f* is that connected with the branches distributed to the capillaries; those capillaries near the vein, over 1, being distended, so that the nerve-fibres are nearly in contact with their walls; while those over 2 are contracted, and a considerable interval is seen to exist between the outer surface of these and the nerve-fibres distributed to them.

The greater part of the nerve-circuit, which I have endeavored to depict, has been demonstrated by actual observation, but there is a break or hiatus as regards the connection of the particular fibres distributed to the artery and those to the capillary, with the nerve-cell. One cannot identify the afferent fibre and the efferent branch connected with the very same cell as is here represented. There is no doubt whatever as regards the existence of two fibres in connection with each nerve-cell in any nerve-centre. Nor, as I have already stated, is there any doubt about the connection of one of these fibres with the fine nerve-fibres which are distributed to the artery, for the continuity has been demonstrated. The ramifications of the fine nerve-fibres upon and amongst the muscular fibres of the artery have also been demonstrated in numerous specimens from representatives of the different classes of Vertebrata. I have not succeeded in tracing the nerve-fibres from capillary vessels to the same identical nerve-cell as that from which the nerve distributed to the little artery which subdivides into the capillaries takes its rise. I consider the arrangement to be as follows: The very fine nerve-fibres which I have shown to be distributed to capillary vessels are probably *afferent.* These transmit centripetally to the nerve-cell impressions from the sides and immediate neighborhood of the capillary vessels, and from the tissues between the capillary vessels. In the cells of the nerve-centre a change takes place whenever the peripheral ramifications of these afferent nerve-fibres from the capillaries are irritated. In consequence of this change effected in the nerve-centre, an impulse to movement is transmitted by the nerves, which are at length distributed to the muscular fibres of the little artery, when the muscular fibres will contract, and the tube of the artery will be reduced in diameter. The calibre of the artery is at once reduced, and the blood stream which flows onward into the capillary vessels is diminished; or, in other words, the quantity of blood passing to a given area of tissue in a given period of time is much reduced.

Under other circumstances the nerve-fibres distributed to the capillary vessels, instead of being irritated, experience a paralyzing influence, in consequence of which a corresponding action is produced in the nerve-centre, and, instead of contraction, we have relaxation of the muscular fibres of the little artery; and the quantity of blood passing through the vessels within a given period of time must be increased to an extent proportionate to the increased diameter of the vessel. Here, then, is a self-regulating nervous mechanism connected with the distribution and regulation of the blood-current in the capillary vessels of the body of a most efficient kind, coming into action on the slightest disturbance of the equilibrium of activity either at the peripheral distribution of the nerves or in the nerve-centres connected with them. The quantity of blood passing through these vessels can be regulated to a nicety. The stream may be increased or diminished suddenly, or an uniform flow maintained for a considerable period of time. These changes are brought about solely by the influence of the nerves in determining the degree of contraction of the muscular fibre cells which encircle the artery.

Let us now apply what we have learned to the phenomena of the flea-bite : When the lancet of the flea, after penetrating the cuticle, reaches the capillaries of the skin, some of the fine nerve-fibres distributed to the capillaries will be severed, others no doubt being stretched or pressed upon by the blood and fluid which escape from the vessels, and in conse-quence of the distention which the latter undergo. The result is a relax-ing or paralyzing action upon the nerve-centre. The efferent nerves being thus influenced, the muscular fibres of the little arteries yield, and become flaccid and elongated. Hence the diameter of the tube of the vessel will become largely increased. A greater quantity of blood will flow into the capillaries, and these vessels will in consequence become distended. This action probably depends partly upon severance of fine nerve-fibres by the cutting action of the lancet of the animal, but it is in part due to the influence of poison expelled at the moment, which spreads for a short distance among the elements of the adjacent tissues, perhaps acting chemically on the nerve-fibres or on their bioplasm, and causing a paralyzing influence.

But what is highly interesting and very remarkable is this : The relax-ing or paralyzing action is exerted *to a definite extent, and maintained without variation at a given point for some time.* The dilatation of the little arteries is effected, and the degree of constriction exerted by the muscular coat is altered for a time. The muscular fibres yield accord-ing to the degree of paralyzing influence produced upon the afferent nerves at the seat of injury. That the degree of dilatation does not vary from moment to moment may be proved in a very simple manner. If you squeeze the little vessels of the congested area of skin by pressing firmly for a second or two with one finger, so as to drive the blood out of the vessels, the whole of the skin subjected to the pressure will be seen at the moment when this is removed, to be uniformly pale. In a few seconds, however, after the pressure has been withdrawn, the blood will re-enter the vessels, and the inflamed area will resume its redness, while the surrounding skin will regain its original tint. The varying degrees of redness observed in different flea-bites are due entirely to the varying degree of dilatation of the hundreds of little arteries which sup-ply the capillary vessels of the inflamed area. The distention of the capillaries varies according to the calibre of the arteries, and is there-fore entirely under nerve control. If complete paralysis of the nerve-fibres distributed to the little arteries, or of the centres from which they emanate, were to occur, the capillaries would become distended to the utmost limit, and the circulation through them would cease. The surrounding tissues deprived of their blood supply would become disorganized, and might at once pass into a gangrenous state, or might slowly degenerate and waste. Such is the nature of the very important vascular phenomena which occur in all cases of inflammation, and which, when affecting a considerable extent of tissue, may cause serious structural changes, and result in the development of chronic disease, or, where certain important organs are affected, may cause even sudden death.

General Vascular Disturbance resulting from Local Injury.—But in many instances, the result of the local injury is much more widely spread. In some cases this is due to poison being introduced into the blood, so that the whole mass of nutrient fluid is poisoned, and, through it, every tissue and organ of the body may suffer. But there are not a few instances in which the facts cannot be thus explained, but seem rather to be due to the same series of changes which occur in an ordinary flea-bite, the action being more intense. The bite of a gnat, the sting of a bee, wasp, or hornet, will occasion phenomena in connection with the vessels of the same kind, but more serious and extensive than the injury inflicted by the lancet of the flea. Such local injuries may cause dilatation of the little arteries and capillaries over a considerable portion of the body. In consequence of the bite of an ordinary gnat, the whole of one arm may become enormously swollen. So large a quantity of exudation may escape from the vessels, that the areolar tissue of the limb may be much distended, the elements of the tissues generally being in a state of tension, their action much deranged or entirely marred. In short, a condition of very acute and serious inflammation may result.

In such a case, I think that the more extensive local mischief is perhaps due to a more severe and more extensive local change having been produced at the seat of injury. Instead of derangement of the action of the vessels of a very limited area of skin, as in the flea-bite, we have evidence of extensive disturbance in the circulation affecting small arteries, capillaries, and veins of the tissues, of part of a limb or of the entire limb. The influence is, however, still limited, and such a case must be distinguished from those in which the tissue-changes result from the whole mass of the blood being poisoned. As a general rule, a gnat-bite does no harm whatever. Most of us have been bitten over and over again ; and I dare say some have carefully watched the interesting operation performed by the insect, and, when the instrument has been carefully inserted through the cuticle, and into the true skin, have felt the pricking sensation which indicates the arrival of its point at the nerve-fibres adjacent to the capillary. Then follows the perforation of the capillary, and soon the blood will be seen to ascend, and you will notice the abdominal cavity of the insect becoming gradually distended by the inflowing blood. In a short time the creature is satisfied, and, after care-fully withdrawing his proboscis, he contentedly flies away, though slowly, for his body will be more than twice as heavy as it was when he first attacked you. With the exception of slight tingling, which lasts for a little while, no further effect, as a general rule, will be produced ; but I know persons who do not escape so easily. Sometimes a single gnat-bite will cause the whole of the hand and arm to swell enormously, and the state of inflammation may last for two or three days, and may be accompanied by much pain. A similar remark applies to the sting of a bee, or wasp or hornet. Some individuals will be seriously affected, while others will escape with very little inconvenience.*

Such facts are not incompatible with the view of the phenomena being essentially due to nerve change, and we have ample evidence that some persons' nerves are much more susceptible to the same degree of irritation, mechanical or chemical, than are those of others. A mechanical injury or a poisonous influence sufficiently severe to cause death in one case might scarcely produce any serious change in another. It is possible that there may be some structural difference in the nervous system of the two persons, but it is perhaps more probable that the cause of difference in the results is deeper, and depends upon some difference in the individuality and powers of the bioplasm of the nerve of a nature not to be rendered evident by physical investigation. We note corresponding peculiarities as regards the action of medicine. I have known instances in which the smallest dose of Morphia will occasion, within three or four hours of its being swallowed, dilatation of the capillary vessels of the greater part of the surface of the body, shown by a diffused red-ness in patches. Less than one-tenth of a grain of Morphia has led to this result, but such a dose, as a general rule, would produce only a very slight effect, or the person might be unconscious that any such drug had been

---

* An interesting fact has been made out by Dr. Manson, in China, with regard to the transference by gnats of embryonic or immature entozoa from the blood of the human organism to water. The minute *Filaria sanguinis hominis* is the entozoon in question. It exists in the blood in certain cases in immense numbers, and has been removed from the circulating medium, and transferred to the situation where it is to undergo further change in the remarkable way just referred to. An excellent *résumé* of what is known concerning this entozoon will be found in a paper read at the Epidemiological Society, by Sir Joseph Fayrer, and published in the " London Lancet " for February 8th, 1879.

We have long known that many infectious diseases may be spread by the agency of insects, but here we have an insect extracting blood from the interior of the vessels, and carrying some of this very same blood, and diffusing any special living particles it may contain into other media, where these organisms may pass another part of their existence, and possibly grow and multiply. It is obvious that other living disease-causing organisms may be distributed far and wide in the same manner, and thus many special fevers, and inflammatory diseases occurring in man and animals, and depending upon a living poison, may be carried to a distance, and preserved for long periods of time, or undergo further development.

given at all. The nerves and the nerve-centres connected with the vascular system exhibit very different degrees of sensitiveness or susceptibility in different persons.

In discussing the probable nature of the actual changes induced by such poisons, which act upon the fine ramifications of the nerves distributed to capillary vessels, we have to consider:—1. The direct local action of the poisonous material on the nerve fibres and other tissues with which it comes at once into contact; and, 2, the local action of the poison on the capillary nerve-fibres in many tissues and organs of the body at a distance from the seat of injury, through the contamination of the whole mass of the blood.

In both cases, whether the action be local or general, circumscribed or diffused, the widest difference as regards the degree of action exerted by the same poison and the same amount of poison on different persons will be observed, and this must be referred to the peculiarity of constitution of the individual, to the degree of tolerance his nerves may have acquired by the influence of previous exposure, and a number of other circumstances. The same amount of poison in the blood may be sufficient to cause the most grave symptoms in one person and not give rise to the slightest change in others.

You see how large a subject is opened for consideration by the demonstration of the nerve-fibres to capillary vessels, and what a number of important and widely separated physiological and pathological actions may be explained and accounted for by the influence of this important part of the nervous system.

OF THE FORMATION OF PUS IN AND NEAR THE CAPILLARIES IN INFLAMMATION AND FEVER.

I have already advanced arguments which, as it seems to me, fully justify the conclusion that fever is a *General Inflammation*, while inflammation is to be regarded as a *Local Fever*. Some among you who have considered the matter may, however, object to this inference, on the ground that what is known as "pus" is a very constant product in inflammations, but is not generally formed in fever. Such an objection will, however, disappear if we study the mode of formation of this living matter, *pus*. Indeed, in most fevers the pathological phenomena are, happily, not sufficiently intense. The changes do not proceed to the extent necessary for the development of pus-corpuscles. There are, however, fevers in which the development of pus is common enough.

In Erysipelas, which may be correctly included under fevers or inflammations, pus, as you are aware, is often formed to an extent sufficient to destroy important tissues and to cause death. Some of you of late years may have been assured that erysipelas, like many other fevers and inflammations, is due to the presence and growth and multiplication of bacteria. The process of suppuration itself, it has been said, is occasioned by these

organisms. I have already treated of this question in " Disease Germs "
and elsewhere. I shall, therefore, only remark here that, in my opinion,
there is no reasonable ground for either hypothesis, and that the facts
can be adequately explained without invoking the aid of bacteria. In
the course of the changes taking place in erysipelas, pus, unfortunately,
is very often formed. You may have suppuration of the tissues in the
greater part of the affected limb. Indeed, in some cases the areolar
tissue extending over a considerable part of the body may be the seat
of the formation and multiplication of pus-corpuscles.

In ordinary fevers life is usually destroyed before that degree of change
which involves the process of suppuration has been reached. If, however, severe fever lasted for a considerable period and life was sustained
for a sufficient time, many of the tissues might pass into the state of
suppuration. Such is, unfortunately, but too frequent in very severe
cases of scarlet fever, in which disease suppuration sometimes occurs in
several of the joints, besides which small abscesses are not unfrequently
developed in many different parts of the body. It is easy to see why
suppuration should be more commonly developed in connection with
intense local inflammation than in the more widely spread, but less intense, action which occurs in fever. In inflammation the change is comparatively circumscribed, and may, therefore, go to a much greater extent
without destroying life than is possible in the case of fever, for the mass
of the blood and every tissue in the body is more or less affected, while
the action of some of the most sensitive organs is seriously deranged
and the organs themselves damaged. Not unfrequently the brain and
some parts of the nervous system seem to be poisoned by the altered
blood. A huge abscess containing pints of pus may be formed in the
course of a fever and the patient nevertheless get perfectly well, if only
his strength can be sufficiently supported and the case be well nursed
and judiciously managed. Anything like general suppuration of all the
tissues of the body is impossible in fever, because death would take
place long before such an event could occur.

The formation of pus, and the manner in which the pus-corpuscles
move and grow and multiply, have been already referred to on p. 223.

**Of the Passage of Blood and Living Particles through the Walls of
Capillary Vessels.—Diapedesis.**—I have now to say a few words about
certain other phenomena of inflammation. When ordinary inflammation
takes place in a part, the vessels, as I have already said, are more or less
distended with blood, and as the walls of these capillary vessels are
stretched and rendered thinner by distention, fluid will more readily
transude through them than when they are in their usual medium state
of tension. Suppose this outline (chalk diagram) to represent the area
of a section of a capillary vessel in the ordinary state, neither contracted
nor stretched. This larger circle with thinner outline (diagram) may
stand for the same capillary vessel, with its walls much thinner and its

calibre greatly increased, as in the state of congestion, which gradually passes into inflammation. Now, it is obvious that, if the walls of this capillary are to be so stretched as to form a tube as much more capacious than the vessel in the ordinary state, as would be the tube of which this circle is the limit, than that indicated by the last outline, great thinning of the walls must take place. Whenever capillary vessels are distended with blood, there must be increased tenuity of their walls. The greater the diameter of the vessel the thinner will be its walls, and the thinner the walls the more readily will fluid permeate them. Now, in Inflammation and Fever, fluid, and often not only fluid, transudes from the blood through the walls of the capillaries of the affected parts into the tissues around the blood-vessels.

The material which is poured out has long been called *Exudation*, and this material varies somewhat in character and composition in different cases. Certain changes taking place in the blood itself may cause the fluid to become more permeable than the ordinary fluid portion (*liquor sanguinis*) of healthy blood. In many forms of disease the quantity of matter dissolved in the fluid which permeates the vascular walls is greatly increased, and probably the fluid itself is otherwise changed. But you must bear in mind that, beside the fluid which transudes through the capillary vessels in inflammation and fever, multitudes of excessively minute and very soft particles also traverse the capillary wall. Of these the great majority are less than the one hundred-thousandth of an inch in diameter, but some are very much larger than this. Indeed, particles as large as a red blood-corpuscle may find their way through the capillary wall without causing any rupture or permanent damage to the vessel, and through openings which it is not easy to demonstrate. Of this, instances have long been known in the case of what has been correctly termed capillary hæmorrhage. After this hæmorrhage has taken place, the stretched and distended vessels may return to their ordinary condition without any deterioration of the structure occurring in the walls which have been stretched. Such phenomena occur in every case of pneumonia.

You will naturally ask how large particles like the red blood-corpuscles pass through the walls of vessels in which no fissures or openings can be discerned. When we study the changes taking place during development, we learn that the walls of the capillary vessels are, as it were, laid down in such manner that the tissue of which they are composed, though exhibiting no definite indication of actual fibres, will tear much more readily in the longitudinal than in the transverse direction. Whenever the capillaries are distended by the accumulation of blood, and their walls stretched by lateral pressure, the fibre net-work, of which they may be supposed to consist, would have its meshes considerably widened in such a way that longitudinal rents or fissures would result, which would be large enough to permit the passage of more than one red blood-cor--

21   Q

puscle at a time through them. The distending force ceasing, the elastic
tissue of the capillary wall would react, and the vessel gradually return
to its ordinary size, the rent slowly closing up.

We can, therefore, readily imagine that a body as large as a blood-
corpuscle would easily escape sideways through one of these fissures and
pass amongst the tissues outside the vessel. Such escape of blood-corpuscles, a few at a time, takes place from the capillaries of the walls of
the air-cells of the lungs in every case of ordinary inflammation of the .
lung tissue, or *Pneumonia*. In cases, however, in which blood extrava-
sates to any great extent, as where blood escapes from a surface in drops,
a free tearing, or other solution of continuity, of the walls of the vessels
undoubtedly occurs. Even where violent hæmorrhage has taken place
from vessels of considerable dimensions, it is often most difficult to
demonstrate the opening. You need not, therefore, be surprised to learn
that it is almost impossible to expose the actual holes, rents, or fissures
in the walls of *capillary vessels* which have allowed the exit of a few
blood-corpuscles. There are cases in which hæmorrhage occurs from a
vast tract of capillary vessels, as for example, of the mucous membrane
of the small intestine, and yet the fissures or rents cannot be detected,
though several pints of blood may have been lost in the course of half
an hour, in consequence of *capillary hæmorrhage*. This may cause faintness and death. In such cases of fatal capillary hæmorrhage, no doubt,
degenerative changes have been taking place in the walls of the capillary
vessels involved, during a considerable period of time previous to the
occurrence of the hæmorrhage. When one comes to examine the mucous
membrane after death, the whole of the surface is found suffused, and
the tissues, so to say, infiltrated with blood which has issued from millions and millions of capillaries, distributed over perhaps as much as six
feet of intestine.

I have seen several instances of death from almost sudden and profuse
capillary hæmorrhage from the mucous membrane, extending over many
feet of the small intestine, consequent upon slow morbid changes proceeding in the liver and resulting in the condition known as *cirrhosis*.
In the course of this disease the circulation through the liver becomes
greatly impeded, and in consequence congestion of the mucous membrane of the intestines ensues, and frequent slight attacks of bleeding
occur, which may at last end in extensive and fatal hæmorrhage. If you
were to inject the vessels in such a case, the injection would ooze from
multitudes of minute openings, but no large aperture would be discovered
in any large or small vein or artery. The case is very different where a
large vessel is opened in the process of ulceration, as frequently occurs
in the course of ulcer of the stomach and in phthisis, or as sometimes
happens in aneurism.

There are certain forms of capillary bleeding or hæmorrhage which
are very common, and not indicative of any actual disease, and which

may fairly be regarded as slight ailments. Bleeding from the mucous membrane of the nose is one of these. Some children frequently suffer from this affection, and in certain instances relief to headache or to a sensation of fulness in the head is afforded by the slight loss of blood which occurs. Hæmorrhage of the same kind may take place from the back of the throat, from the gums, from the stomach, and even from the lungs. Occasionally bleeding takes place from *the rectum*, without producing more than temporary derangement, though, of course, it causes alarm to the patient and his friends.

You must be very careful about giving a too positive opinion concerning the exact nature of many of such cases, for bleeding from one or other of the surfaces above mentioned may be a grave matter, and perhaps the first indication of serious disease. On the other hand, even several teaspoonfuls of blood may escape from capillary vessels without the general health being in any way deranged. After tension has been relieved by this hæmorrhage, the vessels return to their former state and the blood circulates in them as before.

In cases of hæmorrhage from the mucous membrane of the nose, I believe that the capillaries become much congested, and that actual longitudinal rents or fissures are made through which blood escapes. If the attacks are frequent and severe and the patient's strength fails, it may be necessary to adopt remedial measures even in a case of what appears to be ordinary bleeding from the nose. Perfect rest in the half-recumbent posture, the application of cold to the nose externally, sucking small pieces of ice, are usually effectual, but it may be necessary to use styptics or "plug the nostrils" in severe cases. This, however, is not the place to discuss the treatment requisite in cases of such gravity. It should, however, be borne in mind that bleeding not depending upon actual disease may take place from many other organs and surfaces as well as from the mucous membrane of the nose.

Hæmorrhage from minute vessels used to be spoken of as hæmorrhage by exhalation; and the older observers believed the escape of blood from the vessels occurred in some mysterious manner not to be adequately explained. They seemed to think that the blood passed through the walls of vessels in some strange and inscrutable way. By the aid of recent investigations we can form a clear idea of the manner in which the hæmorrhage through the walls of the capillaries may occur without actual rupture. The phenomenon is of great interest, and we may conveniently consider under the same head a process which has been regarded by many observers as essential to more than one general pathological change, and which has been spoken of as *Diapedesis*.

It was proved experimentally by Cohnheim, of Berlin, that colorless blood-corpuscles might pass from the cavity of the peritoneum into the vascular system, and that in the case of the membrane of the frog's foot and other tissues when in a state of inflammation, colorless blood-corpus-

cles made their way through the capillary walls, though no openings could
be seen and the capillaries themselves were not unduly distended.   Cohnheim maintained that this migration of colorless blood-corpuscles was an
ordinary phenomenon ; that it was common, and constantly took place,
to a great extent, in every case of inflammation.   Nay, he went so far
as to insist *that pus itself consisted of colorless blood-corpuscles which
had made their way out of the vessels.*   Of course it occurred to many
that the last proposition was rather difficult to accept, for the number
of pus-corpuscles in an ordinary abscess formed in the course of the
twenty-four hours is so great, that had every colorless blood-corpuscle
in the body made its way into the abscess a mere modicum of the total
quantity of pus present would be thus accounted for.   The pus-corpuscles in a small abscess, or on the surface of an inflamed mucous membrane, outnumber by many times the whole of the colorless blood-
corpuscles in the organism.   Many observers in this country, however,
advocated the above view, and it has in consequence formed a cardinal
doctrine of more than one school of pathology.   Of those who profess
to have *seen* the phenomenon in question, not a few will tell you that
it is easily demonstrated and occurs constantly.   He who proceeds to
study the matter for himself will, I think, find that only very occasionally can he feel at all sure that a colorless blood-corpuscle has actually
passed through the vascular walls.   The careful observer will not unfrequently find that a corpuscle which *seems to pass through the walls of a
vessel* does not really do so, and is, in fact, either in front of the capillary or behind it, and has not come out of the vessel at all.   There is,
however, no doubt that this migration of colorless blood-corpuscles does
occur, but I believe it to be an exceptional, rather than a common or
ordinary, phenomenon, while I feel sure that, in many cases, the process of inflammation may run its course entirely without the escape of a
single blood-corpuscle.

The corpuscles found outside the capillaries in great numbers in cases
of inflammation, are produced not by the passage of colorless corpuscles
from the blood, but by the growth of very minute particles which have
escaped with the transuded fluid.   These particles do not consist of colorless blood-corpuscles, which, as such, have traversed the walls as has
been supposed.   So far from having been colored blood-corpuscles, it is
doubtful whether at any time one of them ever circulated in the blood
as such.   What, then, are these bodies, and how did they attain the
position in which we find them ?

Some years before the above views were published and popularized in
this country, I had described another process of migration, or rather
pouring out, from the blood, suspended in *liquor sanguinis*, of minute
particles of living matter or *bioplasm*, which no doubt play a very important part in the complex phenomenon of inflammation.   I showed
that, if a very thin layer of healthy blood was examined by a high mag-

nifying power, a number of corpuscles, infinitely smaller than either red or colorless corpuscles, were to be detected ; and not only so, but I proved that these minute corpuscles, varying from the one hundred-thousandth to the one ten-thousandth of an inch in diameter, and probably corpuscles still more minute, consisted of bioplasm, or living matter. The blood of man and the higher animals, while circulating in the living body, ought to be regarded as a fluid holding in suspension countless multitudes of minute particles of living matter which, at death, undergo a great change, and become converted into several different substances, among the most important of which is the matter we call fibrin. Similar minute particles of living matter are held in suspension in the circulating and nutrient fluids of every living organism, and are present even in the nutrient fluids of plants.

In the large cells of Vallisneria spiralis, which you may easily grow in a glass jar in your sitting-room, you may see the rotation of the so-called "cell-contents." The most important of these contents being the apparently clear homogeneous fluid which passes round and round the cell, as long as the very minute particles of bioplasm suspended in it, but to be demonstrated only by the aid of very high powers, continue alive. No one has succeeded in accounting for these movements by physical and chemical change, though many have attempted to do so. Many more have affirmed that it can be so explained, and with the confidence and satisfaction characteristic of the new philosophy, have affirmed that, even if the explanation they have given is not quite adequate and satisfactory at this time, it will be found to be so at some future period.

The power of moving resides in the minute particles themselves. As long as the matter of which these consist lives the particles may move, but when it dies the moving power is completely lost. This remarkable *spontaneous movement*, which cannot be explained, which we may see in the pus-corpuscles, in the colorless blood-corpuscles, and in other forms of bioplasm belonging to man, to animals, and to plants, has been attributed to certain reactions between the particles themselves and things in their environment, but if you will only look for yourselves and ponder over what you observe, you will soon be convinced of the incorrectness of the hypothesis. At no period of history have such ridiculous statements been made concerning the nature and actions of living things as in our own time. So far from being in advance of old doctrines, the ancients would have ridiculed much that now passes for philosophy. It must be admitted that the most nonsensical views concerning many things have been received as true because they have been repeatedly urged in the strongest language. When people hear an assertion repeated again and again they think there must be "something in it." So they believe it, or act upon it, as the case may be. The confidence with which physical explanations of purely vital phenomena are insisted upon is most extraordinary. On the one side there is astounding audacity

21 *

and arrogance, on the other meek acquiescence, and an almost incredible credulity. Some teachers do not hesitate to tell the public that they *know* many things which have never been and cannot be proved. They are, we are assured, peculiarly *strong* and "privileged" to prophecy, and to do other out of the way things. Such persons affirm that they discern all sorts of wonderful things, but they cannot tell us how to discern, nor do they explain by what means they have been able to discern. They are "gifted spirits," and do not belong to the class of ordinary mortals. Some prophetic philosophers, without having earnestly studied the phenomena of any living thing in nature, nay, without being even practically skilled in the ordinary methods of investigating the structure of any living thing, dare to wildly assault the whole world of life, and recklessly declare that all living things are produced and built up and worked according to the very same principles and laws by which the non-living world is fettered and confined in eternal helplessness.

Let me persuade you to observe what happens as the simplest of living things grows. Take, for instance, ordinary mildew, which can be obtained easily enough, or which each can grow for himself, for its germs are always present in the air. You may grow it in a little acid urine if you like. By carefully watching it, you will be convinced that it grows by taking up nutrient matter, which is not deposited upon its surface but taken into its very substance, where it becomes converted into living matter, from every particle of which new particles may result. Ask the physicist to explain, if he can do so by any physical laws, the phenomena which have occurred while the organism has been under your observation.

Up to this time, instead of telling us what is going on, instead of describing by what means matter is changed in composition and acquires new properties whenever it is caused to assume the living state, confident physicists assert, and with an air of superiority, what according to their powers of prevision is certainly to be achieved by physicists in the far-off future. Perhaps the materialist gifted with prophetic powers enlarges on the subject of chemical affinity and its possibilities in the future, perhaps he will tell you about properties and attractions, tendencies, molecular forces, potentialities, and evolutions and laws, and discoveries concerning things that may be, or according to him must be, and which he, but no one else, can discern in his imagination. He will *not*, however, tell you what happens whenever lifeless matter is made to live, or when living matter dies. All the assertions made during the last ten years or more on the identity of vital and physical properties have but retarded real advance in biological science. No adequate explanation as regards the nature of the change from non-living to living, and from living to dead, has been discovered in the past. Nothing definite is known to the physicist at the present time, but what is not discovered by him now is, he asserts, to be rendered evident by his successors in the future,—

that future which is now very far off, and which ever gets dimmer and more remote as time passes. The truth is the materialist view of things is a mere absurdity, based on fancies and dicta instead of on facts.

The vital phenomena observed in the case of the mildew or any other simple organism, closely resemble those which are observed in the case of living particles belonging to man and the higher animals, both in health and disease, and can be accounted for only by attributing them to the influence of a peculiar power or agency associated with the matter while it is alive, and which is absolutely distinct from any of the known properties or forces of ordinary matter.

The minute particles of bioplasm or living matter which pass through the walls of the capillary vessels in cases of ordinary inflammation soon begin to undergo alteration. As long as they were being rapidly moved about in the blood-stream these particles would undergo little or no active change; but as soon as they become still and quiescent, by their own inherent power of movement they begin to make their way through the walls of the vessels (p. 240), and soon take up and appropriate the nutrient material which surrounds them in great quantities. While in the blood, probably in those organs where the circulation of the blood goes on very slowly, these minute particles grow and slowly undergo conversion into the bodies known as the colorless blood-corpuscles. When outside the vessels, as in inflammation, the particles grow more quickly, and soon assume the form of the colorless corpuscles which we see in such immense numbers in the interstices of various tissues and just outside the walls of the vessels in inflammation.

1. Under certain circumstances the bioplasts in question soon die, and the products resulting from their death are quickly re-absorbed. 2. Under other conditions they develop a delicate fibrous material. 3. If supplied with plenty of pabulum they may continue to grow and multiply very rapidly until the form of living matter known as pus results. Pus-corpuscles are particles of living matter or bioplasm, which have been developed by direct descent, but with modification in power, from the minute living particles under consideration, or more directly from colorless blood-corpuscles, or from the bioplasm of some tissue. From such particles of bioplasm every form of adventitious fibrous tissue which we find outside the walls of the capillaries and in the interstices of the tissues, in various forms both of acute and chronic inflammation, is produced. The delicate fibrous tissue at first formed loses water, contracts, and gradually becomes condensed. The "thickening" and condensation which you often meet with in tissues which have been inflamed is thus brought about.

As I have already remarked, the minute particles of living matter, or bioplasm, outside the walls of the capillaries may also grow and multiply until multitudes of "pus-corpuscles" result. Even at this time the fact that pus-corpuscles grow and multiply of themselves by the formation of little offsets, outgrowths, or diverticula, which are from time to time detached, is not generally recognized. You may remember, in a former lecture, I described how the bioplasm of a cell might increase in size, and might give off diverticula, which being detached, form separate portions of bioplasm, each of which may grow and give off more processes, until by the growth and multiplication of a few particles millions of the masses of bioplasm known as pus-corpuscles are formed, every one of which may be regarded as the descendant of the bioplasm or nucleus of an epithelial cell. The pus-corpuscles cannot, therefore, be looked upon as an individual colorless blood-corpuscle, which has simply migrated from the blood by traversing the walls of the vessel.

The idea that the formation of pus is in any way dependent upon bacteria or other forms of so-called micro-organisms is negatived by what may be easily seen in the production of pus-corpuscles in epithelial cells. The growth of the bioplasm and its division and subdivision under conditions which involve increased nutrition will convince any one who observes the phenomenon how pus is produced in epithelium ; and as exactly corresponding facts are to be demonstrated by the examination of bioplasm in other tissues, cartilage, fibrous tissue, muscle, nerve, etc., when exposed to the influence of an unusual supply of pabulum, no room is left for doubt as to the exact nature of the pathological process of pus production. I cannot agree with my colleague, Professor Lister, in considering that putrefactive materials may be the cause of suppuration, nor can I admit that this process can be properly attributed to chemical substances or to nervous disturbance. A state of things may be brought about by these which may indirectly occasion the free distribution of nutrient matter to bioplasm to which the production of pus is directly and solely attributable in all cases.

SOME COMMON FORMS OF SLIGHT INFLAMMATION AND OF THEIR TREATMENT.

We will now endeavor to determine what are the essential changes which occur in epithelium and in some other tissue elements in ordinary slight inflammations. These changes do not necessarily lead to any structural alterations ; but if the inflammatory process continues for a certain period of time, it may be followed by tissue degeneration and other pathological phenomena, from which return to the normal state, complete recovery, cannot be looked for. Not a few of the slight inflammations are superficial, involving a very thin layer of the surface tissue only, and although most of them are by no means serious, some are very troublesome and many excessively painful. It is desirable, therefore, not only that you should know how to detect and distinguish them, but you ought to be fully conversant with the exact nature of the minute changes taking place and the methods by which a return to the normal state may be effected.

The treatment of some of the inflammations in question has been already considered, but it seems to me very important that I should do my best to press upon your consideration the character of the changes effected by simple remedies in the vital actions which are proceeding in the inflamed tissue, the effects of some of which have been rendered evident to us by careful microscopical research. He will be most successful in the management of the disease who most nearly succeeds in picturing to himself the wonderful changes which proceed in such marvellous minuteness and detail, and which can only be revealed to those who have long and earnestly studied, and have taken full advantage of, the elaborate means of minute investigation now at their disposal.

The mucous membrane of the nose and its many passages, as has been already stated (p. 214), is very liable to slight inflammation. In the changes which occur during an ordinary cold we have an illustration of the very gradual passage of physiological into pathological actions. There is a particular point in these changes when it would be impossible to decide whether it would be more correct to say that the membrane still remained in a healthy state or had just passed from this into a morbid condition. The difference between certain normal and inflammatory states unquestionably depends only upon an exaggeration of the activity with which normal changes are performed. In suppuration there is too much vital action, too much growth, and too rapid multiplication of living particles.

It is by the careful study of inflammatory changes only moderate in degree that we shall be able to answer the question why in one case the healing, and in another, apparently similar in all general respects, the opposite and destructive process, occurs. A slight wound suppurates which we desire should heal ; an ulcer forms and increases in spite of all our efforts to stop its ravages. The observations made on p. 254. bear upon this most important question ; and while one set of inquirers would attribute the want of repair to some derangement of the nervous system, another set to some chemical poison in the air, another to the presence of bacteria of a malignant type, I would refer it solely to the state of the patient's blood—to the presence in the circulating fluid of an abnormal quantity of material easily appropriated by low forms of bioplasm or living matter, and to the presence of multitudes of minute particles of these—of bioplasm particles, which, passing through the capillary walls, grow and multiply, and actually prevent the slower changes which ordinarily result in the formation of formed material, and which constitute an essential part of the healing process. If the matter upon which these particles live can be removed from the blood, we shall stop the growth and multiplication of the bioplasm particles and cause their death. Hence in cases in which the patient's strength is good, free purgation favors the healing process, and in the case of those who suffer from prostration, alcohol in the blood, and the application of alcohol, and things which act like alcohol to the wound, acts in the same beneficial manner; for this substance interferes with the growth of living matter, and alters the pabulum in such a manner as to render it unfit for the nutrition of the living particles.

Formation of Mucus.—Mucus, as you know, is formed in small quantity in the follicles and glands in connection with the mucous membrane of the nose, even in perfect health. When we suffer from a common "cold in the head," these particles of bioplasm which take part in the formation of the tenacious mucus around them grow and multiply more quickly than they do in the perfectly healthy state. The viscid material (mucus) formed by them is in greater proportion, softer in consistence, perhaps disintegrated and broken down, or actually decomposed, and in it bacteria and low forms of life find materials favorable for their development and eminently suitable for their nutrition.

Mucus-Corpuscle. I have many times spoken of the bioplasm which constitutes the so-called Mucus-corpuscle, but I have not told you how you should proceed to observe the wonderful vital movements which occur during its life, and especially at the commencement of a slight cold, when the activity of the movement is considerably increased. Having obtained, by coughing or sneezing, a small piece of the transparent mucus, about the size of a pin's head, place it on an ordinary microscope plate-glass slide. Next cover it with a piece of the thinnest covering-glass you can obtain, without adding water or any other substance. Gently press down the thin glass cover with the aid of a pin or needle, and place the slide under the microscope, using first of all a quarter of an inch object-glass, and then a twelfth or higher power, if you are fortunate enough to possess one. If not, you can gain the requisite degree of amplifying power in another way, and at the cost of a shilling or two. A piece of brass tubing, of the same diameter as that of the tube of the microscope, and arranged to carry the eye-piece, is fitted to it, sliding in just as the eye-piece does. The total length of the tube, to one end of which the object-glass, and to the other the eye-piece, is attached, is in this way increased to about eighteen inches. The intensity of the illumination being somewhat increased, you will find the little particles of mucus so highly magnified that you will be able to see the slightest changes which take place in their form and contour from moment to moment.

The minute oval particles in the thin layer of transparent mucus, and which consist of living matter or bioplasm, may be said to represent, and indeed correspond to, the "nucleus" of an ordinary epithelial cell, while the mucus—that viscid material which surrounds them—corresponds to the wall of the cell. If the epithelium of other mucous membranes grows unusually fast, a material which not only corresponds to, but resembles, mucus will be formed.

If you select one of the oval corpuscles, the living matter of the mucus, and examine it intently, you will soon observe changes in its outline. Here and there protrusions will occur, portions of the mass moving away from the remainder, and then being withdrawn and incorporated. The movements indeed very closely resemble those seen in an ordinary *amœba*, and are *vital movements* of the same nature. They continue for a considerable period of time—perhaps for twelve hours, or longer, if you can keep the mucus in a moist atmosphere, and so prevent it from drying up. Changes of the same kind occur in bioplasm generally, but it is only here and there that we are able to demonstrate them so satisfactorily as in the case of the living Mucus-corpuscle, Pus-corpuscle, and colorless Blood-corpuscle. In these living particles any one can study, and at any time he desires to do so, the vital movements of bioplasm or living matter.

In an inflamed mucous membrane, besides those prominent derangements, increased redness caused by congestion of the capillaries, and increased dryness consequent upon the defective pouring out of the fluid from the blood to take the place of that which has been quickly removed from the surface by evaporation,—we have to notice important changes in connection with the action of the nerves. Every one who has had a cold knows that the sensation of the part is affected. The mucous membrane is sore and painful, so that his attention is being frequently directed to it. He fancies something is adhering to it which requires to be removed, and is constantly making efforts to get rid of it. In some cases a certain quantity of mucus collects upon the surface and dries, in others the sensation experienced seems rather to be due to the tissues being infiltrated with fluid. Sometimes the mucous membrane, particularly at the margin of the nose, becomes excoriated, or a superficial ulcer may form. In the last case it will be found that the ordinary protective hardened epithelial covering has been here and there removed, and a raw and highly sensitive fissure formed, at the bottom of which are capillaries and nerve-fibres. From the capillaries fluid escapes holding in suspension numerous minute particles of bioplasm, and not unfrequently small quantities of blood itself are poured out. The pain experienced is due to the exposure or incomplete exposure of delicate nerve-fibres. The particular nerves affected are those which are distributed close to the capillary vessels, and which have been described in p. 228. But other nerve-fibres may be involved, for, as I have already mentioned, there are tissues in which nerve-fibres are distributed, although no capillaries exist, which nerve-fibres are concerned in the pain experienced when the tissue is inflamed. At the same time it is probable that the nerves in question belong to the same system as those distributed to capillaries, while there is no doubt that the latter are concerned in transmitting to us the impressions which we call pain. I have already remarked that as regards many tissues to which numbers of nerve-fibres are distributed, we are quite unconscious of their existence so long as the normal or healthy state lasts, but as soon as this gives place to inflammation, pain, it may be of the most exquisite kind, results. The nerves concerned being those of the capillary vessels which belong to that self-regulating system of nerves before referred to (p. 232). These fine nerve-fibres become, as I have said, stretched or pressed upon by the distended capillary vessels, and perhaps otherwise affected by the exudation which takes place. And in consequence of these derangements, this departure from the normal state, as respects the nerve-fibre, and the bioplasm which is connected with it, that disturbance of the nerve-current which we term pain results.

The extreme pain accompanying pleurisy, that caused in the condition we recognize as a rheumatic state of the nerves distributed to the intercostal muscles, and the pain excited during inflammation even of very small portions of the subcutaneous tissues, as in the formation of a boil, or even in the case of a chilblain, are illustrations of the exquisite sensitiveness of nerves in textures, of the existence of which in the normal state we are perfectly unconscious. In all these cases the actual nerve-fibres involved are probably those which run very close to the capillary vessels of the respective tissues.

Eruptions, particularly of a vesicular character, often occur in the course of sensitive nerves, and particularly in the course of nerves which are very commonly the seat of neuralgic pain. Whether the sensitive nerve trunk is directly involved, or whether the fibres distributed to the capillary vessels of the nerve trunk and of the skin situated over the nerve only are affected, it is not possible to say. What, however, seems quite certain is that the vesicles of an eruption which generally is herpetic in its character follow the course of the nerve. The pathological disturbance resulting in the formation of the vesicles may be of a most complex nature, in which reflex nervo-vascular action plays a highly important part. There must be increased nutrition, with pouring out of fluid from the capillary vessels, and this phenomenon is probably due to the relaxation of the muscular fibre-cells of the small arteries and consequent enlargement of their calibre. This change is caused by disturbance in the nerve-centre which governs the arterial contraction and dilatation. The central disturbance may itself be due to impulses emanating from the sensitive nerve itself, or originating in the skin situated over its course and transmitted thence by afferent fibres connected with the centre. In this manner it is very probable that various peculiar eruptions and other disturbances connected with the nutrition of the skin and subjacent structures are occasioned.

But besides the alteration in the sensibility of the mucous membrane in sore throat, important changes take place in connection with reflex nervo-muscular action. You are all no doubt aware that if the fauces be tickled ever so slightly, convulsive movements of swallowing will instantly follow, if the mucous membrane be in a healthy state. In slight "sore throat" it will be found that the response to slight irritation is slow and imperfect, while in severe forms of inflammation no efforts of deglutition can be excited even by severe irritation. The changes in question are due to an alteration in the sensitiveness of the mucous membrane, and probably depend upon pressure or stretching of the delicate nerve-fibres, in consequence of which they cease to conduct impressions from the periphery to the nerve-centres.

The dry state of the surface which is induced by slight inflammation of the mucous membrane may last for a short time and then gradually subside, without any further pathological action. If, however, the dryness and diminished secretion should persist for some weeks, restoration to the ordinary condition takes place very slowly, and before the healthy state can be resumed a condition opposite to that of dryness supervenes. Secretion is poured out, it may be, in very considerable quantity. This tendency to secretion, being once established, may persist for days or weeks, and then begin to diminish in amount. By degrees the glands return to their normal state of slight activity, secreting only a very small amount of transparent viscid mucus.

Counter-action, Counter-irritation.—But we may reduce the secretion consequent upon exaggerated and abnormal action occurring upon a mucous surface by proceeding in another way. Instead of trying to act directly upon the membrane which is the seat of the increased action, we may endeavor to establish increased action of surfaces or organs at a distance, situated in different parts of the body. In this way we may, for example, diminish the inflammation and undue action which are going on in the surface of the nose in many cases of catarrhal inflammation.

I will now direct attention to an important principle connected with the treatment of disease—a principle which has been acted upon for years, or even centuries, and concerning which we are much better informed than our predecessors were. That we can reduce the rate or degree of action in one part of the body by increasing it in another may be proved by a simple experiment. When a cold is coming on, you feel great discomfort about the nose, the mucous membrane of which cavity is so swollen that the nasal passages are obstructed, so that if you try to force air down one nostril, you fail, or only a little air can be forced through if a great effort be made. You are obliged under these circumstances to breathe entirely through the mouth. The discomfort caused by the swollen state of the mucous membrane, depending partly upon exudation into the submucous tissue and partly upon increased nutrition going on in the epithelial covering, may be ameliorated in a very short period of time and in a very simple way. Let the feet be put into water, as hot as you can bear it without severe pain. In the course of a quarter of an hour the disagreeable feeling of fulness and obstruction in the nose will cease. The air will pass through the passages of the nose quite freely. By increasing the flow of blood in the vessels of the skin

22

of the lower extremities, much of the circulating fluid will be diverted, for the time being, from the mucous membrane of the nose.

Many cases of headache are also relieved by putting the feet into hot water. If instead of this a mustard poultice be applied to the back of the neck a similar effect will follow. As soon as the mustard poultice begins to act, the vessels or, more correctly, the nerve-fibres distributed to the capillaries ramifying just beneath the epithelium, after being first irritated and then poisoned by the oil of the mustard, take part in irritating changes, which result in the vessels becoming red and turgid from the increased quantity of blood which is driven into them. The blood in these vessels circulates more slowly and gradually accumulates in them, the surface becoming red and exceedingly painful. Corresponding with this increased action in the healthy part we have reduced action at the seat of the morbid change.

In this way we are able to effect alterations which are of immense importance in the treatment of many different forms of disease. In cases where the morbid action is chronic, we keep up the counter-irritation to a moderate extent, or we repeat the application of the counter-irritant from time to time. Even in very chronic diseases there is good reason for adopting this principle of treatment. In some cases of phthisis, where there was reason to infer that tubercle was limited to a very small extent of pulmonary tissue, benefit seems to have resulted from keeping a small open sore on the skin of the upper part of the chest on the same side of the body. This is a form of " issue." In these days, however, this system of treatment is now rarely, perhaps too seldom, employed.

It is not uncommon to find slight pathological derangements of the skin and mucous membrane of the lips. This surface becomes more or less dry, and the epithelium of the red part of the lip which resembles that covering the skin, only forming a thinner layer, as well as the soft, moist epithelium lining the cavity of the mouth, becomes deranged in its growth. The surface, instead of remaining quite smooth, becomes more or less harsh. Under these circumstances the patient often attempts to make the surface even by rubbing it, so as to remove the little projecting pieces of ragged cuticle. In this way the derangement is kept up or intensified. The cuticle tends to peel off in thin laminæ, and many people cannot resist the temptation to catch at the pieces and tear them away. But then the surface becomes raw and often bleeds. In consequence of the air coming into contact with it, the moisture soon disappears, and the soft, imperfectly-formed cuticle soon gets dry, and the surface becomes corrugated and more painful than ever.

By the irregular growth of epithelium the arrangement of the finest nerve-fibres is disturbed, and constant irritation gives rise to irregular stretching or pressure. The sensations thus caused, and rapidly succeeding one another, excite the patient's constant attention, and in consequence he continually rubs the affected part or keeps constantly picking at any loose portion of cuticle. Immediately around the irritated nerve-fibres are multitudes of particles of living bioplasm actively growing and multiplying, forming a mass of soft, very moist spongy matter, the constituent particles of which are always changing in position. The drying that is proceeding on the surface necessarily disturbs the nerve-fibres, as well as other structures beneath. Schoolboys are very prone to pick their lips when in this state and make them extremely sore, particularly at the line where the thin skin of the lip joins the ordinary skin, and at the angles of the mouth, where little cracks or fissures often form, which may remain for days or weeks, sometimes giving rise to ugly and troublesome sores. It is very desirable to prevent the irritation which so disturbs the patient and causes him to make the sore worse and retard the healing.

Principles of Treatment.—Now, upon what principles should the treatment of such simple excoriations and slight superficial ulcerations be based? Our main object should be to reduce the growth and multiplication of the particles of bioplasm which are instrumental in keeping the fissure moist and open. This cannot be effected by causing them to dry up, because in that case a little crust would soon form, which, in consequence of the contraction produced by desiccation, would afterwards be drawn away from the subjacent parts. In this manner a raw surface again appears, and is perhaps larger than the preceding one. At the same time we must try to prevent this drying up, and to reduce the growth of bioplasm and pouring out from the blood of fresh plasma containing more bioplasm particles. By effecting these objects, certain lotions and other local applications promote healing. Some of them lead to the quick formation of a dry scab, but so thin that it does not become detached. Other applications are employed for the purpose of reducing the rate of growth of the masses of bioplasm on the surface of the sore, which is at the same time kept moist. The formation of the more permanent tissues slowly proceeds beneath this temporary protective covering. This latter process requires a considerable time for its completion. Much formed material has to be slowly produced by the bioplasts of the several tissues, and must subsequently become condensed.

Alcohol.—One of the most potent applications for healing such slight sores as I have referred to is alcohol. The sore place may be painted over once in an hour or so with pretty strong spirit, a camel-hair brush being used for the purpose. Of course, there is a sharp pain at the moment the alcohol comes into contact with the delicate nerve-fibres, but it soon passes off. In many cases it is well to dilute the alcohol with an equal quantity of water or rose-water. It matters little whether you use any of the ordinary spirits or Eau de Cologne, but pure spirits of wine diluted with one-third part of pure water is the best application. By this treatment the thin skin on the surface of the fissure or ulcer becomes hardened, and the soft, new epithelium that is being formed beneath will become condensed, and the new cuticle will gradually assume the usual character of that tissue. Let us consider how alcohol acts advantageously under these circumstances. By its property of coagulating albuminous matters, alcohol tends to retard rapid growth and to interfere with the multiplication of those particles of bioplasm which are growing so rapidly just outside the capillaries. The bioplasm, as I have mentioned, is growing so very fast that there is not time for the development and consolidation of that firm, healthy-formed material which, with living matter within, constitutes a cuticle cell. By applying alcohol, then, you favor the formation of cuticular cells. Wherever the cuticle is thin, by painting it frequently with alcohol, you promote the formation of cuticle and assist the condensation and increase in thickness of the new tissue.

If there should be sores in the mouth; or if the mucous membrane of the gum should be soft and spongy from the infiltration of fluid in the substance of the mucous membrane, the surface of which may be very red and tender, the morbid action may be quickly counteracted by painting the part three or four times a day with spirits of wine, *Spiritus Vini Rectificatus*, or some other form of alcohol, or with spirits of Camphor, *Spiritus Camphoræ*.

Solution of Nitrate of Silver.—Many lotions composed of metallic salts are employed in the treatment of sores. Most of them act by virtue of their property of coagulating and precipitating and forming compounds with albuminous matters. Among these salts is Nitrate of Silver, *Argenti Nitras*, which causes the sores to heal very quickly. With a small camel-hair brush you paint the fissure with a little solution of Nitrate of Silver, consisting of from five to ten grains of the Nitrate in an ounce of Distilled water. This will give pain for the moment, but the soreness soon passes off. The growth and multiplication of the masses of bioplasm are prevented. Time is allowed for the young cells of cuticle to harden. Gradually, new skin is formed, the growth of healthy epithelium is favored, and before long the healing process is completed.

Conjunctiva.—A good illustration of the pathological changes which occur when a complex tissue becomes inflamed is afforded by the mucous membrane which covers the front of the eye and lines the eyelids, the *Conjunctiva*,—when in a state of inflammation. This moist mucous membrane is very highly sensitive, and, as all have occasionally experienced, readily becomes inflamed. If you go out in foggy weather, and afterwards examine the conjunctiva, you will often find many of its vessels distended, and you will observe that it is much redder than it was before it was exposed to the deleterious effects of the irritating substances which are suspended in the air in a fog. The pathological change in question is a reflex action due to disturbance in the nerve-centres induced by the poisonous action of the irritating matter on the pe·ipheral ramifications of the sensitive afferent nerves, and a consequent paralyzing influence upon the nerves of the little arteries. In the case of persons who are in a low state of health who have lived badly for some time, and especially in those who belong to scrofulous families, there is increased liability to inflammation of the conjunctiva, as well as the glands and other structures which are connected with it. When the mucous membrane is inflamed the little glands participate, and from them is poured out an abundant secretion containing numerous particles of bioplasm. The vessels are distended, and that part of the mucous membrane which lines the eyelids and covers the white part (sclerotic) of the eye is reddened and, as I have remarked, in a state which well illustrates the changes taking place in inflammation. The condition is called *Ophthalmia or Conjunctivitis*, and is of great scientific interest, because a transition from the normal or ordinary state of health to the abnormal and temporary state of inflammation may be studied in its gradations. It is easy to examine the membrane from time to time with a lens, and without causing the slightest pain or inconvenience to the patient.

The conjunctiva, especially in ill-fed, ill-nourished scrofulous children, not only readily takes upon itself this exaggerated action, but passes into a state of inflammation which, though slight for a time, may soon become severe, and be accompanied with an abundant formation of a yellowish secretion. If a little of the discharge is examined in the microscope, it will be found to consist of multitudes of particles of living matter, well known as *pus-corpuscles*. Such is the virulence of these particular living particles that if no more of the discharge than can be carried on the point of a needle, be transferred to the surface of the eye of another person, a similar pathological state is quickly established upon it. Serious inflammation is excited, and the same series of phenomena recur. From this case the poison may be transferred to a third, and so on.

Now, if many children in weak health, who for some time previously have been badly managed as regards food, air, exercise, and cleanliness, are allowed to congregate, and especially if they are confined in close, ill-ventilated rooms, the disease may not only arise but soon acquire an extraordinary degree of virulence. It may spread so quickly in such a community of children, that in a short time out of four or five hundred, one-third or even a larger proportion may be suffering from the disease. Of the number affected many will suffer severely, and serious structural changes in the membrane and in subjacent tissues will result. The transparent part of the eye in front, known as the cornea, may ulcerate, and when after some time it heals, the tissue will be so altered that the very transparent texture will become opaque, or the eye itself may be destroyed, blindness of course resulting in either case.

This very virulent poison of purulent ophthalmia may, as I have re-

22 * R

marked, be evolved in the first instance without contagion. The contagious material may originate upon the membrane which during its formation passes from the normal into a pathological condition. A highly contagious poison may also be developed, in the organism of a person suffering from peritonitis and some other inflammatory and febrile diseases. In this case it is to be remarked that the surfaces upon which the changes occur which result in the development of the contagious poison are not, and never have been, exposed to the air. The contagious matter once developed, however, may spread far and wide, and with a rapidity which is quite remarkable. You see, therefore, that an animal poison may be developed of a highly contagious kind, the most minute portion of which, not more than would remain on the point of the finest needle, would establish the same series of pathological phenomena in a comparatively healthy tissue if transferred to it. Probably many of the pus-corpuscles found on the surface of the conjunctiva in a case of purulent ophthalmia do not result from the particle inoculated. Some, no doubt, are formed from the young bioplasts of conjunctival epithelium. There are, therefore, two kinds of bioplasm growing and multiplying at the same time, but so intermingled that it would not be possible to obtain particles of each kind separately.

In inflammation of the conjunctiva, not the least important of the phenomena is the dilatation of the vessels. Of the little arteries, many are dilated to three times their ordinary diameter, and the capillaries are also distended and choked with blood. Capillary vessels so small that hardly a single row of red blood-corpuscles would lie in them and quite invisible in the ordinary state, become so large in inflammation and are so filled with blood that through an ordinary lens they can be seen as distinct dark-red lines. The injection of the vessels may continue for many days and then pass off, or it may become chronic, when other pathological changes take place in consequence. The influence of the nerves and nerve-centre in these vascular changes has been already considered in page 235.

Treatment.—Inflammation of the conjunctiva requires to be carefully treated. It is undesirable to allow this inflammation to go on, especially in children, because it may reach a stage in which there is danger of damage, not only to that very important structure of the eye, the cornea, the clearness of which is essential to distinct vision, but, as before remarked, to the whole organ. Good hygienic conditions are essential in the treatment of the disease as it occurs in children; and it is very important to look for and relieve that preliminary state of inflammation and enlargement of the glands in the membrane, which almost invariably precedes an attack of purulent ophthalmia.

Many astringent substances are of use in the treatment of inflammation of the conjunctiva. These may be applied in various ways. In former days it was the practice to project a small quantity of some astringent powder on the surface of the inflamed conjunctiva, by placing a little of the powder in a quill or piece of straw and blowing it suddenly upon the eye, which was kept open for the moment. These powders were usually made of sugar and the potent substance, in the proportion of from ten parts or more of the former to one part of the latter, the whole being very finely powdered and carefully mixed. *Oxide of Zinc, Nitrate of Potash, Alum, Sulphate of Copper, Nitrate of Silver,* and other substances have been used in this way. But the practice is a bad one, and has been almost entirely abandoned in favor of solutions, which may be applied as drops or by using an eye-glass or an eye-fountain. Strong astringent applications should never be used except under proper advice, or serious damage to the eye may result.

Of Lotions and Eye Waters.—One of the best is a weak solution of Sulphate of Zinc, *Zinci Sulphas*, in water ; or, if you wish to order a more elegant lotion, in Rose Water, *Aqua Rosæ.* As regards the quantity, you may prescribe from a quarter of a grain to a grain to the ounce of water. A very dilute solution will often produce a favorable change in cases of mild inflammation of the conjunctiva, in a few hours. *Sugar of Lead, Plumbi Acetas, or Sulphate of Copper, Cupri Sulphas,* may be used in the same proportion as Sulphate of Zinc; but the latter and *Nitrate of Silver, Argenti Nitras,* are probably the most useful. Of the last, the proportion should be half a grain or less to an ounce of distilled water. If the eye is very painful, a grain of Opium or two or three drops of Laudanum, *Tinctura Opii,* to the ounce of water may be prescribed. In all cases the solution should be carefully filtered before it is applied. A lotion consisting of *Spirits of Wine, Spiritus Vini Rectificatus,* or good brandy, *Spiritus Vini Gallici,* in the proportion of one part to thirty or more parts of water, has also been recommended ; and where the vessels are dilated without any production of pus, the careful application of a weak spirit solution may be useful.

Lotions may be applied to the surface of the eye in two or three different ways. One of he best methods is to seat the patient in a chair and make him throw his head back. You then take a good-sized camel-hair brush which will take up two or three drops of the lotion, which may thus be caused to flow into the inner corner of the affected eye. Of course the patient will instinctively close the eye at the moment, but he must be encouraged to open the lids a little, so that some of the solution may pass in and the surface of the conjunctiva be thoroughly moistened by it in every part.

Another plan is to bathe the eye with an ordinary sponge or rag, but you must always be most careful that the particular sponge or rag is used for no other purpose whatever. Where there are several patients, each must have his own sponge, towel, etc., kept exclusively for his own use.

Another way of applying lotions to the conjunctiva is with the aid of an *Eye-glass.* This is a little glass made something like a small wineglass, the free edge being shaped so as to fit within the margin of the orbit. The eye-glass is half-filled with the lotion, and the patient is directed to hold the glass steadily against the eye, while the head is to be moved about in such a way as to cause the fluid to splash against the surface of the conjunctiva. The glass acts so as to keep the lids open, and in this way you ensure the lotion coming in contact with the surface of the mucous membrane. Lastly, there is the little *Eye-douche or Fountain*, by the aid of which a jet of lotion can be thrown against the eye. All these instruments may be obtained of surgical instrument makers.

Astringent lotions generally by their indirect action upon the nerves of the part, and by their direct action upon the particles of bioplasm which are growing and multiplying, favor the formation of the firm material, upon which the consistence and the protective character of the epithelium depends, and its subsequent condensation. Thus a " raw," or nearly raw, surface again gradually becomes protected with a layer of ordinary slow-growing epithelial tissue.

Sore Throat.—In an early lecture I have adverted to some of the changes which occur in sore throat, but in this place I shall consider one or two questions in connection with the subject which were then passed by. Most of us have suffered more or less from this affection. In the case of those who are susceptible, there frequently occurs a certain amount of congestion and inflammation in the mucous membrane of the fauces, and of the back of the pharynx. If you look at the palate in such a case, you will find it in very much the same state as I described when referring to the mucous membrane of the nose in an ordinary cold. Many of you will have opportunities of making the observation in your own persons. You may easily examine the fauces with the aid of an ordinary looking-glass. Instead of the membrane appearing moist, you will find it nearly dry, and perhaps you may see a piece of half-dry viscid mucus intimately adhering to it. The sensibility of the membrane is also affected. Although it feels sore, you will, however, find that it is less sensitive than in the normal state, while certain of its nerves do not respond so readily to a stimulus as they do in health.

If the throat is perfectly healthy, the process of swallowing, or deglutition, is easily performed, and almost unconsciously—at least without any great effort ; but if the throat is sore, deglutition becomes difficult, and you have to make a very decided effort, perhaps more than one, before the morsel of food can be successfully swallowed.

Then there is another fact of some importance with regard to the action of the mucous membrane. Not only are the nerves which are connected with the capillary vessels, and which are concerned in the sensation of pain and discomfort, obviously affected, but those which are instrumental in exciting by reflex action the contraction of the pharyngeal muscles. If, in the normal state of health, you tickle the soft palate ever so slightly with a feather, if the mucous membrane enjoys its proper sensitiveness, movements of deglutition almost instantly succeed. But if the throat is "sore," the mucous membrane red, and perhaps dry, you may tickle it very decidedly, and only feeble contraction will follow after an interval of time, or no contraction of the muscles will occur. In this action the muscular fibres fail to contract, because the nerve-fibres which carry impressions from the surface of the mucous membrane to the nerve-centre are deranged. Their action for the time being is prevented. There is, as it were, a peripheral paralysis. The motor nerve-fibres, the nerve-centre, and even the afferent trunks themselves, may be all right ; but the fine ramifications of the afferent fibres in the mucous membrane are so affected by the effusion in its substance and other changes, that they do not receive and transmit impressions.

When sore throat attacks persons who have for some time been in a low state of health, or exposed to adverse influences, as sometimes happens in the case of those resident in workhouses, hospitals, jails, and other places, it may run on very quickly to extensive superficial ulceration, which may affect the substance of the tonsil, and progress for several days. The fetid products resulting from the decomposition of the secretion taking place upon or near the ulcerated surface, are sometimes absorbed into the blood and occasion a form of blood-poisoning. If swallowed, the discharges give rise to much disturbance of digestion. It is, therefore, most important in the treatment of such cases to apply substances to the surface which have the effect of completely changing the organic matters and destroying the infecting material.

If Diphtheria exist in the neighborhood, persons in a low state of health, and those already suffering from sore throat, are very likely to take the disease, which sometimes runs its course so very quickly that life is in jeopardy in a few hours after the malady has declared itself, or even before there has been time for the formation of a false membrane, or for the development of any characteristic phenomena of the disease. It is, therefore, of the utmost consequence to very carefully watch cases of sore throat, especially when of an epidemic character. You should see the patient at intervals of a few hours, and you should give quinine and stimulants early, instead of waiting until the patient is very low. In some cases of what is called "hospital sore throat," as well as in Diphtheria, you will be surprised to find that persons may take in twenty-four hours from ten to thirty grains of quinine, and eight or ten ounces of brandy, divided into doses given every two hours, without any indication of the quantity of either remedy being excessive ; and it may be necessary to continue this treatment for many days, giving at the same time plenty of beef-tea or milk.

The Treatment of Sore Throat.—We are often consulted by patients who complain that they are almost constantly suffering from soreness of the throat. It is sometimes better, sometimes worse, but they will tell

you the throat always feels rough and uncomfortable.   Many local applications are of great use.   You may paint the fauces with a solution of
Nitrate of Silver, *Argenti Nitras*, but a stronger solution may be employed than was recommended for applying to the conjunctiva.   A
solution consisting of from five to ten grains to the ounce of distilled
water answers well, or you may employ a mixture of solution of Perchloride of Iron, *Liquor Ferri Perchloridi*, and an equal quantity of
glycerine, *Glycerinum*.   This mixture is very valuable in the treatment
of sore throat, whether it be mild or severe.   The glycerine causes the
Perchloride of Iron to adhere to the surface for a little time, and in that
way increases its beneficial effects.   In forms of sore throat in which
there is a quantity of viscid mucus, accompanied with excoriations or
ulcers on the palate or tonsils, the mixture may be applied every two
hours, or oftener.   The solution is a potent antiseptic, and destroys any
deleterious properties the secretion may possess.   By its application
efforts of vomiting are often excited, and thus much of the secretion is
got rid of.   I have successfully treated in this way many bad forms of
sore throat, which by some would be called "*diphtheritic.*"   The condition is associated with great depression of strength, and, as I have before
said, it is necessary to give quinine and wine or brandy in very decided
doses.   Any of the foul secretion swallowed by accident is rendered
innocuous by the action of the iron.   In this way stomach disturbance,
so apt to ensue in these cases, and which so much increases the risk to
life when it does occur, may be prevented.   Tannin dissolved in glycerine, *Glycerinum Acidi Tannici*, is also a good application.   In applying
such local remedies, whether a solution of Nitrate of Silver, or Glycerine
and Perchloride of Iron, or the Tannin, perhaps the following will prove
to be the best plan.   Take a good large camel's-hair brush, which must
be carefully tied to the end of a stick.   This latter point is important,
because if the brush is simply placed on the stick, it may, unfortunately,
fall off at a critical moment and be swallowed by the patient.   The
possibility of the occurrence of so awkward an accident may be thus
prevented.   The brush is to be thoroughly wetted with the application, and, a few drops being taken up in it, the wet brush is to be well
smeared over the surface of the affected mucous membrane.   After a
quarter of a minute the patient may be allowed to gargle with a little
cold water.

Although severe forms of sore throat cannot certainly be included
among "slight ailments," it is important that your attention should be
directed to the general treatment of the patient.   I have no doubt that
by judicious management many cases are prevented from assuming a
severe form.   If the patient gets low with a quick weak pulse, especially
if ulceration, which may be present, should be extending, and there is
infiltration of the tissues around the tonsils, it is necessary to give wine
or brandy and tonics, such as iron and quinine.   One is often surprised

at the large amount of supporting remedies required in some of these cases. In what used to be called "hospital sore throat," we often find it necessary to give six or eight five-grain doses of quinine in the four-and-twenty hours, and as much as twelve or more ounces of brandy during the same period, and this treatment may have to be maintained during several days.

Gargles.—Various gargles are used in the treatment of sore throat and an inflamed or aphthous (p. 70) state of the mucous membrane of the mouth. The influence of some of these is due to the presence of matter having astringent properties, while others depend for their efficacy upon some form of alcohol.

Port wine is an excellent gargle in cases of ordinary relaxed sore throat ; but some people do not like port or any other kind of wine, and in that case you may order a gargle consisting of one part of spirits of wine to four or five parts of water.

Alum used to be a favorite remedy, dissolved in a little water in the proportion of one drachm to six ounces.

A good gargle may be made by dissolving a drachm of Nitrate of Potash, *Potassæ Nitras*, or Chlorate of Potash, *Potassæ Chloras*, in six or eight ounces of water. An ounce of glycerine or honey may be added. Some like gargles made acid ; for this purpose you may order a drachm of Dilute Acetic, Phosphoric or Hydrochloric acid, to six or eight ounces of water.

Many persons derive benefit from the use of a stimulating gargle, which may be made by adding a little Cayenne pepper, or Tincture of Capsicum, *Tinctura Capsici*, in the proportion of one drachm or less to six ounces of gargle ; but this is not suitable in the case of a very sensitive, irritable mucous membrane, and, indeed, may do harm instead of good.

Common Salt is valuable as a gargle. A weak brine may be made by adding a dessert-spoonful of salt, or less, to half a pint of water. The throat may be gargled with this solution once in two or three hours. In ordering gargles, it is necessary to give the patient exact directions—to tell him to use the gargle frequently, for it is useless to gargle once or twice in the four-and-twenty hours. If the sore throat is at all severe, the gargle should be used once or twice in the hour.

Of exciting increased action in distant parts.—You may sometimes relieve a sore throat, as well as other forms of local inflammation and congestion, by causing increased action in other organs and tissues. The action of a purgative is often followed by the relief of the throat affection. Diuretics and sudorifics may be prescribed with the same object, and counter-irritation may be applied in some other part of the body. A mustard poultice to the neck, by establishing increased action on the cutaneous surface, often reduces the congestion of the mucous membrane of the throat. When slight, and not depending upon a general low state of the system, or altered blood, a sore throat may sometimes be cured in this way in a couple of hours.

Inflammation of the Mucous Membrane of the Air Passages.—Inflammation, as has been already remarked, very commonly affects the mucous membrane of the nose and all the cavities which open into it. There is increased secretion from all the glands and follicles opening upon the surface, increased formation of soft, moist, and imperfectly formed epithelium, taking the form of mucus, and undue turgescence of all the vessels. In consequence there is what is ordinarily called "running from the nose."

When the mucous membrane of the large bronchial tubes is inflamed, and consequently there is an increased formation of mucus on the surface, we have an ordinary catarrh, the phenomena of which have been already referred to. There is in these cases also congestion of the fauces, increased formation of mucus, and increased action of the glands. The transition from the ordinary epithelial cell to the viscid material known as mucus, and from the mucus-corpuscle to the pus-corpuscle, may be observed and studied. In cases in which the inflammation continues for a considerable time, instead of viscid transparent mucus being formed, we meet with ordinary pus, or pus mixed with mucus, which is known as *Muco-pus*, the microscopical characters of which must be carefully studied, as well as those of other kinds of sputum formed in different cases of disease.

What is termed false membrane, or croupous exudation, is frequently formed in cases of inflammation of the mucous membrane of the larynx, trachea, and bronchial tubes. I have seen cases in which a complete and firm membranous cast of these passages was formed on the surface of the mucous membrane, and was expelled entire after much suffering. The firm material consisted entirely of viscid mucus. Casts of the smaller bronchial tubes are also sometimes formed of mucus, but more commonly they will be found to consist of fibrinous material which has been poured out from the blood, and has coagulated in the air-tubes.

Running from the ears is common among children of what is called "a scrofulous habit of body." The epithelium of the meatus undergoes change, and becomes soft, the new epithelium being imperfectly formed, and superabundant. The vessels of the skin are also congested. After the disturbance has existed for some time, the discharge resembles that from an ulcerated surface. Not unfrequently the discharge dries up and forms a crust, which in consequence of the itching and irritation excited, is often picked off by the patient. A raw and very sore surface is exposed, and from this fresh discharge escapes, which in turn dries, and then follows a repetition of the process. The condition is often very obstinate and difficult to cure. In most instances constitutional treatment by iron and other tonics and cod-liver oil is absolutely requisite.

As the health improves, the discharge begins to diminish, and at last ceases altogether.

Inflammation of the Mucous Membrane of the Stomach and Intestinal Canal.—The mucous membrane of the stomach is very liable to conges- tion and inflammation, much more so, I think, than is generally supposed. From time to time these pathological changes probably affect small patches of mucous membrane, last for a time, and then pass off if the mucous membrane is soothed and allowed to rest from active work for a few days.

In all our best works on Medicine, the subject of Ulcer of the stomach is fully treated of, but there is a state of things allied to ulcer, and lead- ing to it, to which reference is seldom made. The state of mucous mem- brane to which I allude is not so serious as ulcer, but it is much more common, and, if not-relieved, may be succeeded by the formation of an ulcer. The mucous membrane of the stomach, like the nasal and bron- chial mucous membrane, "takes cold." It becomes red and less moist than in the normal state. There is often great discomfort and very fre- quently severe pain. The glands are more or less affected, and the func- tions of the stomach are very seriously disturbed. The secretion of gastric juice is interfered with and its qualities changed. Digestion is of course deranged, and sometimes completely checked. There may be much flatulence, which adds to the distress. Many patients, instead of allowing the stomach to rest for a while, are too prone to call for food when they experience any uneasiness. They feel exhausted, and think a good meat meal will certainly relieve their discomfort. This they take, and very soon find they have made a mistake, for their pain is increased. If they are fortunate, vomiting will be excited, and all that has been taken, with perhaps other matters already in the stomach, will be rejected, when considerable relief will be experienced. When you have reason to think that a patient is suffering from this slight inflammation, it is de- sirable to at once carry out measures for his relief, and effect a return to the healthy state as soon as possible, for the stomach is an organ whose work cannot be suspended for long at a time without the whole organism suffering. You order, therefore, nutritious, but unirritating, soft or liquid food for a while, and then take care that for the next few weeks only food of a soothing character, and which will be very easily digested, passes into the stomach. The patient must on no account be allowed to take ordinary diet, and you must tell him not to touch beer, and enjoin him not to take very cold or very hot liquids of any kind. Every form of alcohol should, as a general rule, be withheld, because in a great many instances alcohol only irritates, and sometimes greatly increases the pain. It may do much harm, though it must be admitted that not unfrequently it relieves for the moment the discomfort and sinking feeling which some- times distress the patient. For this reason it is imperative to be cautious in such cases. We ought never to give people any excuse for perma-

23

nently damaging their tissues, by acquiring the habit of taking too much alcohol.

The digestion of meat almost entirely depends upon the secretion formed by the stomach glands. When this secretion is temporarily deranged, it is better to allow the mucous membrane of the stomach to do as little work as possible. Meat and fish should, therefore, be withheld for a time. The patients should be put on a milk diet. You may order them to take bread and milk, or arrowroot and milk, or rice, sago, tapioca, maccaroni, vermicelli, and cooked in such a manner as to make a very soft moist food. By adopting this course, the patient applies something like a poultice to the disturbed mucous membrane of his stomach, and in many other cases, with great and immediate benefit. It does no one any harm to live on soft food of a farinaceous kind for a few days or a week. Indeed, not a few would gain in health if they systematically adopted such a diet for a week or two once in every two or three months. A very good substance to recommend patients to eat under these circumstances, only you will find many will refuse to eat it, is lentil flour, well boiled and made thick like gruel.

Any part of the mucous membrane of the small or large intestine may be affected by congestion and catarrhal inflammation. There are many cases in which there is severe pain " in the stomach," as the patient says, but which depends upon derangement of some part of the small or large intestine. The mucous membrane may be congested in patches, and the action of the follicles and of the villi for a time, becomes seriously disturbed. By taking care that only bland substances. and as little as possible of these, pass along the small intestine for a time, the mucous membrane will be soon restored to its normal state. It is important to check such disturbances as soon as possible. Though according to the patient himself, he may be suffering only from pain " in the stomach," —if he do not take complete rest, what is only a slight ailment may soon become a grave malady. In such cases, diet is of more consequence than medicine, but if the pain is very severe, it may be necessary to give small doses of sedatives. Advantage also results from employing mild counter-irritants over the belly. The best counter-irritant is a poultice made of half mustard and half linseed-meal. This may be applied to the surface, near the seat of pain, and it unquestionably relieves the inflammation. A mustard leaf is more easily prepared, but a piece of writing-paper should intervene between it and the skin, or the action will be too strong, and the patient will remove it before there has been time for the counter-irritant to have done good.

The external application of warmth greatly relieves pain which results from a congested or inflamed state of the mucous membrane of the intestinal canal. A linseed poultice, or flannels wrung out in hot water, will be of service. If, however, this does not soon afford relief, the surface of the poultice or the flannel may be sprinkled with turpentine. The thick India-rubber bottle for hot water should find a place in every traveller's trunk. It is most useful in the treatment of abdominal and other pain. I have already referred to it on p. 151.

Stimulating liniments are, as a general rule, not advisable. You do not want to move the bowels about in the least degree, or to disturb the parts at all. If you allow people to rub things in, the chances are they add to the sufferings of the patient, and do harm to tissues already tender and irritable, and in a state verging upon actual disease. This rubbing in of liniments is often adopted most injudiciously for every kind of pain, and you not unfrequently find a self-constituted and most self-confident medical adviser "rubbing away!" the pain of an inflamed joint. Many nurses and ladies having a turn for doctoring require to be cautioned on this head, for many conditions are made worse by rubbing, and in some instances very serious inflammation may be excited by the operation.

Congestion and inflammation of a portion of the mucous membrane of the large bowel is not uncommon. There is in such cases severe pain and the action of the bowel is much deranged. The condition may pass on to ulceration, which may endanger life. Ulcers frequently form in the lower part of the small intestines in cases of Typhoid fever, the healing of which is always a very slow process. Every case of Typhoid fever requires the most careful management and constant attention, not only at the time ulcers are forming and the sloughs separating, but during the healing process. Though this disease cannot be included among "slight ailments," it is very desirable that you should know that health is only very slowly restored, and that three months sometimes pass before a patient suffering from Typhoid can with safety be allowed to resume his usual diet and habits of life. All attempts to hasten convalescence are unwise, and every now and then a patient is lost in consequence. Full time must always be allowed for the healing of ulcers in any part of the alimentary canal.

There happens to be just now a case of mild dysentery under my care in the hospital. The man suffers much pain, and from the usual symptoms. He passes liquid motions with a good deal of mucus. In this case we are adopting, with the greatest benefit, a mode of treatment which may be considered "empirical," (ϵμπειρία, experience;) for, although the remedy employed is undoubtedly useful, we do not know precisely how it acts. Ipecacuanha powder is of the greatest value in many such cases—not only where there is actual ulceration of the mucous membrane of the colon, but where there is an approach or tendency to this condition. In India this drug is much used in the treatment of dysenteric affections. You may begin with doses of two or three grains of Ipecacuanha, in the form of a powder or pill, and you may increase the dose up to twenty grains or more, twice or three times a day; or five or ten grains may be given with a half a grain or less of opium, which will prevent its emetic action. Some persons cannot take opium, and in this case the Ipecacuanha must be given at first in small doses. The medicine may be continued until the symptoms are greatly relieved. In many cases the patient is completely cured in a month or six weeks.

If you desire to study the mode of action of an emetic in your own organism, there will be no harm in trying the experiment with this drug. You may take twenty grains of Ipecacuanha powder, *Pulvis Ipecacuanhæ* (not *Pulvis Ipecacuanhæ Compositus*), suspended in half a tumbler of warm or lukewarm water. The dose may be followed by one or two tumblers of warm water, and in the course of ten minutes or a quarter of an hour, you will have an opportunity of studying the violent contraction of the muscular coat of the stomach, which will be excited by reflex action consequent upon the irritating effect of the Ipecacuanha upon the afferent nerve-fibres of the mucous membrane of the organ. Ipecacuanha is one of the most potent, and in action one of the least disagreeable, of emetic remedies.

Congestion and inflammation occur in connection with other mucous membranes, as well as those to which I have specially drawn your attention. Thus, the gall-bladder and gall-ducts may suffer congestion, and inflammation of the mucous membrane of the urinary bladder, of the ureters, and of the pelvis of the kidney are unfortunately frequently met with, but these cannot, I regret to say, be classed among slight ailments, and they will come under our consideration in another part of the course.

Chilblains.—This troublesome and often very painful affection is due to local changes in the vessels of the skin of parts of the body most distant from the large vessels, notably the fingers and toes, and occasionally the ears and nose. These parts are more exposed to cold than the rest of the body, and to them the blood will be driven into the ramifications of the arteries with less force than elsewhere. Anything that retards the return of the blood towards the heart, such as the pressure on the superficial veins by tight gloves or shoes or garters, increases the tendency to chilblains. On the other hand, anything that promotes the circulation, large and easy boots and gloves lined with wash-leather or other warm material, may prevent their occurrence in persons predisposed to the malady.

Chilblains seldom occur in the adult, and they are far more common among ill-fed, weak children than among strong and healthy ones. Insufficient exercise, especially in the case of those, and in towns they are very numerous, who suffer from weak heart's action, sitting in cold rooms and sleeping in chilly bedrooms favor the development of chilblains, which are also encouraged by insufficient clothing. Warm woollen undergarments down to the wrists and ankles often prevent the occurrence of chilblains in those who have been subject to them. Exposure to cold, more especially when the vessels of the skin have been for some time previously subjected to pressure, is usually the immediate cause of an attack.

In the capillaries of the affected skin the blood flows slowly and remains too long in the vessels. The composition of the stagnant blood is probably altered by being too long exposed to the influence of cold, and in consequence does not flow onwards towards the veins. Soluble matters transude through the walls of the vessels, and the skin and subjacent textures in consequence become swollen. The afferent nerve-fibres running with the capillaries are necessarily affected, and their action becomes sluggish, and the muscular fibres encircling the minute arteries soon undergo relaxation. When the force of the heart's action becomes greater, and the activity of the circulation temporarily increased, as occurs after meals or when the patient gets warm in the evening or in bed, a rush of blood occurs to the extremities. The relaxed arteries and thin capillaries become greatly distended, the temperature of the part rising several degrees. The sensitive nerves at the same time being disturbed in such a way as to occasion the intense itching and discomfort experienced by the patient.

In some cases there is little or no itching, but, nevertheless, the congested state of the vessels, and consequent soddening of the tissues, may result in damage to the cuticle which may be raised in bullæ, which soon rupture, and the formation of troublesome sores, which heal very slowly, and add to the patient's suffering. In bad cases the skin around the vesicles becomes dark and soddened, and sloughs of considerable size may be formed, which often leave deep and bad ulcers, requiring a considerable time for healing.

Treatment.—Chilblains often give rise to very severe suffering, and are difficult to cure. Appearing to be a purely local affection, the disease is too often treated by purely local measures only. In a great many instances it will, however, be found that improvement in the general health and strength is followed by a cessation of the painful inflammation. Tonics, especially preparations of Bark and of Iron, should be given. One or two tablespoonfuls of wine daily often effect great improvement without any local treatment whatever, and if this plan is adopted early in the winter season, the subjects of chilblains will sometimes escape an attack.

Great care should be taken to clothe all children who are tortured with chilblains in woollen next the skin. The rooms in which they live should be well warmed in winter, and everything done to assist the weak and very likely slow circulation. Gradual cooling down is likely to do more harm in the case of those subject to chilblains than sudden exposure to cold for a short time only.

Local Treatment of Chilblains.—If the skin is not very tender, it may be painted with Tincture of Iodine, or very gently smeared with a lini-

23 *

ment composed of equal parts of Soap Liniment, *Linimentum Saponis*, and Tincture of Iodine, *Tinctura Iodi*. Smearing the inflamed skin with a little Turpentine, *Oleum Terebinthinæ*, or Acetic Acid, *Acidum Aceticum*, or the Liniment of Turpentine and Acetic Acid, *Linimentum Terebinthinæ Aceticum*, or Camphorated Spirit, *Spiritus Camphoræ*, undoubtedly much relieves the itching; but if the cuticle is tender or sore, such remedies do harm instead of good. In this case the tender part is to be painted over with several layers of Collodion, or the *Collodion flexile*, made of Collodion, Canada Balsam, and Castor-oil. In this way a sort of artificial cuticle is made, by which the tender parts beneath are protected until they recover their healthy condition, and time has been allowed for the formation of new cuticular cells beneath, and for the hardening process to be carried out by which the protective property of the cuticle is established. If the skin is actually broken, a small poultice is to be applied with or without some stimulating substance, such as Resin Ointment, *Unguentum Resinæ*, or Peruvian Balsam, *Balsamum Peruvianum*. The health must at the same time be well sustained by good food, wine, Quinine, and Cod-Liver Oil. When the sloughing process has ceased, a stimulating zinc lotion, one or two grains to an ounce of water, or carbolic acid lotion, or one part of absolute Phenol to forty parts of water, may be used, or Lister's antiseptic gauze may be applied.

Boils, although brought about by very different circumstances, some unimportant, others indicative of grave disease, may be fairly included among "slight ailments." The old name for boil is *Furunculus*.

This affection played a more formidable part during and anterior to the middle ages than since and than it does now. In former days many very serious and fatal febrile conditions were characterized by the formation of boils. Although in these days boils may be associated with certain forms of blood-poisoning, usually fatal, they are much more common in states of the system due to temporary derangement of the blood than they are in serious blood diseases which soon destroy life.

Pathologically the boil is of great interest, as the inflammation begins in one spot and quickly involves a number of tissues, including nerves, blood-vessels, and lymphatics, as well as all the textures forming the true skin. A small portion of the complex tissue is destroyed, in fact it dies, and is cast off as a slough of dead decomposing tissue, the removal of which is soon followed by the healing process.

The local inflammation thus ending in mortification and removal of a portion of the skin and subjacent structures, starts from within. It is difficult to decide whether the local change begins in a capillary or lymphatic vessel; but in most cases it is probably in the capillary, which is the seat of the changes which result in the formation of the boil. Particles, probably of living matter, adhere to the wall of the capillary, and grow and multiply until the vessel is occluded partly by accumulation of matter caused by the growth and multiplication of these tiny particles, and partly by fibrin from the blood. The capillary being thus plugged, exudation takes place from the adjacent capillary vessels; and with the fluid poured out minute particles of living matter also escape, and these multiply in the surrounding tissue. In this way the ordinary nutrition of the part suffers, and the usual flow of fluid to and from the living matter of the several tissues which takes place in health is stopped. The nerves of the capillaries and other parts are stretched and pressed upon in consequence, and considerable pain is experienced. The rapid growth and multiplication of living matter, which occurs in every part of the affected region, as usual is associated with the increased development of heat. The inflamed tissues constituting the boil are sensibly warmer than the surrounding healthy tissues.

A certain amount of pus is formed between the core of dead tissue and the surrounding healthy structures. By this process the disintegration of the affected tissues is assisted, and the separation of the slough of dead tissue from the surrounding healthy part is expedited.

Boils may be caused by a poison developed within the system or introduced into the blood from without. The inhalation of infected air, eating diseased meat, over-eating, insufficient and bad food, too much animal food, may establish a state of health favorable to the formation of boils. An actual alteration, no doubt, takes place in the blood, although it is not possible to determine its exact nature. Boils are liable to occur after recovery or partial recovery from fevers, and are very common in cases of diabetes; but the precise influence exerted by the diabetic state upon the tissue, which results in the development of the boil, has not yet been ascertained. The bites of mosquitos, if numerous, may occasion blood-poisoning and considerable derangement of the health, lasting for a considerable time, and ending in the formation of boils of an obstinate kind in different parts of the body.

Carbuncle, Anthrax, is closely allied to boils, but is more serious from the much larger area and depth of the inflamed tissue, and from the more serious constitutional disturbance. The inflammation is more diffused; the slough formed is often so very large that the patient's strength is exhausted before its separation is effected, and the reparative process can begin. This affection cannot properly be included among "slight ailments," and I therefore only refer to it as a farther development of the boil.

Treatment.—As regards the treatment of boils, the best advice I can give you is to leave them alone. Incisions are not needed, and any attempt to expedite the removal of the slough does harm by breaking down the temporary separation between the slough and the healthy tissue, thus causing some of the irritating discharge to pass into the surrounding areolar tissue, starting therein a similar inflammatory action leading to sloughing over a wider area. It is important, however, to prevent the boil from being rubbed or pressed upon by the clothes. A small piece of thick Amadou plaster-like felt may be taken, and a hole cut large enough to receive the boil, the summit of which may be partially covered by a piece of ordinary plaster. Yeast has been highly recommended internally, but its efficacy is doubtful. Quinine, mineral acids, and tonics of various kinds seem to be useful. Wine may be given in the case of patients whose strength has been worn out by prolonged exhausting disease, but in ordinary cases more harm than good results from stimulants.

It has been remarked several times, in these introductory lectures on Slight Ailments, that illnesses which apparently come on suddenly are themselves but the consequence of prior changes which have been going on for some time previous to the attack. These preliminary changes are a necessary and essential part of the illness, and, but for them, the attack could not have occurred. The invasion, it is true, *seems* to be sudden, but the apparently rapid passage from comparative health to decided illness is deceptive, for derangement even of a serious character has certainly existed for some time, though the patient may not have been aware of it. In many cases very great disturbance only gives rise to mere discomfort, and the patient himself can form no conception of the serious changes which are going on in his tissues. In not a few instances, especially persons about or past the middle period of life, the nerves are more or less numbed owing to structural changes in them. They do not respond as readily as they should do, and in consequence their owner does not experience the pain and discomfort which ought to warn him of the occurrence of derangement in action or alteration in structure.

By paying attention to the signs and symptoms of derangements which may be correctly termed slight, and relieving them as soon as possible, we may succeed in preventing the occurrence of grave pathological changes. You will remark that many persons who will tell you they do not know what it is to feel well, have not in the whole course of their lives once been seriously ill, and such lives you will often find will be exceptionally long. The nerves are sound, and their peripheral ramifications in a healthy and highly sensitive condition, so that the slightest change in their neighborhood is made evident to their owner by pain and discomfort, or by some form of nerve disturbance. The man who experiences slight derangements of health oftentimes takes steps to relieve his discomfort, and, by acting thus, very likely succeeds in removing the condition which precedes the development of actual disease. It is also probable that the very means taken to remove slight symptoms are also effective in bringing about a state of the system which is not favorable to the development of severe illness, or the invasion of morbid poisons. It would seem as if some preparatory changes were necessary to render the organism fitted either for the reception of morbid poisons, or for the initiation of the majority of morbid changes in tissues and organs. Even in the case of many purely local lesions it is probable that, for some considerable time before any actual structural change has occurred, there have been congestion and disturbed action. But for the persistence of these, the local disease would not have manifested itself. How important it is, therefore, that we should search for evidence of preliminary change, in order that, by altering the conditions of life for a time, by relieving local congestion, by promoting excretion, or by establishing some increased local action, we may succeed in bringing about a return to physiological health before any of those grave morbid conditions, which will occupy much of our attention in this course of lectures on the Principles and Practice of Medicine, can be established.

I have already drawn your attention to the preliminary changes which occur in the conjunctiva and glands connected with it, by which it becomes fitted for the reception and propagation of the minute particle of that specific and poisonous bioplasm which is concerned in the development of a most formidable and destructive kind of inflammation. Although, undoubtedly, there are a few living poisons which are so virulent in their properties, and have such extraordinary power of vitality that almost every one exposed to their influence is attacked with the disease they engender, this is so decidedly exceptional that one may fairly venture to advance the conclusion that it is at least conceivable that individual human or animal organisms may exist, upon which the great majority of contagious poisons known to invade might beat in vain. And, as time goes on, I think I shall convince you that the prospect of our being successful in discovering the means of enabling the individual organism to resist the assaults of contagion is far brighter than that of our discovering how to exterminate contagion itself, and to prevent new forms of contagious living matter from springing into life.

The poison instrumental in carrying ophthalmia undoubtedly spares some exposed to its influence, and, amongst those attacked, varying degrees of severity of the disease will be observed. Even ringworm, and many other diseases invariably associated with the growth and multiplication of a special vegetable organism, will not invade every individual indiscriminately, and those who have been long under bad influence as regards bodily health, are sure to be the first attacked, and to suffer most severely and for the longest time from the disease. Of a number of persons swallowing the poison of typhoid, or exposed for the same period of time to its baneful influence, some will escape altogether, some will be violently assaulted by the poison, but will escape without the specific disease being developed in consequence of a sharp attack of diarrhœa, some will pass through a mild form of the disease, and a small number will be severely attacked, of which perhaps one-eighth will be destroyed by the fever or its consequences.

S

So, too, with regard to acute inflammations and various diseases of a non-contagious character, what seems to be a sudden illness is probably but the climax of a series of changes which have been going on for a considerable time, although the patient may not have been aware that anything was wrong. An attack of acute rheumatism is always referred to exposure to wet and cold, or to sleeping in a damp bed, or to a long drive or walk in the rain, or to some single unfortunate circumstance or want of caution on the part of the patient. But how many of us are exposed, over and over again, to adverse conditions of precisely the same kind with perfect impunity. The peculiar state of the blood which precedes the attack of illness, and which alone renders the attack possible, has been produced after a prolonged course of pathological changes. But if this special state of blood exists not, instead of the person exposed to the adverse influences being attacked by acute rheumatism or pneumonia, or pleurisy, or some other acute inflammation, he experiences, perhaps, a sharp rigor, accompanied possibly by local pain and general discomfort, succeeded in two or three hours by profuse sweating, probably diarrhœa, and the secretion of urine rich in urates, uric acid, and other matters. In the course of a day or two, except feeling a little weak, the patient regains his normal state of health. Perhaps, indeed, for some time afterwards he may even feel exceptionally well and vigorous. He has, in fact, been relieved by the removal of various substances which had been for some time accumulating in his blood to his detriment, and which at any moment might have been instrumental in the development of local disease in some important organ. These considerations, supported by many more to which I might advert, suggest the general conclusion that the maintenance of each individual organism in a good state of health, the careful attention on the part of the practitioner to slight ailments, and the recognition by him of any symptoms that may indicate slight derangement of function or action, are of far greater consequence than the hunting after and extermination of various species of hypothetical pathological organisms, even though it were actually possible to catch and exterminate legions.

I believe that if the organism be in a proper state, almost all disease germs coming in contact with it, or entering it, will certainly die, instead of growing and multiplying and deranging or destroying important constituents of the blood and tissues. Many of the poisons in question are round about us—in the food we eat—in the water we drink. The foot of a fly will carry enough poisonous matter to infect a household. It is, therefore, vain to be always seeking to annihilate contagion which you can only destroy to a most limited and probably useless extent. On the other hand, it seems exceedingly reasonable, and especially on the part of nurses and ourselves, who must be continually exposed to the assaults of disease germs, to do all that is possible to promote and improve the resisting power of the body. We always notice that of those exposed to the same adverse conditions, but a very small percentage will be seriously ill. A moderate number only after suffering exposure will catch cold or experience some slight derangement. The majority will entirely escape. No doubt such facts may, in part, be explained on the supposition of the existence of difference in constitution in the different individuals. Allowing amply for this, however, there is good ground for concluding that it is possible to preserve the body in such a state of health as would enable it to resist attacks of contagious poisons, to any one of which, in a different condition, it would certainly succumb. In other words, there is good reason for the conclusion that it is possible to resist the onslaught of contagious poisons, and, therefore, that it is possible to still increase the health of the community. By detecting and treating slight derangements, I have no doubt whatever that we frequently succeed in establishing a state of the system which renders the supervention of serious disease almost impossible.

The comparative immunity of those who are frequently troubled with various slight derangements of health has been frequently noticed. Perhaps it is to be explained by the existence, in particular individuals, of a highly sensitive and exceptionally active state of those nerve-fibres, and that part of the nervous system which is intimately connected with the healthy action of the circulating and digestive systems. In some persons these nerves respond to the slighest stimulus, and the least departure from the ordinary state at once occasions inconvenience or discomfort ; while in others, considerable variation, as regards temperature, quality and quantity of food, make little or no impression, and occasion no immediate disturbance or derangement. But, in the latter case, pathological changes may take place, and may result in grave structural alteration, without the patient having experienced the least discomfort, or even being made aware that any departure from health had occurred in his system before the supervention of the serious illness which you are asked to investigate and treat. Perhaps, in some such manner, we may attempt to account for the fact that certain individuals are suddenly struck down by terrible disease while they seem to be in good health, and others, who never feel well, or look well, reach old age without experiencing one single attack of any illness so serious as to endanger life. Such persons, it must be noted, are often obliged to be very careful, as regards diet, and the feeling of tiredness, after great exertion, is in them so distinct that it must be yielded to. Thus they are forced to take rest before any damage whatever has been done to their organs. It is not probable that careful attention to the process of excretion, as well as to the quality and quantity of food that is taken, brings about and preserves a state of blood in which disease germs, instead of growing and multiplying, would die? How many ailments may not be prevented by judicious starving, or by living for a day or two now and then on low diet? How thoroughly may not the blood be depurated by a sharp purge given, perhaps, just before *liquor sanguinis* was about to escape from the vessels, to be poured, perhaps, into the air-cells of the lung? Might not the purgation be fairly considered to have prevented an impending attack of acute Pneumonia or Inflammation of the Lung, and thus to have really "cut short" the disease? May not moderate doses of Bicarbonate of Potash or Soda, taken in solution twice or three times a day for a week or two, avert an attack of acute rheumatism? Will not a small dose of certain preparations of Mercury, now and then, prevent attacks of gout or rheumatism or sick headache or dyspepsia or biliousness? Is it not reasonable to conclude that certain salts, by their action on the bowels and kidneys, by promoting free elimination, establish a general state of the tissues, which may for the time render it impossible that certain morbid changes of serious consequence should occur?

I have endeavored, in these few lectures, to show you why we should not fail to devote some attention to the study of those slight departures from the normal state which possibly, in these days, are sometimes passed over by the practitioner, although, on the one hand, their import may be strangely exaggerated, or, on the other, hardly noticed by the patient himself. As I have tried to impress upon you many times, slight derangements sometimes afford the first and only indications of commencing disease of a serious character. There is good reason for thinking that by judicious management, not only may some troublesome though slight ailments be entirely relieved, but further and progressive morbid changes may be prevented or retarded.

The principles upon which the treatment of many slight ailments may be successfully conducted, are the same as those upon which the management of more marked developments of morbid phenomena is based. I have given illustrations of the simplest and slightest ailments, and have endeavored to show how their treatment may be most simply and successfully carried out, and I have attempted to lead you on by degrees to consider more highly complex pathological changes, and to explain the principles upon which more complex methods of treatment are based. In no way, I believe, can you so quickly acquire that sound knowledge of pathological processes, and of the means of checking or modifying them, which are daily required in practice, as by adopting the course I have advocated. Let me, therefore, conclude by again impressing upon you the importance of not neglecting the study of the nature and treatment of "Slight Ailments" now, or at any period of your professional career.

INDEX.

ABSORPTION of fluid in constipation, 117.
Acid application to liver, 167.
—— drinks in sick headache, 179.
—— eructations, 147.
—— of the stomach, 95.
Action, increased, its effects in treatment, 253.
Acute Jaundice, 166.
Afferent nerves of capillaries, 235.
Ague fit, 212.
Ailments beginning like a cold, 203.
Air-passages, inflammation of, 264.
Albuminous matters, effects of alcohol on, 256.
Alcohol, bad effects of, 81.
—— causing vertigo, 156.
—— in dyspepsia, 81.
—— its use in the treatment of fissures and ulcerations, 255.
Alkalies in rheumatism, 198.
Aloes in cases of offensive breath, 74.
—— preparations of, in constipation, 138.
Alum as a gargle, 263.
—— spray in sore throat, 69.
Ammonia, chloride of, 191.
Amœba, 251.
Anæmia, state of tongue in, 62.
Anorexia, 75.
Anthrax, 271.
Appetite, impaired, 75.
—— voracious, 77.
Apples in constipation, 128.
Aphthæ, 70.
Ardor ventriculi, 90.
Area of redness in flea-bite, 225.
Arsenic, 191.
Arteries, alteration of, in flea-bite, 225.
Artery with nerve-fibres distributed to it, 227, 230.
Artificial teeth, value in dyspepsia, 101.
Ascarides, 154.
Ascaris lumbricoides, 154.
Astringents in ophthalmia, 260.
—— in the treatment of diarrhœa, 151.
—— in the treatment of piles, 122.
Aural vertigo, 157.

BACTERIA in blood in health, 50.
—— as a cause of disease, 51.
—— in intestine of infant, 49.
Balsam, Peruvian, 270.
Baptistin, 163.

Bat's wing, nerves to, 233.
Beef-tea, peptonized, 109.
Bilious diarrhœa, 150.
Biliousness, 157.
—— treatment of, 161.
Bioplasm changes in outside capillaries, 247.
—— growth of, in inflammation, 222.
—— minute particles in blood, 245.
Bite, flea, 222.
—— gnat, 237.
Black tongue, 64.
Blood in fever and inflammation, 221.
—— filaria in, 144.
—— in constipation, 121.
—— passing through vessels in fever, 222.
—— state of, in sick headache, 171.
Blue pill in biliousness, 161.
Body-heat in fever, 222.
—— in man and animals, 206.
Borax and honey for thrush, 71.
Borborygmi, 93.
Brain, overworking, 188.
—— and stomach, 155.
Bread, 127.
Breath, odor of, 72.
Bright red tongue, 63.
Bromide of potassium in rheumatism, 199.
Bronchitis kettle, 68.
Brow ague, 168.
Brown bread, 113, 127.
Bulimia, 78.

CÆCUM affected in sick headache, 171.
Calibre of small artery, maintenance of, at a given point, 227.
Calomel in dyspepsia, 93.
—— effect on secretion of saliva, 61.
Camphorated spirits in the treatment of chilblains, 270.
Capillaries in flea-bite, 225.
—— in inflammation, 222.
—— passage of corpuscles through wall; of, 240.
Capillary hæmorrhage, 224.
—— capillary vessels, nerves of, 230.
Carbolic acid as a gargle, 69.
—— in cases of offensive breath, 73.
Carbuncle, 271.
Cardialgia, 90.
Carlsbad water, 143.
Castor-oil for constipation, 135.
—— for diarrhœa, 146.

Catarrh, 214.

Catarrhal inflammation of stomach, 266.

Catching cold, 202.

Catechu, 151.

Cayenne pepper in nausea, 86.

Cells, changes in epithelial, in a flea-bite, 222.

—— of liver in biliousness, 160.

Chaff, 113.

Chalk mixture, 152.

Changes, minute, in fever and inflammation, 219.

Charcoal powder in cases of offensive breath, 72, 73.

Cheltenham water, 142.

Chilblains, 268.

Children, constipation in, 120.

—— high temperature in slight ailments, 217.

Chlorate of potash in sore throat, 69.

—— as a gargle, 263.

Chloride of sodium in sore throat, 69.

Chloral hydrate, 192.

—— its dangers, 186.

Chlorodyne, 94.

Cholera, 145, 211.

Chronic rheumatism, treatment of, 196.

Citrate of magnesia, 143.

Circulation, intermolecular, 39.

—— capillary, mechanism for governing, 232.

Civilization, slight ailments, 18.

Clothing, warm, importance of, 99.

Cleaning of tongue, 65.

Clinical thermometer, 209.

Clyster, 123.

Coffee in constipation, 128, 135.

COHNHEIM, on migration of blood corpuscles, 243.

Cold bath in constipation, 125.

—— catching, 202.

—— causing a febrile attack, 221.

—— influence of, on blood and tissues, 221.

—— its influence in diarrhœa, 149.

—— sick headache, 178.

—— stage in fever, 210.

—— treated by counter-irritation, 253.

—— treatment of a, 214.

Collodion, 270.

Colon, tenderness of, 149.

Color of the tongue, 42.

Complexion in those who suffer from constipation, 118.

Condiments, 97.

CONDY'S fluid, gargle of, 65.

—— in offensive breath, 73.

Congestion of capillaries in flea-bite, 224.

—— of mucous membrane of bowel, 267.

Conjunctiva, inflammation of, 256.

Connective-tissue formed by bioplasm, 247.

Constipation, 111.

—— in jaundice, 165.

—— in sick headache, 171.

—— treatment of, 109, 131.

Contagion, 275.

Contagious disease, 46.

Contractile power of bowel, loss of, 116.

Contraction of minute arteries, 228.

Co-ordinating power in vertigo, 156.

Corpuscles, mucus, 250.

—— blood, passage through vascular walls, 241.

—— outside capillaries in inflammation, 244.

Coryza, 214.

Counter-irritation, 253.

—— in sick headache, 178.

—— in stomach, 266.

Cracks and fissures of tongue, 65.

—— on lips, 254.

Critics subject to constipation, 115.

Croakings, flatulent, 93.

Croton-chloral-hydrate, 192.

—— oil in constipation, 140.

Croupous membrane, 264.

Curry powder in nausea, 80.

—— in dyspepsia, 97.

DEATH-carrying bacteria, 54.

Decay, part played in by fungi, 44.

Decillionths of grains, 29.

Degeneration of muscles in rheumatism, 196.

Demonstrating nerves distributed to capillaries, 232.

Deranged action of glandular organs, 89.

Diabetes, 77.

—— causing boils, 271.

Diagnosis, importance of being cautious in making, 217.

Diapedesis, 240, 243.

Diarrhœa, 144.

—— treatment of, 151.

Diathesis, 76.

Diet in constipation, 117.

—— in rheumatism, 211.

—— in diarrhœa, 150.

—— in hot and cold climates, 98.

—— in indigestion, 93.

Digestion, artificial, 109.

—— in jaundice, 167.

—— non-nutritious matters in, 113.

—— in rheumatism, 205.

Digestion in sick headache, 169.

Dilatation of capillary vessels in fever and inflammation, 222, 232.

Diluents in a cold, 218.

Diphtheria, 261.

Disease germs, 275.

Disks for hypodermic injection, 192.

Dispensaries, self-supporting, 35.

Dissection of nerves of intestines, 87.

Diuretics in a cold, 215.

Dorsum of tongue, 43.

Douche, eye, 260.

Dover's powder, 191.

Dried apples in constipation, 129.

Drowsiness, 184.

Dry mouth and fauces, 67.

Dry tongue, 58.
—— brown tongue, 63.
Dust and disease, 50.
Dysentery, 267.
Dyspepsia, 84
—— treatment of, 94.

EAST wind causing biliousness, 162.
Eau de Cologne in treatment of cracks and fissures of lips, 255.
Efferent nerves to arteries, 236.
Effervescing citrate of magnesia, 143
—— saline purgatives, 143.
Elaterium in constipation, 140.
Emetics, 92, 268.
Empirical treatment, 267.
Endurance, powers of, in sufferers from sick headache, 172.
Enemata, action of, 123.
Epilepsy and sick headache, 174.
Epithelial cells of tongue, 43, 44, 45.
Epithelium, irregular growth of, 254.
—— pus formed in, 224.
Epsom salts, 141.
Eructations, acid, 147.
Eruption in fever, 221.
Eruptions, 252.
Examining mucus-corpuscle, 249.
Excess of urea, 208.
Excoriations, treatment of, 255.
Excretion, importance of, 204.
Exercise in constipation, 125.
External applications in indigestion, 96.
Exudation, 241.
—— in fever and inflammation, 222.
—— in rheumatism, 195.
Eye-glass, 259.
Eye waters, 259.

FÆCAL matter, impaction of, 116.
False membrane, 264.
Fasting girls, 77.
Fauces, dryness of, 67.
Febrile diseases, 203.
Fever, local, 222.
—— and inflammation, 207, 219.
Feverish and inflammatory state, 202.
Feverishness produced by irritation of stomach, 146.
Feverishness, secretion in, 213.
Fevers, formation of pus in, 239.
Fibrin, bacteria in, 50.
Fibrous matter, formed from bioplasts, 247.
Filaria sanguinis hominis, 238.
Filiform papillæ, 43.
Fissures and cracks of tongue, 65.
Flannel for warm clothing, 99.
Flatulence, 92.
Flea-bite, 222.
Fluid, quantity of, to be taken, 83.
—— importance of taking, in constipation, 117, 129.
Fog, its effects on conjunctiva, 256.
Food, abstention from, in sick headache, 177.

Food, importance of not taking too much, 19, 79.
Fountain, eye, 260.
FOWLER, DR., his case of the fasting girl, 77.
Friedrichshall water, 142.
Fruit causing diarrhœa, 145.
—— in constipation, 128.
Fungi, germs of, 45.
—— growth and multiplication of, 45.
—— on tongue, 44.
Fungiform papillæ, 43.
Furred tongue, 61.
Furunculus, 270.

GALL stones, 166.
Gamboge, 140.
Ganglia, 89.
—— regulating calibre of small arteries 227.
Gargles, 263.
Gastric glands, nerves of, 87.
Gastralgia, 89.
Gastric juice, variation in quantity of, 57.
Gastrodynia, 89.
General changes from local injury, 237.
Germs of fungi, 44
—— in every part of body, 48.
—— on tongue, 44.
Giddiness, 154.
Glands of conjunctiva, inflamed, 257.
—— exciting action of, in offensive breath, 73.
—— gastric, wasting of, 100.
Glauber salts, 141.
Glycerine and water, 64.
Gnat-bite, changes resulting from, 237.
Gout and sick headache, 174.
Granulated effervescing salines, 143.
Gravedo, 214.
Gray powder, 61, 70, 102, 167, 176.
Growth of fungi, 47.
Guarana in sick headache, 181.
Guiacum in rheumatism, 199.

HÆMORRHAGE, 65.
—— capillary, 224.
Hæmorrhoids or piles, 120.
Hair-like processes of papillæ of tongue, 44.
HALLIER on fungi, 53.
Headache, treatment of, 175.
—— sick, 167.
Healing process disturbed in constipation, 119.
Healthy individuals rare, 19.
Heartburn, 90.
Heat of body, 206.
—— in fever, 206.
Hemicrania, 168.
Homœopaths, 28.
Honey and borax in aphthæ, 71.
Horse radish, 60.
Hospital, out-patients, 36.
Hot climates, diet in, 97.

Hot stage in fever, 210.
—— water, India-rubber bottle for, 151.
Humbug, medical, 26.
Hunyadi Janos water, 143.
Hydrocyanic acid in nausea, 85.
Hygienic treatment of constipation, 125.
Hypodermic injection, 186, 191.
Hyposulphite of soda, 65.
Hydrochloric acid, external application of, to liver, 167.
Hydrocyanic acid, its effects, 24.
Hyla, nerve-cells of, 228.
—— artery of, 228.
Hysterical loss of appetite, 76.

IMMUNITY to severe disease of those suffering from slight ailments, 275.
Impaction of fæcal matter, 116.
India-rubber bottle for hot water, 151.
Indian corn flour, 127.
Indigestion, 84.
—— in old age, 100.
—— resulting from loss of teeth, 100.
—— treatment of, 94.
—— warm clothing in, 100.
Infant, growth of fungi in intestine of, 49.
Infantile diarrhœa, treatment of, 146.
Ingluvin, 108.
Inflammation, 202, 219.
—— heat of blood in, 207.
—— minute particles of bioplasm passing through vessels, 247.
—— slight, 248.
Inhalers, 68.
Injection, 123.
—— hypodermic, 192.
Injury in case of a flea-bite, 226.
Intercostal muscles, pain in, 194.
Intermolecular circulation, 39.
Intestinal canal, ganglia and nerves of, 228.
—— nerves of, 86.
—— inflammation of, 265.
—— worms, 152.
Iodide of potassium in cracks of tongue, 66.
—— in rheumatism, 199.
Iodine in chilblains, 269.
Ipecacuanha as an emetic, 92.
—— in ulcers of colon, 267.
Iron, its influence in darkening the motions, 150.
—— tincture of, in sore throat, 262.
—— muriated tincture of, in thrush, 71.
—— in neuralgia, 191.
Irritability in biliousness, 158.
—— of dyspeptic persons, 94.
Irritation of mucous membrane, 253.
—— of stomach causing diarrhœa, 145.
Issue, 254.
Itching in chilblains, 269.

JALAP in constipation, 136.
Jaundice, 163.
Joints, state of, in rheumatism, 195.
Juglandin, 163.

KETTLE, bronchitis, 68.
Kino, 151.
Kneading the bowels, 127.
Krameria, 151.

LARGE intestine deranged in sick headache, 171.
Lavement, 123.
Leaves, fungi of, 46.
Lemon-juice when mouth dry, 60.
Lentils, 266.
Leptothrix buccalis, 45.
Licorice powder, compound, in constipation, 137.
Lime-water in diarrhœa, 147.
Liquid taken, its influence on action of bowels, 117.
Liquor sanguinis, 241.
—— bioplasm in, 222.
Lips, vascularity of, 255.
Literary men, constipation of, 115.
Liver, its deranged action in biliousness, 160.
—— exciting action of, in offensive breath, 73.
—— in sick headache, 171.
Living matter, changes in, 247.
—— particles, passage of, through vessels, 241.
Local injury, vascular disturbances from, 237.
Logwood, 151.
Loss of appetite, 76.
Lotion for eyes, 260.
Lozenges, bismuth, in dyspepsia, 96.
Lumbago, 194.
Lungs, capillary hæmorrhage from the, 241.

MANAGEMENT of patients, 21.
Manson, Dr., on filaria, 238.
Mastication, defects of, 100.
Materies morbi, 54.
Meat in inflamed mucous membrane of stomach, 266.
—— little required by bilious people, 161.
—— too much, 98.
Mechanism for governing calibre of arteries, 232.
—— for regulating capillary circulation, 232.
Ménière's disease, 157.
Mercury in sick headache, 175.
—— its use in offensive breath, 74.
Metallic taste in mouth, 70.
Micrococci, 45.
Microscopic ganglia, 70.
—— observation, 38.
Mildew, vital phenomena of, 246.
Milk and lime-water, 147.
Mind in sick headache, 170.
Mindererus, 215.
Misery and despair in biliousness, 159.
Moist application to bowels in constipation, 120.

Molecular circulation, 39.
Morphia, its influence on the circulation, 238.
Mortification, 223.
—— following boils, 270.
Movements of mucus-corpuscles, 250.
—— vital, 223.
Mouth, aphthæ in, 70.
—— dryness of, 58.
Muco-pus, 264.
Mucous membrane, inflamed, 249, 264.
—— of stomach, inflamed, 265.
Mucus corpuscle, 250.
—— evacuations, 148.
—— formation of, 250.
—— of pig's stomach as pepsine, 105.
—— secreted in a cold, 253.
Muscular fibre cells of intestine, 86.
—— of small artery, 227, 235.
—— rheumatism, 195.
Mustard as an emetic, 92.
—— leaf, mode of using, 266.
Myrrh, tincture of, in cases of offensive breath, 73.

NARES, dryness of, 67.
Natural history of disease, 37.
Nausea, 79.
—— in sick headache, 168.
Nerve, action of, determining calibre of arteries, 227.
—— cells and fibres governing capillary circulation, 228.
—— circuit, 236.
—— derangement in sick headache, 173.
—— disorders, relation of fever to, 220.
—— disturbance in chilblains, 269.
—— fibres concerned in pain, 251.
—— eruptions in course of, 252.
—— of stomach and intestine, 85.
—— storms, 174.
Nerves of digestive system, 55.
—— to capillary vessels, 230.
—— and ganglia, stomach, 85.
—— of hyla, 228.
—— of intestinal canal, 86.
Nervous excitement producing diarrhœa, 144.
Nervousness, 187.
Neuralgia, 189.
—— treatment of, 190.
Neuralgia and gouty affections, and sick headache, 174.
Nitrate of silver in sore throat, 68.
—— in treating sores on lips, 256.
Nose, hæmorrhage from, 243.
Nucleus of a cell, 250.
Nutritive matters, 113.
Nux vomica in constipation, 137.

OATMEAL in constipation, 113, 127.
Odor of the breath, 72.
Offensive breath, 72.
Oidium albicans, 45.

Old age, accumulation of fæcal matter in, 116.
—— indigestion in, 100.
Olive oil, 146.
Oozing of blood from capillaries, 241.
Operation, fever after, treatment of, 119.
Ophthalmia, 257.
—— poison of, 273.
Opium in diarrhœa, 152.
—— homœopathic doses, 28.
Ostrich-pepsine, 107.
Outgrowths from bioplasm, 247.
Out-patient department of hospitals, 35.
Over-sensitiveness in sick headache, 173.
Oxidation not increased in fever and in flammation, 207, 222.

PAIN, 85,
—— conducting nerve-fibres, 88.
—— nerve-fibre concerned in, 151.
—— neuralgic, 190.
—— pleuritic, 252.
—— in the stomach, 266.
—— rheumatic, 193, 197.
Palate, soft, dryness of, 67.
Papillæ of tongue, filiform, and fungiform, 43.
Paralyzing action of nerve-centres and fibres, 236.
Pathological changes, nature of, 52.
Peculiarity of dress, 28.
Pepsine, and its uses, 102.
—— of the pig, 105.
—— of the ostrich, 107.
Peptones, 110.
Pericarditis, pain in, 88.
Periodical sick headaches, 173.
Peripheral paralysis, 261.
Peritonitis, 88.
Perspiration, free, in rheumatism, 197.
Peruvian balsam, 270.
Petechiæ, 224.
Pharynx, changes in mucous membrane, of, 68.
Phosphate of soda, 142.
Physical views of vital action, 246.
Phytolaccin, 163.
Pig, pepsine of, 105.
Piles or hæmorrhoids, 120.
Pleurisy, pain in, 89, 251.
Plexuses, nerve, 87.
Pneumonia, 274.
—— increased oxidation in, 208.
Podophyllin in constipation, 139.
Poison of disease, 274.
Pork, its dethronement in America, 189.
Port wine as a gargle, 263.
Poultice, its use in treatment of ulcer of stomach, 266.
—— in dyspepsia, 97.
Preliminary changes in febrile attacks, 204.
—— various diseases, 273.
Pressure in causing chilblains, 268.

Principles of treatment of slight and severe ailments, 35.
Prescribing, 36.
Prunes in constipation, 128.
Prussic acid in nausea, 83.
Pullna water, 142.
Purgative enemata, 123.
Purgatives in cases of offensive breath, 74.
—— in a cold, 215.
—— in constipation, 131.
—— in indigestion, 93.
Pus from bioplasm of epithelium, 223.
—— corpuscles, formation of, 223.
—— in boils, 271.
—— not altered blood-corpuscles, 240.
—— formation of, in and near capillaries, 239.
Putrid fluids, bacteria in, 47.
Pyrethrum, 60.
Pyrosis, 90.

QUACKERY, 27.
—— its consequences, 32.
Quinine, action of, 40.

RASH in fever, 220.
Reabsorption of fluids from intestine, 117.
Rectum, bleeding from the, 243.
Redness of skin in fever, 220.
—— in flea bite, 224.
Regularity of action, importance of, 96.
Reputation of quacks, 33.
Rest, importance of, 57.
—— in sick headache, 177.
—— importance of, in treatment, 266.
Restlessness, 185.
Rhatamy, tincture of, 152.
Rheumatic pains, 193.
Rheumatism, tongue in, 61.
—— causes of, 274.
—— treatment of, 196.
Rhubarb in constipation, 132, 135.
Rigors, 210.
Rubbing in constipation, 126.
—— in liniments, 267.
Running from the ear, 264.
Rochelle salts, 142.

SALICINE, 191.
Saline purgatives in constipation, 140.
Salines, action of, 57.
Saliva, exciting flow of, 60.
Salt as a gargle, 263.
Santonin, 154.
Sarcina ventriculi, 45.
Scammony in constipation, 137.
Scarlet fever, rash in, 220.
Scepticism, 31.
Scrofulous children, ophthalmia in, 257.
Sea-side causing biliousness, 163.
Secretion, free, 213.
—— importance of, in preventing illness, 273.

Self-supporting dispensaries, 35.
Senses disturbed in sick headache, 173.
Sensitiveness of inflamed mucous membrane, 251.
—— of peritoneum, 88.
Serious diseases, 36.
Serous membranes, pain in, when inflamed, 88.
Shampooing in rheumatism, 197.
Shrinking of muscles in rheumatism, 195.
Shivering and rigors, 203.
Sialogues, 60.
Sick headache, 167.
—— treatment of, 175.
Slight inflammation, 248.
Smoking as a remedy for constipation, 131.
Sordes, 64.
Sore on lips, 254.
—— on mouth, 70.
—— throat, 260.
—— state of mucous membrane in, 252.
Spirit of Mindererus, 215.
Spray in treating sore throat, 68.
Starving in sick headache, 177.
Steel, tincture of, 71.
Stings or bites of gnats, 237.
Stimulants in sick headache, 173, 176.
Stomach, derangement of, in sick headache, 170.
—— poulticing the, 266.
—— acids of, 91.
—— capillary hæmorrhage from the, 244.
—— fungi in, 48.
—— irritation of, producing fever, 146.
—— of pig, 105.
—— ulcer of, 265.
—— wind in the, 92.
Sudden illness, 274.
Sulphate of magnesia and soda, 141.
Sulphurous acid gargle, 65.
Swallowing, 260.
Sweating in rheumatism, 200.
—— stage in fever, 210.
Sycophants, 27.
Sympathetic system, nerves of, 86.
Syringes for injections, 124.

TACT and treatment, 25.
Tannic acid, glycerine of, in sore throat, 68.
Tannin, use in sore throat, 262.
Tapeworm, 154.
Tartar emetic, 80.
Tartrate of soda and potash, 142.
Taste, metallic, in the mouth, 70.
Tasteless salt, 141.
Tea-drinking in sick headache, 179.
Tectotalism, 82.
Teeth, loss of, causing dyspepsia, 100.
Temperature of body, ascertaining, 209.
—— rise of, in febrile states, 206.
Temporary jaundice, 164.
Tendons in rheumatism, 195.
Thermometer, use of, 209.

Thickening and condensation of connective tissue, 247.

Thirst, 83.

Thought in sick headache, 170.

Threadworms, 153.

Thrush, 70.

Tissues, changes of, in inflammation, 219.

Tobacco, a cause of vertigo, 156.

Tobacco-smoking in constipation, 131.

Tongue, 42.

—— cracks and fissures of, 65.

—— dry and moist, 58.

—— in various derangements, 55.

—— in vegetable organisms on, 45.

Tonics, in chilblains, 269.

Toothache, 190.

Trades, constipation dependent on various, 114.

Transudation of fluid through vessels, 145.

Treatment of aphthæ, 71.

—— of boils, 271.

—— of chilblains, 269.

—— of a cold, 214.

—— of drowsiness, 185.

—— empirical, 267.

—— of inflamed mucous membrane, 255.

—— of rheumatism, 196.

—— of sick headache, 175.

—— of slight ailments, principles of, 36.

—— of sore throat, 261.

Turkish bath in rheumatism, 197.

Turpentine in chilblains, 270.

ULCER of bowel, 267.

—— of stomach, 265.

—— in mouth, 70.

—— of mucous membrane, 249.

Urea, excess of, in fever, 208.

Urine in sick headache, 173.

VALLISNERIA, bioplasm of cells of, 245.

—— cells of leaf of, 47.

Vapor-bath in rheumatism, 197.

Vascular disturbance resulting from local injury, 237.

Veins, state of, in hæmorrhoids, 121.

Vertigo, 154.

Vessels in fever and inflammation, 220.

Villi, nerves of, 87.

Virulent pus-corpuscles, 257.

Vital movements, 250.

Vomiting, 80.

—— in sick headache, 168, 180.

Voracious appetite, 77.

Vulgarity of manner, 28.

WAKEFULNESS, 185.

Warm-blooded animals, 206.

Warm clothing, importance of, 99, 202.

Warmth, importance of, 149, 151, 202.

—— chilblains treated by, 268.

—— in sick headache, 178.

—— in treating pain in the stomach, 266.

Wasting of muscles in rheumatism, 195.

Water in treating biliousness, 162.

Waterbrash, 90.

Weakness as a consequence of dyspepsia, 102.

White moist furred tongue, 61.

Wind in the stomach, 92.

Woollen clothing, importance of, 99.

Worms, intestinal, 152.

Wounds do not heal in constipation, 119.

—— not healing in sick headache, 170.

YAWNING in sick headache, 169.

Yeast in treating boils, 272.

Yellow atrophy of liver, 166.

THE END.

| CATALOGUE
No. 1. | | JANUARY 1898. |

CATALOGUE

OF

MEDICAL, DENTAL,

Pharmaceutical, and Scientific Publications,

WITH A SUBJECT INDEX,

OF ALL BOOKS PUBLISHED BY

P. BLAKISTON, SON & CO.

(SUCCESSORS TO LINDSAY & BLAKISTON),

PUBLISHERS, IMPORTERS, AND BOOKSELLERS,

1012 WALNUT ST., PHILADELPHIA.

SPECIAL NOTE.

The prices as given in this catalogue are absolutely net, no discount will be allowed retail purchasers under any consideration. This rule has been established in order that everyone will be treated alike, a general reduction in former prices having been made to meet previous retail discounts. Upon receipt of the advertised price any book will be forwarded by mail or express, all charges prepaid.

We keep a large stock of Miscellaneous Books relating to Medicine and Allied Sciences, published in this country and abroad. Inquiries in regard to prices, date of edition, etc., will receive prompt attention.

The following Catalogues sent free upon application:—

CATALOGUE No. 1.—A complete list of the titles of all our publications on Medicine, Dentistry, Pharmacy, and Allied Sciences, with Classified Index.

CATALOGUE No. 2.—Medical Books. Illustrated with portraits of prominent authors and figures from special books.

CATALOGUE No. 3.—Pharmaceutical Books.

CATALOGUE No. 4.—Books on Chemistry and Technology.

CATALOGUE No. 5.—Books for Nurses and Lay Readers.

CATALOGUE No. 6.—Books on Dentistry and Books used by Dental Students.

CATALOGUE No. 7.—Books on Hygiene and Sanitary Science; Including Water and Milk Analysis, Microscopy, Physical Education, Hospitals, etc.

SPECIAL CIRCULARS.—Morris' Anatomy; Gould's Medical Dictionaries; Moullin's Surgery; Books on the Eye; The ? Quiz Compends ? Series, Visiting Lists, etc. We can also furnish sample pages of many of our publications.

P. Blakiston, Son & Co.'s publications may be had through booksellers in all the principal cities of the United States and Canada, or any book will be sent, postpaid, upon receipt of the price, or forwarded by express, C. O. D. No discount can be allowed retail purchasers under any circumstances. Money should be remitted by express or post-office money order, registered letter, or bank draft.

CLASSIFIED LIST, WITH PRICES,

OF ALL BOOKS PUBLISHED BY

P. BLAKISTON, SON & CO., PHILADELPHIA.

When the price is not given below, the book is out of print or about to be published.
Cloth binding, unless otherwise specified.   For full descriptions see following Catalogue.

ANATOMY.

Ballou. Veterinary Anat. $0 80
Campbell. Dissector -   1.00
Heath. Practical. 7th Ed.   4.25
Holden. Dissector.   -   2.50
—— Osteology.   5.25
—— Landmarks. 4th Ed.   1.00
Macalister's Text-Book.   5.00
Marshall's Phys. and Anat.
 Diagrams.   40.00 and 60.00
Morris. Text-Book of. 791 Illus,
 Clo, 6.00; Sh , 7.00; ½ Rus., 8.00
Potter. Compend of.   5th
 Ed. 133 Illustrations.   .80
Wilson's Anatomy 11th Ed. 5.00
Windle. Surface Anatomy. 1.00

ANESTHETICS.

Buxton. Anæsthetics. -
Turnbull. 4th Ed.   2.50

BRAIN AND INSANITY.

Blackburn. Autopsies. -   1.25
Gowers. Diagnosis of Dis-
 eases of the Brain. 2d Ed. 1.50
Horsley. Brain and S. Cord. 2.50
Ireland. Mental Diseases of
 Children.   -
Lewis (Bevan). Mental
 Diseases. 2d Ed.   -
Mann's Psychological Med. 3.00
Régis. Mental Medicine.   2.00
Stearns. Mental Dis Illus. 2.75
Tuke. Dictionary of Psycho-
 logical Medicine. 2 Vols. 10.00
Wood. Brain and Overwork. .40

CHEMISTRY.

See Technological Books, Water.
Allen. Commercial Organic
 Analysis. 2d Ed. Volume I.   ——
—— Volume II. -   ——
—— Volume III. Part I.   ——
—— Volume III. Part II. 4.50
—— Volume III. Part III. 4.50
—— Volume III. Part IV.   ——
Bartley. Medical and Phar-
 maceutical. 4th Ed.   2.75
Bloxam's Text-Book. 8th Ed. 4.25
Caldwell. Qualitative and
 Quantitative Analysis.   1.50
Clowes. Qual. Analysis. - 1.25
Groves and Thorp. Chemi-
 cal Technology Vol. I. Fuels 5.00
—— Vol. II. Lighting. - 4.00
Holland. Urine, Gastric Con-
 tents, Poisons and Milk Anal-
 ysis. 5th Ed.   1.00
Leffmann's Compend.   .80
—— Progressive Exercises. 1.00
—— Milk Analysis. -   1.25
—— Structural Formulæ. - 1.00
Muter. Pract. and Anal.   1.25
Oettel. Electro-Chem.   .75
—— Electro-Chem. Exper. .75
Richter's Inorganic. 4th Ed. 1.75
—— Organic. 2d Ed.   4.50
Smith. Electro-Chem. Anal. 1.25
Smith and Keller. Experi-
 ments. 3d Ed. Illus.   .60
Stammer. Chem Problems. .50
Sutton. Volumetric Anal.   2.00
Symonds. Manual of.   2.00
Watts. (Fowne's) Inorg.   2.00
—— (Fowne's) Organ.   2.00
Woody. Essentials of. 4th Ed. ——

CHILDREN.

Cautley. Feeding of Infants. 2.00
Hale. Care of.   .50
Hatfield. Compend of.   .80
Ireland. Mental Dis. of.   ——
Meigs. Milk Analysis.   .50
Money. Treatment of.   2.50
Power. Surgical Diseases of. 2.50
Starr. Digestive Organs of. 2.00
—— Hygiene of the Nursery. 1.00
Taylor and Wells. Manual. ——

CLINICAL CHARTS.

Griffiths. Graphic. Pads. $0.50
Keen. Outline Drawings of
 Human Body   -   1.00
Temperature Charts, Pads. .50

COMPENDS

And The Quiz-Compends.
Ballou. Veterinary Anat.   .80
Brubaker's Physiol. 8th Ed. .80
Gould and Pyle. The Eye. .80
Hall. Pathology. Illus.   .80
Hatfield. Children.   .80
Horwitz. Surgery. 5th Ed. .80
Hughes. Practice. 2 Pts. Ea. .80
Landis. Obstetrics. 5th Ed. .80
Leffmann's Chemistry. 4th Ed. .80
Mason. Electricity.   .75
Potter's Anatomy. 5th Ed. .80
—— Materia Medica. 6th Ed. .80
Schamberg. Skin Diseases. .80
Stewart. Pharmacy. 5th Ed. .80
Warren. Dentistry. 2d Ed. .80
Wells. Gynæcology.   .80

CONSUMPTION.

Harris and Beale. Pulmo-
 nary Consumption. -   2.50
Powell. Diseases of Lungs,
 including Consumption. - 4.00
Tussey. High Altitude Treatment of.   1.50

DEFORMITIES.

Reeves. Bodily Deformities
 and their Treatment. Illus. 1.75

DENTISTRY.

Barrett. Dental Surg. -   1.00
Blodgett. Dental Pathology. 1.25
Flagg. Plastic Filling. -   4.00
Fillebrown. Op. Dent. Illus. 2.25
Gorgas. Dental Medicine. 4.00
Harris. Principles and Prac. 6.00
—— Dictionary of. 5th Ed. 4.50
Heath. Dis. of Jaws. -   4.50
—— Lectures on Jaws. Bds. .50
Richardson. Mech. Dent.   5.00
Sewell. Dental Surg.   2.00
Taft. Operative Dentistry.   ——
——, Index of Dental Lit.   2.00
Talbot. Irregularity of Teeth. 3.00
Tomes. Dental Surgery.   4.00
—— Dental Anatomy.   ——
Warren's Compend of.   .80
—— Dental Prosthesis and
 Metallurgy. Illus.   1.25
White. Mouth and Teeth. .40

DIAGNOSIS.

Fenwick. Medical. 8th Ed. 2.50
Tyson's Manual. 3d Ed. Illus. ——

DICTIONARIES.

Gould's Illustrated Dictionary
 of Medicine, Biology, and Al-
 lied Sciences, etc. Leather,
 Net, $12.00; Half Russia,
 Thumb Index,   -   *Net,* 12 00
Gould's Student's Medical Dic-
 tionary. ½ Lea., 10th Ed.,
 3.25; ½ Mor., Thumb Index. 4.00
Gould's Pocket Dictionary,
 12,000 medical words. Lea.,
 1.00; Thumb Index,   -   1.25
Harris' Dental. Clo. 4.50; Shp. 5.50
Longley's Pronouncing.   .75
Maxwell. Terminologia Med-
 ica Polyglotta.   3.00
Treves. German-English.   3.25

EAR.

Burnett. Hearing, etc.   .40
Dalby. Diseases of. 4th Ed. 2.50
Hovell. Treatise on. -   5.00
Pritchard. Diseases of. 3d Ed. 1.50
Woakes. Deafness, Giddi-
 ness, and Noises in the Head. 2.00

ELECTRICITY

Bigelow. Plain Talks on Medical Electricity. 43 Illus.   1 00

[Electricity, continued]

Mason's Electricity and its
 Medical and Surgical Uses. $ .75
Jones. Medical Electricity.
 2d Ed. Illus. -   2.50

EYE.

Arlt. Diseases of. -   1.25
Donders. Refraction.   ——
Fick. Diseases of the Eye. 4.50
Gould and Pyle. Compend. 0.80
Gower's Ophthalmoscopy. 4.00
Harlan. Eyesight. -   .40
Hartridge. Refraction. 8th Ed. 1.50
——Ophthalmoscope. 3d Ed. 1.50
Hansell and Bell. Clinical
 Ophthalmology. 120 Illus. 1.50
Macnamara. Diseases of.   3.50
Morton. Refraction. 6th Ed. 1.00
Ohlemann. Ocular Therap. ——
Phillips. Spectacles and Eye-
 glasses. 49 Illus. 2d Ed. 1.00
Swanzy's Handbook. 6th Ed. 3.00
Thorington. Retinoscopy.   ——
Walker. Student's Aid.   1.50

FEVERS.

Collie. On Fevers. -   2.00
Goodall and Washbourn. 3.00

HEADACHES.

Day. Their Treatment, etc. 1.00

HEALTH AND DOMESTIC MEDICINE.

Bulkley. The Skin.   .40
Burnett. Hearing. -   .40
Cohen. Throat and Voice. .40
Dulles. Emergencies. 5th Ed. 1.00
Harlan. Eyesight. -   .40
Hartshorne. Our Homes.   .40
Osgood. Dangers of Winter. .40
Packard. Sea Air, etc.   .40
Richardson's Long Life.   .40
Westland. The Wife and
 Mother.   1.50
White. Mouth and Teeth. .40
Wilson. Summer and its Dis. .40
Wood. Overwork.   .40

HISTOLOGY.

Stirling. Histology. 2d Ed. 2.00
Stöhr's Histology Illus. - 3.00

HYGIENE.

Canfield. Hygiene of the Sick-
 Room. -   -   1.25
Coplin and Bevan. Practi-
 cal Hygiene. Illus. - 3.25
Fox. Water, Air, Food.   3.50
Kenwood. Public Health
 Laboratory Guide.   2.00
Lincoln. School Hygiene. .40
McNeill. Epidemics and Iso-
 lation Hospitals. -   3.50
Notter and Firth.   7.00
Parkes' (E.). See "Notter."
—— (L. C.), Manual.   2.50
—— Elements of Health. 1.25
Starr. Hygiene of the Nursery. 1.00
Stevenson and Murphy. A
 Treatise on Hygiene. In 3
 Vols. *Circular*   Vol. I. 6.00
 upon application. Vol. II, 6.00
    Vol. III, 5.00
Wilson's Handbook. 8th Ed. ——
Weyl. Coal-Tar Colors,   1.25

MASSAGE.

Kleen and Hartwell. -   2.25
Murrell. Massage. 5th Ed. 1.25
Ostrom. Massage. 87 Illus. 1.00

MATERIA MEDICA.

Biddle. 13th Ed. Cloth,   4.00
Bracken. Materia Med.   2.75
Davis. Essentials of Materia
 Med and Pres. Writing.   1.50
Gorgas. Dental. 5th Ed.   4.00
Heller. Essentials of.   1.50
Potter's Compend of. 5th Ed. .80
Potter's Handbook of. Sixth
 Ed. Cloth, 4.50; Sheep,   5.50

Sayre. Organic Materia Med.
and Pharmacognosy. - $4.00
White & Wilcox. Mat. Med.,
Pharmacy, Pharmacology,
and Therapeutics. 3d Ed.
Enlarged. Cloth, 2.75; Sh. 3.25

MEDICAL JURISPRUDENCE.
Mann. Forensic Med. 6.50
Reese. Medical Jurisprudence
& Toxicology,4th Ed.3.00; Sh. 3.50

MICROSCOPE.
Beale. How to Work with. 6.50
—— In Medicine. 6.50
Carpenter. The Microscope.
7th Ed. 800 Illus. 5.50
Lee. Vade Mecum of. - 4.00
MacDonald. Examination of
Water and Air by. 2.50
Reeves. Med. Microscopy. 2.50
Wethered. Medical Micros-
copy. Illus. - 2.00

MISCELLANEOUS.
Black. Micro-organisms. .75
Burnet. Food and Dietaries. 1.50
Duckworth. On Gout. 6.00
Garrod. Rheumatism, etc. 5.00
Gould. Borderland Studies. 2.00
Gowers. Dynamics of Life. .75
Haig. Uric Acid. 3.00
Hare. Mediastinal Disease. 2.00
Hemmeter. Dis. of Stomach. 6.00
Henry. Anæmia. - .50
Leffmann. Coal Tar Products. 1.25
Lizars. On Tobacco .40
rshall. Women's Med. Col. 1.50
New Sydenham Society's
Publications, each year. 8.00
Parrish. Inebriety. - 1.00
St. Clair. Medical Latin. 1.00
Sansom. Dis. of Heart. - 6.00
Treves. Physical Education. .75

NERVOUS DISEASES, Etc.
Beevor. Nervous Diseases. ——
Gowers. Manual of. 2d Ed.
530 Illus. Vol. 1, 3.00; Vol. 2, 4.00
—— Syphilis and the Ner-
vous System. - - 1.00
—— Diseases of Brain. 1.50
—— Clinical Lectures. 2.00
—— Epilepsy. New Ed. ——
Horsley. Brain and Spinal
Cord. Illus. - - 2.50
Obersteiner. Central Nervous
System. - - 5.00
Ormerod. Manual of. 1.00
Osler. Cerebral Palsies. 2.00
—— Chorea. - 2.00
Preston. Hysteria. Illus. 2.00
Watson. Concussions. 1.00

NURSING.
Brown. Physiology for Nurses. .75
Canfield. Hygiene of the Sick-
Room. - - - 1.25
Cuff. Lectures to Nurses. 1.00
Cullingworth. Manual of. .75
—— Monthly Nursing. .40
Domville's Manual. 8th Ed. .75
Fullerton. Obst. Nursing. 1.00
—— Nursing in Abdominal
Surg. and Dis. of Women, 1.50
Humphrey. Manual 15th Ed 1.00
Shawe. District Nursing. 1.00
Starr. Hygiene of the Nursery. 1.00
Temperature Charts. - .50
Voswinkel. Surg. Nursing. 1.00

OBSTETRICS.
Bar. Antiseptic Midwifery. 1.00
Cazeaux and Tarnier. Text-
Book of. Colored Plates. 4.50
Davis. Obstetrics. Illus. 2.00
Jellett. Midwifery. - 1.75
Landis. Compend. 5th Ed. .80
Schultze. Obstetric Diagrams.
20 Plates, map size. *Net*, 26.00
Strahan. Extra-Uterine Preg. .75
Winckel's Text-book. 5.00

PATHOLOGY.
Barlow. General Pathology——
Blackburn Autopsies. 1.25

Blodgett. Dental Pathology $1.25
Coplin. Manual of. 265 Illus. 3.00
Gilliam. Essentials of. .75
Hall. Compend. Illus. .80
Virchow. Post-mortems. .75
Whitacre. Lab. Text-book. 1.50

PHARMACY
Beasley's Receipt-Book. 2.00
—— Formulary. - 2.00
Coblentz. Manual of Pharm. 3.50
Proctor. Practical Pharm. 3.00
Robinson. Latin Grammar of. 1.75
Sayre. Organic Materia Med.
and Pharmacognosy. - 4.00
Scoville. Compounding. 2.50
Stewart's Compend. 5th Ed. .80
U. S. Pharmacopœia. 7th
Revision. Cl. 2.50; Sh., 3.00
Select Tables from U. S. P. .25

PHYSIOLOGY.
Brown. Physiol. for Nurses. .75
Brubaker's Compend. Illus-
trated. 8th Ed. - .80
Kirke's New 14th Ed. (Halli-
burton.) Cloth, 3.25; Sh., 4.00
Landois' Text-book. 845 Illus-
trations. - - ——
Starling. Elements of. - 1.00
Stirling. Practical Phys. 2.00
Tyson's Cell Doctrine. - 1.50
Yeo's Manual. 254 Ill. 6th Ed. 2.50

POISONS.
Murrell. Poisoning. - 1.00
Reese. Toxicology. 4th Ed. 3.00
Tanner. Memoranda of. .75

PRACTICE.
Beale. Slight Ailments. 1.25
Charteris. Guide to. 2.00
Fowler's Dictionary of. 3.00
Hughes. Compend. 2 Pts. ea. .80
—— Physicians' Edition.
1 Vol. Morocco, Gilt edge. 2.25
Roberts. Text-book. 9th Ed. 4.50
Taylor's Manual of. - 2.00
Tyson. The Practice of Medi-
cine. Illus. Cl. 5.50; Sheep, 6.50

PRESCRIPTION BOOKS.
Beasley's 3000 Prescriptions. 2.00
—— Receipt Book. 2.00
Davis. Materia Medica and
Prescription Writing. 1.50
Pereira's Pocket-book. .75
Wythe's Dose and Symptom
Book. 17th Ed. - - .75

SKIN.
Bulkley. The Skin. - .40
Crocker. Dis. of Skin. Illus. 4.50
Impey. Leprosy. - 3.50
Schamberg. Compend. 80
Van Harlingen. Diagnosis
and Treatment of Skin Dis.
3d Ed. 60 Illus. 2.75

SURGERY AND SURGICAL DISEASES
Caird and Cathcart. Sur-
geon's Pocket-Book. Lea. 2.50
Deaver. Appendicitis. 3.50
—— Surgical Anatomy. ——
Dulles. Emergencies. 1.00
Hacker. Wounds. - .50
Heath's Minor. 10th Ed. 1.25
—— Diseases of Jaws. 4.50
—— Lectures on Jaws. .50
Horwitz. Compend. 5th Ed. .80
Jacobson. Operations of. - 3.00
Macready on Ruptures 6.00
Maylard. Surgery of the Ali-
mentary Canal. - 7.50
Moullin. Complete Text-
book. 3d Ed. by Hamilton,
600 Illustrations and Colored
Plates. Cl. 6.00; Sh. 7.00
Roberts' Fractures. - 1.00
Smith. Abdominal Surg. 10.00
Swain. Surgical Emer. 1.75

Voswinkel. Surg Nursing. $1.00
Walsham. Practical Surg. 2.00
Watson's Amputations. 5.50

TECHNOLOGICAL BOOKS.
Cameron. Oils & Varnishes. 2.25
—— Soap and Candles. 2.00
Gardner. Brewing, etc. 1.50
Gardner. Bleaching and
Dyeing. - - - 1.50
Groves and Thorp. Chemi-
cal Technology. Vol. 1.
Mills on Fuels. Cl. 5.00
Vol. II. Lighting. 4.00
Vol. III. Lighting Contin'd. ——

THERAPEUTICS.
**Allen, Harlan, Harte, Van
Harlingen.** Local Thera. 3.00
Biddle. 13th Edition - 4.00
Field. Cathartics and Emetics. 1.75
Mays. Theine. - 50
Napheys' Therapeutics. Vol.
1. Medical and Disease of
Children. - Cloth, 4.00
——Vol. 2. Surgery, Gynæc.
& Obstet. - Cloth, 4.00
Potter's Compend. 5th Ed. .80
—— Handbook of. 4.50; Sh. 5.50
Waring's Practical. 4th Ed. 2.00
White and Wilcox. Mat.
Med., Pharmacy, Pharmacol-
ogy, and Thera. 3d Ed. 2.75

THROAT AND NOSE.
Cohen. Throat and Voice. .40
Hall. Nose and Throat. - 2.50
Hutchinson. Nose & Throat. ——
Mackenzie. Throat Hospital
Pharmacopœia. 5th Ed. 1.00
McBride. Clinical Manual,
Colored Plates. 2d Ed. - 6.00
Potter. Stammering, etc. 1.00
Woakes. Post-Nasal Catarrh. 1.00

URINE & URINARY ORGANS.
Acton. Repro. Organs. 1.75
Allen. Diabetic Urine. 2.25
Brockbank. Gall-Stones. 2.25
Beale. Urin. Deposits. Plates. 2.00
Holland. The Urine, Milk and
Common Poisons. 5th Ed. 1.00
Memminger. Diagnosis by
the Urine. Illus. - 1.00
Moullin. The Prostate. 1.50
Thompson. Urinary Organs. 3.00
Tyson. Exam. of Urine. 1.25
Van Nüys. Urine Analysis. 1.00

VENEREAL DISEASES.
Cooper. Syphilis. 2d Ed. - 5.00
Gowers. Syphilis and the
Nervous System. - - 1.00
Jacobson. Diseases of Male
Organs. Illustrated. - 6.00

VETERINARY.
Armatage. Vet. Rememb. 1.00
Ballou. Anat. and Phys. .80
Tuson. Pharmacopœia. 2.25

VISITING LISTS.
Lindsay & Blakiston's Reg-
ular Edition. 1.00 to 2.25
—— Perpetual Ed. 1.25 to 1.50
—— Monthly Ed. .75 to 1.00
Send for Circular.

WATER.
Fox. Water, Air, Food. 3.50
Leffmann. Examination of. 1.25
MacDonald. Examination of. 2.50

WOMEN, DISEASES OF.
Byford (H. T.). Manual. 2d
Edition. 341 Illustrations. 3.00
Byford (W. H.). Text-book. 3.00
Dührssen. Gynecological
Practice. 105 Illustrations. 1.50
Lewers. Dis. of Women. 2.50
Wells. Compend. Illus. .80
Winckel, by Parvin. Manual
of. Illustrated. 3d Ed. - ——

P. BLAKISTON, SON & CO.'S
Medical and Scientific Publications,

No. 1012 Walnut St., Philadelphia.

ACTON. The Functions and Disorders of the Reproductive Organs in Childhood, Youth, Adult Age and Advanced Life, considered in their Physiological, Social and Moral Relations. By Wm. ACTON, M.D., M.R.C.S. 8th Edition. Cloth, $1.75

ALLEN, HARLAN, HARTE, VAN HARLINGEN. Local Therapeutics. A Handbook of Local Therapeutics, being a practical description of all those agents used in the local treatment of diseases of the Eye, Ear, Nose, Throat, Mouth, Skin, Vagina, Rectum, etc., such as Ointments, Plasters, Powders, Lotions, Inhalations, Suppositories, Bougies, Tampons, and the proper methods of preparing and applying them. By HARRISON ALLEN, M.D., Laryngologist to the Rush Hospital for Consumption; late Surgeon to the Philadelphia and St. Joseph's Hospitals. GEORGE C. HARLAN, M.D., late Professor of Diseases of the Eye in the Philadelphia Polyclinic and College for Graduates in Medicine; Surgeon to the Wills Eye Hospital, and Eye and Ear Department of the Pennsylvania Hospital. RICHARD H. HARTE, M.D., Surgeon to the Episcopal and St. Mary's Hospital; Ass't Surg. University Hospital; and ARTHUR VAN HARLINGEN, M.D., Professor of Diseases of the Skin in the Philadelphia Polyclinic and College for Graduates in Medicine; late Clinical Lecturer on Dermatology in Jefferson Medical College; Dermatologist to the Howard Hospital. In One Handsome Compact Volume. Cloth, $3.00; Sheep, $4.00; Half Russia, $5.00

ALLEN. Commercial Organic Analysis. A Treatise on the Modes of Assaying the Various Organic Chemicals and Products employed in the Arts, Manufactures, Medicine, etc., with Concise Methods for the Detection of Impurities, Adulterations, etc. Second Edition. Revised and Enlarged. By ALFRED ALLEN, F.C.S.

    Vol. I. Alcohols, Ethers, Vegetable Acids. Starch, etc. *Out of Print.*

    Vol. II. Fixed Oils and Fats, Hydrocarbons and Mineral Oils, Phenols and their Derivatives, Coloring Matters, etc. *Out of Print.*

    Vol. III—Part I. Acid Derivatives of Phenols, Aromatic Acids, Tannins, Dyes, and Coloring Matters. 8vo. *Out of Print.*

    Vol. III—Part II. The Amines, Pyridine and its Hydrozines and Derivatives. The Antipyretics, etc. Vegetable Alkaloids, Tea, Coffee, Cocoa, etc. 8vo. Cloth, $4.50

    Vol. III—Part III. Vegetable Alkaloids, Non-Basic Vegetable Bitter Principles. Animal Bases, Animal Acids, Cyanogen Compounds, etc. Cloth, $4.50

    Vol. III—Part IV. The Proteids and Albuminoid Compounds. *In Press.*

    Chemical Analysis of Albuminous and Diabetic Urine. Illus. Cloth, $2.25

ARLT. Diseases of the Eye. Clinical Studies on Diseases of the Eye. Including the Conjunctiva, Cornea and Sclerotic, Iris and Ciliary Body. By Dr. FERD. RITTER VON ARLT, University of Vienna. Authorized Translation by LYMAN WARE, M.D., Surgeon to the Illinois Charitable Eye and Ear Infirmary, Chicago. Illustrated. 8vo. Cloth, $1.25

ARMATAGE. The Veterinarian's Pocket Remembrancer: being Concise Directions for the Treatment of Urgent or Rare Cases, embracing Semeiology, Diagnosis, Prognosis, Surgery, Treatment, etc. By GEORGE ARMATAGE, M.R.C.V.S. Second Edition. 32mo. Boards, $1.00

BALLOU. Veterinary Anatomy and Physiology. By Wm. R. BALLOU, M.D., Prof. of Equine Anatomy, New York College of Veterinary Surgeons, Physician to Bellevue Dispensary, and Lecturer on Genito-Urinary Surgery, New York Polyclinic, etc. With 29 Graphic Illustrations. 12mo. *No. 12 ? Quiz-Compend? Series.* Cloth, .80. Interleaved, for the addition of Notes, $1.25

BAR. Antiseptic Midwifery. The Principles of Antiseptic Methods Applied to Obstetric Practice. By Dr. PAUL BAR, Obstetrician to, formerly Interne in, the Maternity Hospital, Paris. Authorized Translation by HENRY D. FRY, M.D., with an Appendix by the author. Octavo. Cloth, $1.00

BARRETT. Dental Surgery for General Practitioners and Students of Medicine and Dentistry. Extraction of Teeth, etc. By A. W. BARRETT, M.D. Third Edition. 86 Illustrations. 12mo. Cloth, $1.00

BARTLEY. Medical and Pharmaceutical Chemistry. Fourth Edition. A Text-book for Medical and Pharmaceutical Students. By E. H. BARTLEY, M.D., Professor of Chemistry and Toxicology at the Long Island College Hospital; Dean and Professor of Chemistry, Brooklyn College of Pharmacy; President of the American Society of Public Analysts; Chief Chemist, Board of Health, of Brooklyn, N. Y. Revised and Enlarged. With Illustrations, Glossary and Complete Index. 12mo. 711 pages. Cloth, $2.75; Leather, $3.25

BEALE. On Slight Ailments; their Nature and Treatment. By LIONEL S. BEALE, M.D., F.R.S., Professor of Practice, King's Medical College, London. Second Edition. Enlarged and Illustrated. 8vo. Cloth, $1.25

The Use of the Microscope in Practical Medicine. For Students and Practitioners, with full directions for examining the various secretions, etc., in the Microscope. Fourth Edition. 500 Illustrations. 8vo. Cloth, $6.50

How to Work with the Microscope. A Complete Manual of Microscopical Manipulation, containing a full description of many new processes of investigation, with directions for examining objects under the highest powers, and for taking photographs of microscopic objects. Fifth Edition. Containing over 400 Illustrations, many of them colored. 8vo. Cloth, $6.50

One Hundred Urinary Deposits, on eight sheets, for the Hospital, Laboratory, or Surgery. New Edition. 4to. Paper, $2.00

BEASLEY'S Book of Prescriptions. Containing over 3100 Prescriptions, collected from the Practice of the most Eminent Physicians and Surgeons—English, French, and American; a Compendious History of the Materia Medica, Lists of the Doses of all Officinal and Established Preparations, and an Index of Diseases and their Remedies. By HENRY BEASLEY. Seventh Edition. Cloth, $2.00

Druggists' General Receipt Book. Comprising a copious Veterinary Formulary; Recipes in Patent and Proprietary Medicines, Druggists' Nostrums, etc.; Perfumery and Cosmetics; Beverages, Dietetic Articles and Condiments; Trade Chemicals, Scientific Processes, and an Appendix of Useful Tables. Tenth Edition. Revised. *Just Ready.* Cloth, $2.00

Pocket Formulary and Synopsis of the British and Foreign Pharmacopœias. Comprising Standard and Approved Formulæ for the Preparations and Compounds Employed in Medical Practice. Eleventh Edition. Cloth, $2.00

BEEVOR. Diseases of the Nervous System and Their Treatment. By CHAS. EDWARD BEEVOR, M.D., F.R.C.P., Physician to the National Hospital for Paralyzed and Epileptic; Formerly Assistant Physician University College Hospital, London. 12mo. *Nearly Ready.*

BIDDLE'S Materia Medica and Therapeutics. Including Dose List, Dietary for the Sick, Table of Parasites, and Memoranda of New Remedies. By Prof. JOHN B. BIDDLE, M.D., Late Prof. of Materia Medica in Jefferson Medical College, Philadelphia. Thirteenth Edition, thoroughly revised in accordance with new U. S. P., by CLEMENT BIDDLE, M.D., Assistant Surgeon, U. S. Navy. With 64 Illustrations and a Clinical Index. Octavo. Cloth, $4.00; Sheep, $5.00

BIGELOW. Plain Talks on Medical Electricity and Batteries, with a Therapeutic Index and a Glossary. Prepared for Practitioners and Students of Medicine. By HORATIO R. BIGELOW, M.D., Fellow of the British Gynæcological Society; of the American Electro-Therapeutic Association; Member American Medical Association, etc. 43 Illus., and a Glossary. 2d Ed. 12mo. Cloth, $1.00

BLACK. Micro-Organisms. The Formation of Poisons. A Biological study of the Germ Theory of Disease. By G. V. BLACK, M.D., D.D.S. Cloth, .75

BLACKBURN. Autopsies. A Manual of Autopsies, Designed for the use of Hospitals for the Insane and other Public Institutions. By I. W. BLACKBURN, M.D., Pathologist to the Government Hospital for the Insane, Washington, D. C. With ten Full-page Plates and four other Illustrations. 12mo. Cloth, $1.25

BLODGETT'S Dental Pathology. By ALBERT N. BLODGETT, M.D., Late Prof. of Pathology and Therapeutics, Boston Dental Coll. 33 Illus. 12mo. Cloth, $1.25

BLOXAM. Chemistry, Inorganic and Organic. With Experiments. By CHARLES L. BLOXAM. Edited by J. M. THOMPSON, Professor of Chemistry in King's College, London, and A. G. BLOXAM, Head of the Chemistry Department, Goldsmiths' Institute, London. Eighth Edition. Revised and Enlarged. 281 Engravings, 20 of which are new. 8vo. Cloth, $4.25 ; Leather, $5.25

BRACKEN. Outlines of Materia Medica and Pharmacology. By H. M. BRACKEN, Professor of Materia Medica and Therapeutics and of Clinical Medicine, University of Minnesota. Cloth, $2.75

BROCKBANK. On Gall-Stones or Cholelithiasis. By EDWARD MANSFIELD BROCKBANK, M.D., M.R.C.P., London, Late Resident Medical Officer, Manchester Royal Infirmary, etc. 12mo. Cloth, $2.25

BROWN. Elementary Physiology for Nurses. By MISS FLORENCE HAIG BROWN. Late in Charge Nurse Department, St. Thomas' Hospital, London. With many Illustrations. Cloth, .75

BRUBAKER. Physiology. A Compend of Physiology, specially adapted for the use of Students and Physicians. By A. P. BRUBAKER, M.D., Demonstrator of Physiology at Jefferson Medical College, Prof. of Physiology, Penn'a College of Dental Surgery, Philadelphia. Eighth Edition. Revised, Enlarged, and Illustrated. *No. 4, ?Quiz-Compend? Series.* 12mo. Cloth, .80 ; Interleaved, $1.25

BULKLEY. The Skin in Health and Disease. By L. DUNCAN BULKLEY, M.D., Attending Physician at the New York Hospital. Illustrated. Cloth, .40

BURNET. Foods and Dietaries. A Manual of Clinical Dietetics. By R. W. BURNET, M.D., M.R.C.P., Physician to the Great Northern Central Hospital. With Appendix on Predigested Foods and Invalid Cookery. Full directions as to hours of taking nourishment, quantity, etc., are given. Second Edition. 12mo. Cloth, $1.50

BURNETT. Hearing, and How to Keep It. By CHAS. H. BURNETT, M.D., Prof. of Diseases of the Ear at the Philadelphia Polyclinic. Illustrated. Cloth, .40

BUXTON. On Anesthetics. A Manual. By DUDLEY WILMOT BUXTON, M.R.C.S., M.R.C.P., Ass't to Prof. of Med., and Administrator of Anesthetics, University College Hospital, London. Third Edition, Illustrated. 12mo. *In Press.*

BYFORD. Manual of Gynecology. A Practical Student's Book. By HENRY T. BYFORD, M.D., Professor of Gynecology and Clinical Gynecology in the College of Physicians and Surgeons of Chicago ; Professor of Clinical Gynecology, Women's Medical School of Northwestern University, and in Post-Graduate Medical School of Chicago, etc. Second Edition, Enlarged. With 341 Illustrations, many of which are from original drawings and several of which are colored. 12mo. 596 pages. Cloth, $3.00

BYFORD. Diseases of Women. The Practice of Medicine and Surgery, as applied to the Diseases and Accidents Incident to Women. By the late W. H. BYFORD, A.M., M.D. Fourth Edition. 306 Illustrations. Octavo
Cloth, $2.00 ; Leather, $2.50

CAIRD AND CATHCART. Surgical Handbook. By F. M. CAIRD, F.R.C.S., and C. W. CATHCART, F.R.C.S. Eighth Edition, Revised. 208 Illustrations. 12mo. 321 pages. Full Red Morocco, Gilt Edges, and Round Corners, $2.50

CALDWELL. Chemical Analysis. Elements of Qualitative and Quantitative Chemical Analysis. By G. C. CALDWELL, B.S., PH.D., Professor of Agricultural and Analytical Chemistry in Cornell University, Ithaca, New York, etc. Third Edition. Revised and Enlarged. Octavo. Cloth, $1.50

CAMERON. Oils and Varnishes. A Practical Handbook, by JAMES CAMERON, F.I.C. With Illustrations, Formulæ, Tables, etc. 12mo. Cloth, $2.25
    Soap and Candles. A New Handbook for Manufacturers, Chemists, Analysts, etc. 54 Illustrations. 12mo. Cloth, $2.00

CAMPBELL. Outlines for Dissection. To be Used in Connection with Morris's Anatomy. By W. A. CAMPBELL, M.D., Demonstrator of Anatomy, University of Michigan. Octavo. Cloth, $1.00

CANFIELD. Hygiene of the Sick-Room. A book for Nurses and others. Being a Brief Consideration of Asepsis, Antisepsis, Disinfection, Bacteriology, Immunity, Heating and Ventilation, and kindred subjects, for the use of Nurses and other Intelligent Women. By WILLIAM BUCKINGHAM CANFIELD, A.M., M.D., Lecturer on Clinical Medicine and Chief of Chest Clinic, University of Maryland, Physician to Bay View Hospital and Union Protestant Infirmary, Baltimore. 12mo. Cloth, $1.25

CARPENTER. The Microscope and Its Revelations. By W. B. CARPENTER, M.D., F.R.S. Seventh Edition. By Rev. DR. DALLINGER, F. R. S. Revised and Enlarged, with 800 Illustrations and many Lithographs. Octavo. 1100 Pages. Cloth, $5.50

CAUTLEY. Feeding of Infants and Young Children by Natural and Artificial Methods. By EDMUND CAUTLEY, M.D., Physician to the Belgrave Hospital for Children, London. 12mo. Cloth, $2.00

CAZEAUX and TARNIER'S Midwifery. With Appendix, by Mundé. The Theory and Practice of Obstetrics, including the Diseases of Pregnancy and Parturition, Obstetrical Operations, etc. By P. CAZEAUX. Remodeled and re-arranged, with revisions and additions, by S. TARNIER, M.D. Eighth American, from the Eighth French and First Italian Edition. Edited by ROBERT J. HESS, M.D., Physician to the Northern Dispensary, Phila., etc., with an Appendix by PAUL F. MUNDÉ, M.D., Professor of Gynecology at the New York Polyclinic. Illustrated by Chromo-Lithographs, Lithographs, and other Full-page Plates and numerous Wood Engravings. 8vo. Cloth, $4.50; Full Leather, $5.50

CHARTERIS. Practice of Medicine. The Student's Guide. By M. CHARTERIS, M.D., Professor of Therapeutics and Materia Medica, Glasgow University, etc. Sixth Edition, with Therapeutical Index and many Illustrations. Cloth, $2.00

CLOWES AND COLEMAN. Elementary Practical Chemistry and Qualitative Analysis. Adapted for Use in the Laboratories of Schools and Colleges. By FRANK CLOWES, D.SC., Professor of Chemistry, University College, Nottingham, and J. BERNARD COLEMAN, Demonstrator of Chemistry, Nottingham, England. 54 Illustrations. Cloth, $1.25

COBLENTZ. Manual of Pharmacy. A Text-Book for Students. By VIRGIL COBLENTZ, A.M., PH.G., PH.D., Professor of Theory and Practice of Pharmacy; Director of Pharmaceutical Laboratory, College of Pharmacy of the City of New York. Second Edition, Revised and Enlarged. 437 Illustrations. Octavo. 572 pages. Cloth, $3.50; Sheep, $4.50; Half Russia, $5.50

COHEN. The Throat and Voice. By J. SOLIS-COHEN, M.D. Illus. 12mo. Cloth, .40

COLLIE, On Fevers. A Practical Treatise on Fevers, Their History, Etiology, Diagnosis, Prognosis, and Treatment. By ALEXANDER COLLIE, M.D., M.R.C.P., Lond., Medical Officer of the Homerton and of the London Fever Hospitals. With Colored Plates. 12mo. Cloth, $2.00

COOPER. Syphilis. By ALFRED COOPER, F.R.C.S., Senior Surgeon to St. Mark's Hospital; late Surgeon to the London Lock Hospital, etc. Edited by EDWARD COTTERELL, F.R.C.S., Surgeon London Lock Hospital, etc. Second Edition. Enlarged and Illustrated with 20 Full-Page Plates containing many handsome Colored Figures. Octavo. Cloth, $5.00

COPLIN. Manual of Pathology. Including Bacteriology, the Technic of Post-Mortems, and Methods of Pathologic Research. By W. M. LATE COPLIN, M.D., Professor of Pathology and Bacteriology, Jefferson Medical College; Pathologist to Jefferson Medical College Hospital and to the Philadelphia Hospital; Bacteriologist to the Pennsylvania State Board of Health. Being the Second Edition of the author's "Lectures on Pathology." Rewritten and Enlarged. 265 Illustrations, many of which are original. 12mo. 638 pages. Cloth, $3.00

COPLIN and BEVAN. Practical Hygiene. By W. M. L. COPLIN, M.D., and D. BEVAN, M.D., Ass't Department of Hygiene, Jefferson Medical College; Bacteriologist, St. Agnes' Hospital, Philadelphia, with an Introduction by Prof. H. A. HARE, and articles on Plumbing, Ventilation, etc., by Mr. W. P. Lockington. 138 Illustrations, some of which are in colors. 8vo.

Cloth, $3.25; Sheep, $4.25; Half Russia, $5.25

CROCKER. Diseases of the Skin. Their Description, Pathology, Diagnosis, and Treatment, with special reference to the Skin Eruptions of Children. By H. RADCLIFFE CROCKER, M.D., Physician to the Dept. of Skin Diseases, University College Hospital, London. 92 Illustrations. Second Edition. Enlarged. 987 pages. Octavo. Cloth, $4.50; Sheep, $5.50; Half Russia, $6.50

CUFF. Lectures on Medicine to Nurses. By HERBERT EDMUND CUFF, M.D., Late Ass't Medical Officer, Stockwell Fever Hospital, England. With 25 Illustrations. Cloth, $1.00

CULLINGWORTH. A Manual of Nursing, Medical and Surgical. By CHARLES J. CULLINGWORTH, M.D., Physician to St. Thomas' Hospital, London. Third Revised Edition. With Illustrations. 12mo. Cloth, .75
    A Manual for Monthly Nurses. Third Edition. 32mo. Cloth, .40

DALBY. Diseases and Injuries of the Ear. By SIR WILLIAM B. DALBY, M.D., Aural Surgeon to St. George's Hospital, London. Illustrated. Fourth Edition. With 38 Wood Engravings and 8 Colored Plates. Cloth, $2.50

DAVIS. A Manual of Obstetrics. Being a complete manual for Physicians and Students. By EDWARD P. DAVIS, M.D., Professor of Obstetrics and Diseases of Infancy in the Philadelphia Polyclinic, Clinical Lecturer on Obstetrics, Jefferson Medical College; Professor of Diseases of Children in Woman's Medical College, etc. Second Edition, Revised. With 16 Colored and other Lithograph Plates and 134 other Illustrations. 12mo. Cloth, $2.00

DAVIS. Essentials of Materia Medica and Prescription Writing. By J. AUBREY DAVIS, M.D., Ass't Dem. of Obstetrics and Quiz Master in Materia Medica, University of Pennsylvania; Ass't Physician, Home for Crippled Children, Philadelphia. 12mo. $1.50

DAY. On Headaches. The Nature, Causes, and Treatment of Headaches. By WM. H. DAY, M.D. Fourth Edition. Illustrated. 8vo. Cloth, $1.00

DOMVILLE. Manual for Nurses and others engaged in attending to the sick. By ED. J. DOMVILLE, M.D. Eighth Edition. Revised. With Recipes for Sickroom Cookery, etc. 12mo. Cloth, .75

GRIFFITH'S Graphic Clinical Chart. Designed by J. P. CROZER GRIFFITH, M.D., Instructor in Clinical Medicine in the University of Pennsylvania. *Printed in three colors.* Sample copies free. Put up in loose packages of 50, .50
    Price to Hospitals, 500 copies, $4.00; 1000 copies, $7.50. With name of Hospital printed on, 50 cents extra.

GROVES AND THORP. Chemical Technology. A new and Complete Work. The Application of Chemistry to the Arts and Manufactures. Edited by CHARLES E. GROVES, F.R.S., and WM. THORP, B.SC., F.I.C., assisted by many experts. In about eight volumes, with numerous illustrations. *Each volume sold separately.*
    Vol. I. FUEL AND ITS APPLICATIONS. 607 Illustrations and 4 Plates. Octavo.
                            Cloth, $5.00; Half Morocco, $6.50
    Vol. II. LIGHTING. Illustrated. Octavo. Cloth, $4.00; Half Morocco, $5.50
    Vol. III. LIGHTING—Continued. *In Press.*

GOWERS. Manual of Diseases of the Nervous System. A Complete Text-book. By WILLIAM R. GOWERS, M.D., F.R.S., Physician to National Hospital for the Paralyzed and Epileptic; Consulting Physician, University College Hospital; formerly Professor of Clinical Medicine, University College, etc. Second Edition. Revised, Enlarged and in many parts rewritten. With many new Illustrations. Two Volumes. Octavo.
    VOL. I. **Diseases of the Nerves and Spinal Cord.** 616 pages.
                  Cloth, $3.00; Sheep, $4.00; Half Russia, $5.00
    VOL. II. **Diseases of the Brain and Cranial Nerves; General and Functional Diseases.** 1069 pages.
                  Cloth, $4.00; Sheep, $5.00; Half Russia, $6.00
    ***This book has been translated into German, Italian, and Spanish. It is published in London, Milan, Bonn, Barcelona, and Philadelphia.

    Syphilis and the Nervous System. Being a revised reprint of the Lettsomian Lectures for 1890, delivered before the Medical Society of London. 12mo. Cloth, $1.00

    Diagnosis of Diseases of the Brain. 8vo. Second Ed. Illus. Cloth, $1.50

    Medical Ophthalmoscopy. A Manual and Atlas, with Colored Autotype and Lithographic Plates and Wood-cuts, comprising Original Illustrations of the changes of the Eye in Diseases of the Brain, Kidney, etc. Third Edition. Revised, with the assistance of R. MARCUS GUNN, F.R.C.S., Surgeon, Royal London Ophthalmic Hospital, Moorfields. Octavo. Cloth, $4.00

    The Dynamics of Life. 12mo. Cloth, .75

    Clinical Lectures. A new volume of Essays on the Diagnosis, Treatment, etc., of Diseases of the Nervous System. Cloth, $2.00

    Epilepsy and Other Chronic Convulsive Diseases. Second Edition. *In Press*

HACKER. Antiseptic Treatment of Wounds, Introduction to the, according to the Method in Use at Professor Billroth's Clinic, Vienna. By Dr. VICTOR R. V. HACKER, Assistant in the Clinic Billroth, Professor of Surgery, etc. Translated by Surgeon-Captain C. R. KILKELLY, M.B. 12mo. Cloth, .50

HAIG. Causation of Disease by Uric Acid. A Contribution to the Pathology of High Arterial Tension, Headache, Epilepsy, Gout, Rheumatism, Diabetes, Bright's Disease, etc. By ALEX. HAIG, M.A., M.D. (Oxon)., F.R.C P., Physician to Metropolitan Hospital, London. Illustrated. *Fourth Edition.* $3.00

HALE. On the Management of Children in Health and Disease. Cloth, .50

HALL. Compend of General Pathology and Morbid Anatomy. By H. NEWBERY HALL, PH.G., M.D., Professor of Pathology and Medical Chemistry; Post-Graduate Medical School; Surgeon to the Emergency Hospital, Chicago; Chief Ear Clinic, Chicago Medical College, etc. With 91 Illustrations. *No. 15 ? Quiz-Compend ? Series.* Cloth, .80. Interleaved for Notes, $1.25

HALL. **Diseases of the Nose and Throat.** By F. DE HAVILLAND HALL, M.D., F.R.C.P. (Lond.), Physician in charge Throat Department Westminster Hospital; Joint Lecturer on Principles and Practice of Medicine, Westminster Hospital Medical School, etc. Two Colored Plates and 59 Illus. 12mo. Cloth, $2.50

HANSELL and BELL. **Clinical Ophthalmology, Illustrated.** A Manual for Students and Physicians. By HOWARD F. HANSELL, A.M., M.D., Lecturer on Ophthalmology in the Jefferson College Hospital, Philadelphia, etc., and JAMES H. BELL, M.D., late Member Ophthalmic Staff, Jefferson College Hospital; Ophthalmic Surgeon, Southwestern Hospital, Phila. With Colored Plate of Normal Fundus and 120 Illustrations. 12mo. Cloth, $1.50

HARE. **Mediastinal Disease.** The Pathology, Clinical History and Diagnosis of Affections of the Mediastinum other than those of the Heart and Aorta. By H. A. HARE, M.D. (Univ. of Pa.), Professor of Materia Medica and Therapeutics in Jefferson Medical College, Phila. 8vo. Illustrated by Six Plates. Cloth, $2.00

HARLAN. **Eyesight,** and How to Care for It. By GEORGE C. HARLAN, M.D., Prof. of Diseases of the Eye, Philadelphia Polyclinic. Illustrated. Cloth, .40

HARRIS'S Principles and Practice of Dentistry. Including Anatomy, Physiology, Pathology, Therapeutics, Dental Surgery and Mechanism. By CHAPIN A. HARRIS, M.D., D.D.S., late President of the Baltimore Dental College, Author of "Dictionary of Medical Terminology and Dental Surgery." Thirteenth Edition. Revised and Edited by FERDINAND J. S. GORGAS, A.M., M.D., D.D.S., Author of "Dental Medicine;" Professor of the Principles of Dental Science, Oral Surgery, and Dental Mechanism in the University of Maryland. 1250 Illustrations. 1180 pages. 8vo. Cloth, $6.00; Leather, $7.00; Half Russia, $8.00

    Dictionary of Dentistry. Fifth Edition, Revised. Including Definitions of such Words and Phrases of the Collateral Sciences as Pertain to the Art and Practice of Dentistry. Fifth Edition. Rewritten, Revised and Enlarged. By FERDINAND J. S. GORGAS, M.D., D.D.S., Author of "Dental Medicine;" Editor of Harris's "Principles and Practice of Dentistry;" Professor of Principles of Dental Science, Oral Surgery, and Prosthetic Dentistry in the University of Maryland. Octavo. Cloth, $4.50; Leather, $5.50

HARRIS and BEALE. **Treatment of Pulmonary Consumption.** By VINCENT DORMER HARRIS, M.D. (Lond.), F.R.C.P., Physician to the city of London Hospital for Diseases of the Chest; Examining Physician to the Royal National Hospital for Diseases of the Chest, Ventnor, etc., and E. CLIFFORD BEALE, M.A., M.B. (Cantab.), F.R.C.P., Physician to the City of London Hospital for Diseases of the Chest, and to the Great Northern Central Hospital, etc. A Practical Manual. 12mo. Cloth, $2.50

HARTRIDGE. **Refraction.** The Refraction of the Eye. A Manual for Students. By GUSTAVUS HARTRIDGE, F.R.C.S., Consulting Ophthalmic Surgeon to St. Bartholomew's Hospital; Ass't Surgeon to the Royal Westminster Ophthalmic Hospital, etc. 98 Illustrations and Test Types. Eighth Edition. Revised and Enlarged by the Author. Cloth, $1.50

    On The Ophthalmoscope. A Manual for Physicians and Students. Third Edition. With Colored Plates and 68 Wood-cuts. 12mo. Cloth, $1.50

HARTSHORNE. **Our Homes.** Their Situation, Construction, Drainage, etc. By HENRY HARTSHORNE, M.D. Illustrated. Cloth, .40

HATFIELD. **Diseases of Children.** By MARCUS P. HATFIELD, Professor of Diseases of Children, Chicago Medical College. With a Colored Plate. Second Edition. *Being No. 14, ? Quiz-Compend ? Series.* 12mo. Cloth, .80
                           Interleaved for the addition of notes, $1.25

HELLER. **Essentials of Materia Medica, Pharmacy, and Prescription Writing.** By EDWIN A. HELLER, M.D., Quiz-Master in Materia Medica and Pharmacy at the Medical Institute, University of Pennsylvania. 12mo. Cloth, $1.50

HEATH. **Minor Surgery and Bandaging.** By CHRISTOPHER HEATH, F.R.C.S., Holme Professor of Clinical Surgery in University College, London. Tenth Edition. Revised and Enlarged. With 158 Illustrations, 62 Formulæ, Diet List, etc. 12mo. Cloth, $1.25

    Practical Anatomy. A Manual of Dissections. Eighth London Edition. 300 Illustrations. Cloth, $4.25

    Injuries and Diseases of the Jaws. Fourth Edition. Edited by HENRY PERCY DEAN, M.S., F.R.C.S., Assistant Surgeon London Hospital. With 187 Illustrations. 8vo. Cloth, $4.50

    Lectures on Certain Diseases of the Jaws, delivered at the Royal College of Surgeons of England, 1887. 64 Illustrations. 8vo. Boards, .50

HEMMETER. **Diseases of the Stomach.** Their Special Pathology, Diagnosis, and Treatment. With Sections on Anatomy, Analysis of Stomach Contents, Dietetics, Surgery of the Stomach, etc. By JOHN C. HEMMETER, M.D., PHILOS.D., Clinical Professor of Medicine at the Baltimore Medical College, Consultant to the Maryland General Hospital, etc. With Colored and other Illustrations.
Cloth, $6.00 ; Leather, $7.00 ; Half Russia, $8.00

HENRY. **Anæmia.** A Practical Treatise. By FRED'K P. HENRY, M.D., Physician to Episcopal Hospital, Philadelphia. Half Cloth, .50

HOLDEN'S Anatomy. Sixth Edition. A Manual of the Dissections of the Human Body. By JOHN LANGTON, F.R.C.S., Surgeon to, and Lecturer on Anatomy at, St. Bartholomew's Hospital. Carefully Revised by A. HEWSON, M.D., Demonstrator of Anatomy, Jefferson Medical College, etc. 311 Illustrations. 12mo. 800 pages. Cloth, $2.50 ; Oil-cloth, $2.50 ; Leather, $3.00

    Human Osteology. Comprising a Description of the Bones, with Colored Delineations of the Attachments of the Muscles. The General and Microscopical Structure of Bone and its Development. 7th Ed., carefully Revised. With Lithographic Plates and Numerous Illustrations. Cloth, $5.25

    Landmarks. Medical and Surgical. 4th Edition. 8vo. Cloth, $1.00

HOLLAND. **The Urine, the Gastric Contents, the Common Poisons and the Milk.** Memoranda, Chemical and Microscopical, for Laboratory Use. By J. W. HOLLAND, M.D., Professor of Medical Chemistry and Toxicology in Jefferson Medical College, of Philadelphia. Fifth Edition, Enlarged. Illustrated and Interleaved. 12mo. Cloth, $1.00

HORSLEY. **The Brain and Spinal Cord.** The Structure and Functions of. Being the Fullerian Lectures on Physiology for 1891. By VICTOR A. HORSLEY, M.B., F.R.S., etc., Assistant Surgeon, University College Hospital, Professor of Pathology, University College, London, etc. With numerous Illustrations. Cloth, $2.50

HORWITZ'S Compend of Surgery, including Minor Surgery, Amputations, Fractures, Dislocations, Surgical Diseases, and the Latest Antiseptic Rules, etc., with Differential Diagnosis and Treatment. By ORVILLE HORWITZ, B.S., M.D., Professor of Genito-Urinary Diseases, late Demonstrator of Surgery, Jefferson Medical College. Fifth Edition. Very much Enlarged and Rearranged. Over 300 pages. 167 Illustrations and 98 Formulæ. 12mo. *No. 9 ? Quiz-Compend ? Series.*
Cloth, .80. Interleaved for notes, $1.25

HOVELL. **Diseases of the Ear and Naso-Pharynx.** A Treatise including Anatomy and Physiology of the Organ, together with the treatment of the affections of the Nose and Pharynx which conduce to aural disease. By T. MARK HOVELL, F.R.C.S. (Edin.), M.R.C.S. (Eng.), Aural Surgeon to the London Hospital, to Hospital for Diseases of the Throat, and to British Hospital for Incurables, etc. 122 Illustrations. Octavo. Cloth, $5.00

HUMPHREY. **A Manual for Nurses.** Including general Anatomy and Physiology, management of the sick-room, etc. By LAURENCE HUMPHREY, M.A., M.B., M.R.C.S., Assistant Physician to, and Lecturer at, Addenbrook's Hospital, Cambridge, England. Sixteenth Edition. 12mo. Illustrated. Cloth, $1.00

HUGHES. Compend of the Practice of Medicine. Fifth Edition. Revised and Enlarged. By DANIEL E. HUGHES, M.D., Chief Resident Physician Philadelphia Hospital; formerly Demonstrator of Clinical Medicine at Jefferson Medical College, Philadelphia. In two parts. *Being Nos. 2 and 3, ? Quiz-Compend? Series.*

PART I.—Continued, Eruptive and Periodical Fevers, Diseases of the Stomach, Intestines, Peritoneum, Biliary Passages, Liver, Kidneys, etc., and General Diseases, etc.

PART II.—Diseases of the Respiratory System, Circulatory System and Nervous System; Diseases of the Blood, etc.

Price of each Part, in Cloth, .80; interleaved for the addition of Notes, $1.25

Physicians' Edition.—In one volume, including the above two parts, a section on Skin Diseases, and an index. *Fifth revised, enlarged Edition. 568 pages.* Full Morocco, Gilt Edge, $2.25

" Carefully and systematically compiled."—*The London Lancet.*

HUTCHINSON. The Nose and Throat. A Manual of the Diseases of the Nose and Throat, including the Nose, Naso-Pharynx, Pharynx and Larynx. By PROCTER S. HUTCHINSON, M.R.C.S., Ass't Surgeon to the London Hospital for Diseases of the Throat. Illustrated by Lithograph Plates and 40 other Illus., many of which have been made from original drawings. 12mo. 2d Ed. *In Press.*

IMPEY. A Handbook on Leprosy. By S. P. IMPEY, M.D., M.C., Late Chief and Medical Superintendent, Robben Island Leper and Lunatic Asylums, Cape Colony, South Africa. Illustrated by 37 Plates and a Map. Octavo. Cloth, $3.50

IRELAND. The Mental Affections of Children. Idiocy, Imbecility, Insanity, etc. By W. W. IRELAND, M.D. (Edin.), of the Home and School for Imbeciles, Mavisbush, Scotland; late Medical Supt. Scot. National Institute for Imbecile Children; Author of "The Blot on the Brain," etc. 300 pages. *In Press.*

JACOBSON. Operations of Surgery. By W. H. A. JACOBSON, B.A. (Oxon.), F.R.C.S., (Eng.); Ass't Surgeon, Guy's Hospital; Surgeon at Royal Hospital for Children and Women, etc. With over 200 Illust. Cloth, $3.00; Leather, $4.00

Diseases of the Male Organs of Generation. 88 Illustrations. Cloth, $6.00

JELLETT. The Practice of Midwifery. Embodying the Treatment adopted in the Rotunda Hospital, Dublin. By HENRY JELLETT, B.A., M.D., Assistant Master, Rotunda Hospital, with a Preface by W. J. SMYLY, M.D., F.R.C.P.I., Late Master. With many Illustrations and an Appendix containing Statistics of the Hospital. 12mo. Cloth, $1.75

JONES. Medical Electricity. A Practical Handbook for Students and Practitioners of Medicine. By H. LEWIS JONES, M.A., M.D., M.R.C.P., Medical Officer in Charge Electrical Department, St. Bartholomew's Hospital. Second Edition of Steavenson and Jones' Medical Electricity. Revised and Enlarged. 112 Illustrations. 12mo. Cloth, $2.50

KEEN. Clinical Charts. A series of seven Outline Drawings of the Human Body, on which may be marked the course of any Disease, Fractures, Operations, etc. By W. W. KEEN, M.D., Professor of the Principles of Surgery and Clinical Surgery, Jefferson Medical College, Philadelphia. Put up in pads of 50, with explanations. Each pad, $1.00. Each Drawing may also be had separately gummed on back for pasting in case book. 25 to the pad. Price, 25 cents.

* Special Charts will be printed to order. Samples free.

KIRKE'S Physiology. (*14th Authorized Edition. 12mo. Dark Red Cloth.*) A Handbook of Physiology. Fourteenth London Edition, Revised and Enlarged. By W. D. HALLIBURTON, M.D., F.R.S., Professor of Physiology King's College, London. Thoroughly Revised and in many parts Rewritten. 661 Illus., many of which are printed in Colors. 851 pages. 12mo. Cloth, $3.25; Leather, $4.00

IMPORTANT NOTICE. This is the identical Fourteenth Edition of "Kirke's Physiology," as published in London by John Murray, the sole owner of the book. It is the only edition containing the revisions and additions of Dr. Halliburton, and the new and original illustrations included at his suggestion. It is the edition of which the London *Lancet* speaks in its issue of October 17, 1896, as follows: " The book as now presented to the student may be regarded as a thoroughly reliable exposition of the present state of physiological science."

KENWOOD. Public Health Laboratory Work. By H. R. KENWOOD, M.B., D.P.H., F.C.S., Instructor in Hygienic Laboratory, University College, late Assistant Examiner in Hygiene, Science and Art Department, South Kensington, London, etc. With 116 Illustrations and 3 Plates. Cloth, $2.00

KLEEN. Handbook of Massage. By EMIL KLEEN, M.D., PH.D., Stockholm and Carlsbad. Authorized Translation from the Swedish, by EDWARD MUSSEY HART-WELL, M.D., PH.D., Director of Physical Training in the Public Schools of Boston. With an Introduction by Dr. S. WEIR MITCHELL, of Philadelphia. Illustrated with a series of Photographs made specially by Dr. KLEEN for the American Edition. 8vo. Cloth, $2.25

LANDIS' Compend of Obstetrics ; especially adapted to the Use of Students and Physicians. By HENRY G. LANDIS, M.D. Fifth Edition. Revised by WM. H. WELLS, M.D., Ass't Demonstrator of Clinical Obstetrics, Jefferson Medical College ; Member Obstetrical Society of Philadelphia, etc. Enlarged. With Many Illustrations. *No. 5 ? Quiz-Compend ? Series.*
Cloth, .80 ; interleaved for the addition of Notes, $1.25

LANDOIS. A Text-Book of Human Physiology ; including Histology and Microscopical Anatomy, with special reference to the requirements of Practical Medicine. By DR. L. LANDOIS, Professor of Physiology and Director of the Physiological Institute in the University of Greifswald. Fifth American, translated from the last German Edition, with additions, by WM. STIRLING, M.D., D.SC., Brackenbury Professor of Physiology and Histology in Owen's College, and Professor in Victoria University, Manchester ; Examiner in Physiology in University of Oxford, England. With 845 Illustrations, many of which are printed in Colors. 8vo. *In Press.*

LAZARUS-BARLOW. General Pathology. By W. S. LAZARUS-BARLOW, M.D., Demonstrator of Pathology at the University of Cambridge, England.
In Preparation.

LEE. The Microtomist's Vade Mecum. Fourth Edition. A Handbook of Methods of Microscopic Anatomy. By ARTHUR BOLLES LEE, formerly Ass't in the Russian Laboratory of Zoology, at Villefranche-sur-Mer (Nice). 887 Articles. Enlarged and Revised, and in many portions greatly extended. 8vo. Cloth, $4.00

LEFFMANN'S Compend of Medical Chemistry, Inorganic and Organic. Including Urine Analysis. By HENRY LEFFMANN, M.D., Prof. of Chemistry in the Woman's Medical College in the Penna. College of Dental Surgery and in the Wagner Free Institute of Science, Philadelphia ; Pathological Chemist Jefferson Medical College. *No. 10 ? Quiz-Compend ? Series.* Fourth Edition. Rewritten. Cloth, .80. Interleaved for the addition of Notes, $1.25

    The Coal-Tar Colors, with Special Reference to their Injurious Qualities and the Restrictions of their Use. A Translation of Theodore Weyl's Monograph. 12mo. Cloth, $1.25

    Progressive Exercises in Practical Chemistry. A Laboratory Handbook. Illustrated. Third Edition, Revised and Enlarged. 12mo. Cloth, $1.00

    Examination of Water for Sanitary and Technical Purposes. Third Edition. Enlarged. Illustrated. 12mo. Cloth, $1.25

    Analysis of Milk and Milk Products. Arranged to suit the needs of Analytical Chemists, Dairymen, and Milk Inspectors. Second Edition, Revised and Enlarged, with Illustrations. 12mo. Cloth, $1.25

    Handbook of Structural Formulæ for the Use of Students, containing 180 Structural and Stereo-chemic Formulæ. 12mo. Interleaved. Cloth, $1.00

LEWERS. On the Diseases of Women. A Practical Treatise. By Dr. A. H. N. LEWERS, Assistant Obstetric Physician to the London Hospital ; and Physician to Out-patients, Queen Charlotte's Lying-in Hospital ; Examiner in Midwifery and Diseases of Women to the Society of Apothecaries of London. With 146 Engravings. Fifth Edition, Revised. Cloth, $2.50

LINCOLN. School and Industrial Hygiene. By D. F. LINCOLN, M.D. Cloth, .40

LEWIS (BEVAN). Mental Diseases. A text-book having special reference to the Pathological aspects of Insanity. By BEVAN LEWIS, L.R.C.P., M.R.C.S., Medical Director, West Riding Asylum, Wakefield, England. 18 Lithographic Plates and other Illustrations. Second Edition. 8vo. *In Press.*

LIZARS (JOHN). On Tobacco. The Use and Abuse of Tobacco. Cloth, .40

LONGLEY'S Pocket Medical Dictionary for Students and Physicians. Giving the Correct Definition and Pronunciation of all Words and Terms in General Use in Medicine and the Collateral Sciences, with an Appendix, containing Poisons and their Antidotes, Abbreviations Used in Prescriptions, and a Metric Scale of Doses. By ELIAS LONGLEY. Cloth, .75; Tucks and Pocket, $1.00

MACALISTER'S Human Anatomy. 800 Illustrations. A New Text-book for Students and Practitioners. Systematic and Topographical, including the Embryology, Histology and Morphology of Man. With special reference to the requirements of Practical Surgery and Medicine. By ALEX. MACALISTER, M.D., F.R.S., Professor of Anatomy in the University of Cambridge, England. 816 Illustrations. Octavo. Cloth, $5.00; Leather, $6.00

MACDONALD'S Microscopical Examinations of Water and Air. With an Appendix on the Microscopical Examination of Air. By J. D. MACDONALD, M.D. 25 Lithographic Plates, Reference Tables, etc. Second Ed. 8vo. Cloth, $2.50

MACKENZIE. The Pharmacopœia of the London Hospital for Diseases of the Throat. By SIR MORELL MACKENZIE, M.D. Fifth Edition. Revised and Improved by F. G. HARVEY, Surgeon to the Hospital. Cloth, $1.00

MACNAMARA. On the Eye. A Manual. By C. MACNAMARA, M.D. Fifth Edition, Carefully Revised; with Additions and Numerous Colored Plates, Diagrams of Eye, Wood-cuts, and Test Types. Demi 8vo. Cloth, $3.50

MACREADY. A Treatise on Ruptures. By JONATHAN F. C. H. MACREADY, F.R.C.S., Surgeon to the Great Northern Central Hospital; to the City of London Hospital for Diseases of the Chest; to the City of London Truss Society, etc. With 24 full-page Plates and numerous Wood-Engravings. Octavo. Cloth, $6.00

MANN. Forensic Medicine and Toxicology. A Text-Book by J. DIXON MANN, M.D., F.R.C.P., Professor of Medical Jurisprudence and Toxicology in Owens College, Manchester; Examiner in Forensic Medicine in University of Manchester, etc. Illustrated. Octavo. Cloth, $6.50

MANN'S Manual of Psychological Medicine and Allied Nervous Diseases. Their Diagnosis, Pathology, Prognosis and Treatment, including their Medico-Legal Aspects; with chapter on Expert Testimony, and an abstract of the laws relating to the Insane in all the States of the Union. By EDWARD C. MANN, M.D. With Illustrations. Octavo. Cloth, $3.00

MARSHALL. The Woman's Medical College of Pennsylvania. An Historical Outline. By CLARA MARSHALL, M.D., Dean of the College. 8vo. Cloth, $1.50

MARSHALL'S Physiological Diagrams, Life Size, Colored. Eleven Life-size Diagrams (each 7 feet by 3 feet 7 inches). Designed for Demonstration before the Class. By JOHN MARSHALL, F.R.S., F.R.C.S., Professor of Anatomy to the Royal Academy; Professor of Surgery, University College, London, etc.

In Sheets, $40.00   Backed with Muslin and Mounted on Rollers, $60.00
Ditto, Spring Rollers, in Handsome Walnut Wall Map Case (Send for Special Circular), ... $100.00
Single Plates, Sheets, $5.00; Mounted, $7.50; Explanatory Key, 50 cents.
No. 1—The Skeleton and Ligaments. No. 2—The Muscles and Joints, with Animal Mechanics. No. 3—The Viscera in Position. The Structure of the Lungs. No. 4—The Heart and Principal Blood-vessels. No. 5—The Lymphatics or Absorbents. No. 6—The Digestive Organs. No. 7—The Brain and Nerves. Nos. 8 and 9—The Organs of the Senses. Nos. 10 and 11—The Microscopic Structure of the Textures and Organs. (*Send for Special Circular.*)

MASON'S Compend of Electricity, and its Medical and Surgical Uses. By CHARLES F. MASON, M.D., Assistant Surgeon U. S. Army. With an Introduction by CHARLES H. MAY, M.D., Instructor in the New York Polyclinic. Numerous Illustrations. 12mo. Cloth, .75

MAXWELL. Terminologia Medica Polyglotta. By Dr. THEODORE MAXWELL, assisted by others in various countries. 8vo. Cloth, $3.00

The object of this work is to assist the medical men of any nationality in reading medical literature written in a language not their own. Each term is usually given in seven languages, viz.: English, French, German, Italian, Spanish, Russian and Latin.

MAYLARD. The Surgery of the Alimentary Canal. By ALFRED ERNEST MAYLARD, M.B., B.S., Senior Surgeon to the Victoria Infirmary, Glasgow. With 27 Full-Page Plates and 117 other Illustrations. Octavo. Cloth, $7.50

MAYS' Theine in the Treatment of Neuralgia. By THOMAS J. MAYS, M.D. 16mo. ½ bound, .50

McBRIDE. Diseases of the Throat, Nose and Ear. A Clinical Manual for Students and Practitioners. By P. McBRIDE, M.D., F.R.C.P. (Edin.), Surgeon to the Ear and Throat Department of the Royal Infirmary; Lecturer on Diseases of Throat and Ear, Edinburgh School of Medicine, etc. With Colored Illustrations from Original Drawings. 2d Edition. Octavo. Handsome Cloth, Gilt top, $6.00

McNEILL. The Prevention of Epidemics and the Construction and Management of Isolation Hospitals. By DR. ROGER McNEILL, Medical Officer of Health for the County of Argyll. With numerous Plans and other Illustrations. Octavo. Cloth, $3.50

MEIGS. Milk Analysis and Infant Feeding. A Treatise on the Examination of Human and Cows' Milk, Cream, Condensed Milk, etc., and Directions as to the Diet of Young Infants. By ARTHUR V. MEIGS, M.D. 12mo. Cloth, .50

MEMMINGER. Diagnosis by the Urine. The Practical Examination of Urine, with Special Reference to Diagnosis. By ALLARD MEMMINGER, M.D., Professor of Chemistry and of Hygiene in the Medical College of the State of S. C.; Visiting Physician in the City Hospital of Charleston, etc. 23 Illus. 12mo. Cloth, $1.00

MONEY. On Children. Treatment of Disease in Children, including the Outlines of Diagnosis and the Chief Pathological Differences between Children and Adults. By ANGEL MONEY, M.D., M.R.C.P., Ass't Physician to the Hospital for Sick Children, Great Ormond St., London. 2d Edition. 12mo. Cloth, $2.50

MORRIS. Text-Book of Anatomy. 791 Illustrations, many in Colors. A complete Text-book. Edited by HENRY MORRIS, F.R.C.S., Surg. to, and Lect. on Anatomy at, Middlesex Hospital, assisted by J. BLAND SUTTON, F.R.C.S., J. H. DAVIES-COLLEY, F.R.C.S., WM. J. WALSHAM, F.R.C.S., H. ST. JOHN BROOKS, M.D., R. MARCUS GUNN, F.R.C.S., ARTHUR HENSMAN, F.R.C.S., FREDERICK TREVES, F.R.C.S., WILLIAM ANDERSON, F.R.C.S., and Prof. W. H. A. JACOBSON. One Handsome Octavo Volume, with 791 Illustrations, 214 of which are printed in colors. Cloth, $6.00; Leather, $7.00; Half Russia, $8.00

"Taken as a whole, we have no hesitation in according very high praise to this work. It will rank, we believe, with the leading Anatomies. The illustrations are handsome and the printing is good."—*Boston Medical and Surgical Journal.*

"The work as a whole is filled with practical ideas, and the salient points of the subject are properly emphasized. The surgeon will be particularly edified by the section on the topographical anatomy, which is full to repletion of excellent and useful illustrations."—*The Medical Record, New York.*

Handsome circular, with sample pages and colored illustrations, and list of schools where it has been recommended, will be sent free to any address.

MORTON on Refraction of the Eye. Its Diagnosis and the Correction of its Errors. With Chapter on Keratoscopy, and Test Types. By A. MORTON, M.B. Sixth Edition, Revised and Enlarged. Cloth, $1.00

MOULLIN. Surgery. Third Edition, by Hamilton. A Complete Text-book. By C. W. MANSELL MOULLIN, M.A., M.D. (Oxon.), F.R.C.S., Surgeon and Lecturer on Physiology to the London Hospital; formerly Radcliffe Traveling Fellow and Fellow of Pembroke College, Oxford. Third American Edition. Revised and edited by JOHN B. HAMILTON, M.D., LL.D., Professor of the Principles of Surgery and Clinical Surgery, Rush Medical College, Chicago; Professor of Surgery, Chicago Polyclinic; Surgeon, formerly Supervising Surgeon-General, U. S. Marine Hospital Service; Surgeon to Presbyterian Hospital; Consulting Surgeon to St. Joseph's Hospital and Central Free Dispensary, Chicago, etc. 600 Illustrations, over 200 of which are original, and many of which are printed in Colors. Royal Octavo. 1250 pages.

Handsomely bound in Cloth, $6.00; Leather, $7.00; Half Russia, $8.00
" The aim to make this valuable treatise practical by giving special attention to questions of treatment has been admirably carried out. Many a reader will consult the work with a feeling of satisfaction that his wants have been understood, and that they have been intelligently met. He will not look in vain for details, without proper attention to which he well knows that the highest success is impossible."— *The American Journal of Medical Sciences.*

Handsome circular, with sample pages and colored illustrations, will be sent to any address upon application.

  Enlargement of the Prostate. Its Treatment and Radical Cure. Illustrated. Octavo. Cloth, $1.50

MURRELL. Massotherapeutics. Massage as a Mode of Treatment. By WM. MURRELL, M.D., F.R.C.P., Lecturer on Pharmacology and Therapeutics at Westminster Hospital. Fifth Edition. Revised. 12mo. Cloth, $1.25
  What To Do in Cases of Poisoning. Seventh Edition, Enlarged and Revised. 64mo. Cloth, $1.00

MUTER. Practical and Analytical Chemistry. By JOHN MUTER, F.R.S., F.C.S., etc. Fourth Edition. Revised, to meet the requirements of American Medical Colleges, by CLAUDE C. HAMILTON, M.D., Professor of Analytical Chemistry in University Med. Col. and Kansas City Col. of Pharmacy. 51 Illus. Cloth, $1.25

NAPHEYS' Modern Therapeutics. Ninth Revised Edition, Enlarged and Improved. In Two Handsome Volumes. Edited by ALLEN J. SMITH, M.D., Professor of Pathology, University of Texas, Galveston, late Ass't Demonstrator of Morbid Anatomy and Pathological Histology, Lecturer on Urinology, University of Pennsylvania; and J. AUBREY DAVIS, M.D., Ass't Demonstrator of Obstetrics, University of Pennsylvania; Ass't Physician to Home for Crippled Children, etc.
  VOL. I.—**General Medicine and Diseases of Children.**
Handsome Cloth binding, $4.00
  VOL. II.—**General Surgery, Obstetrics, and Diseases of Women.**
Handsome Cloth binding, $4.00

NEW SYDENHAM SOCIETY Publications. Three to Six Volumes published each year. *List of Volumes upon application.* Per annum, $8.00

NOTTER and FIRTH. The Theory and Practice of Hygiene. A Complete Treatise by J. LANE NOTTER, M.A., M.D., F.C.S., Fellow and Member of Council of the Sanitary Institute of Great Britain; Professor of Hygiene, Army Medical School; Examiner in Hygiene, University of Cambridge, etc., and R. H. FIRTH, F.R.C.S., Assistant Professor of Hygiene, Army Medical School, Netly. Illustrated by 10 Lithographic Plates and 135 other Illustrations, and including many Useful Tables. Octavo. 1034 pages. Cloth, $7.00
*_** This volume is based upon Parkes' Practical Hygiene, which will not be published hereafter.

OBERSTEINER. **The Anatomy of the Central Nervous Organs.** A Guide to the study of their structure in Health and Disease. By Professor H. OBERSTEINER, of the University of Vienna. Translated and Edited by ALEX. HILL, M.A., M.D., Master of Downing College, Cambridge. 198 Illustrations. 8vo. Cloth, $5.50

OETTEL. **Practical Exercises in Electro-Chemistry.** By DR. FELIX OETTEL. Authorized Translation by EDGAR F. SMITH, M.A., Professor of Chemistry, University of Pennsylvania. Illustrated. Cloth, .75

    Introduction to Electro-Chemical Experiments. Illustrated. By same Author and Translator. Cloth, .75

OHLEMANN. **Ocular Therapeutics** for Physicians and Students. By M. OHLE-MANN, M.D. Translated and Edited by CHARLES A. OLIVER, A.M., M.D., Attending Surgeon to Wills Eye Hospital, Ophthalmic Surgeon to the Philadelphia and to the Presbyterian Hospitals, Fellow of the College of Physicians of Philadelphia, etc. *In Press.*

ORMEROD. **Diseases of Nervous System,** Student's Guide to. By J. A. ORMEROD, M.D. (Oxon.), F.R.C.P. (Lond.), Mem. Path., Clin., Ophth., and Neurol. Societies, Physician to National Hospital for Paralyzed and Epileptic and to City of London Hospital for Diseases of the Chest, Dem. of Morbid Anatomy, St. Bartholomew's Hospital, etc. With 66 Wood Engravings. 12mo. Cloth, $1.00

OSGOOD. **The Winter** and Its Dangers. By HAMILTON OSGOOD, M.D. Cloth, .40

OSLER. **Cerebral Palsies of Children.** A Clinical Study. By WILLIAM OSLER, M.D., F.R.C.P. (Lond.), Professor of Medicine, Johns Hopkins University, etc. 8vo. Cloth, $2.00

    Chorea and Choreiform Affections. 8vo. Cloth, $2.00

OSTROM. **Massage and the Original Swedish Movements.** Their Application to Various Diseases of the Body. A Manual for Students, Nurses and Physicians. By KURRE W. OSTROM, from the Royal University of Upsala, Sweden; Instructor in Massage and Swedish Movements in the Hospital of the University of Pennsylvania, and in the Philadelphia Polyclinic and College for Graduates in Medicine, etc. Third Edition. Enlarged. Illustrated by 94 Wood Engravings, many of which were drawn especially for this purpose. 12mo. Cloth, $1 00

PACKARD'S Sea Air and Sea Bathing. By JOHN H. PACKARD, M.D. Cloth, .40

PARKES' Practical Hygiene. By EDWARD A. PARKES, M.D. Superseded by "Notter and Firth" Treatise on Hygiene. See previous page.

PARKES. **Hygiene and Public Health.** A Practical Manual. By LOUIS C. PARKES, M.D., D.P.H. London Hospital; Assistant Professor of Hygiene and Public Health at University College, etc. Fifth Edition, Enlarged and Revised. 80 Illustrations. 12mo. Cloth, $2.50

    The Elements of Health. An Introduction to the Study of Hygiene. Illustrated. Cloth, $1.25

PARRISH'S Alcoholic Inebriety. From a Medical Standpoint, with Illustrative Cases from the Clinical Records of the Author. By JOSEPH PARRISH, M.D., President of the Amer. Assoc. for Cure of Inebriates. Cloth, $1.00

PEREIRA'S Prescription Book. Containing Lists of Terms, Phrases, Contractions and Abbreviations used in Prescriptions, Explanatory Notes, Grammatical Construction of Prescriptions, Rules for the Pronunciation of Pharmaceutical Terms. By JONATHAN PEREIRA, M.D. Sixteenth Edition. Cloth, .75; Tucks $1.00

PHILLIPS. **Spectacles and Eyeglasses,** Their Prescription and Adjustment. By R. J. PHILLIPS, M.D., Instructor on Diseases of the Eye, Philadelphia Polyclinic, Ophthalmic Surgeon, Presbyterian Hospital. Second Edition, Revised and Enlarged. 49 Illustrations. 12mo. Cloth, $1.00

PHYSICIAN'S VISITING LIST. Published Annually. Forty-sixth Year (1897) of its Publication.

Hereafter all styles will contain the interleaf or special memoranda page, except the Monthly Edition, and the sizes for 75 and 100 Patients will come in two volumes only. The Sale of this Visiting List increased over ten per cent. in 1896.

REGULAR EDITION.

For 25 Patients weekly.				Tucks, pocket and pencil, Gilt Edges,					$1.00
50	"	"		"	"	"	"	"	1.25
50	"	" 2 vols.	{ Jan. to June } { July to Dec. }	"	"	"	"	"	2.00
75	"	" 2 vols.	{ Jan. to June } { July to Dec. }	"	"	"	"	"	2.00
100	"	" 2 vols.	{ Jan. to June } { July to Dec. }	"	"	"	"	"	2.25

Perpetual Edition, without Dates and with Special Memorandum Pages.
For 25 Patients, interleaved, tucks, pocket and pencil, ... $1.25
50 " " " " 1.50

Monthly Edition, without Dates. Can be commenced at any time and used until full. Requires only one writing of patient's name for the whole month. Plain binding, without Flap or Pencil, .75. Leather cover, Pocket and Pencil, $1.00

EXTRA Pencils will be sent, postpaid, for 25 cents per half dozen.

☞ This List combines the several essential qualities of strength, compactness, durability and convenience. It is made in all sizes and styles to meet the wants of all physicians. It is not an elaborate, complicated system of keeping accounts, but a plain, simple record, that may be kept with the least expenditure of time and trouble—hence its popularity. A special circular, descriptive of contents will be sent upon application.

POTTER. **A Handbook of Materia Medica, Pharmacy, and Therapeutics,** including the Action of Medicines, Special Therapeutics of Disease, Official and Practical Pharmacy, and Minute Directions for Prescription Writing, etc. Including over 600 Prescriptions and Formulæ. By SAMUEL O. L. POTTER, M.A., M.D., M.R.C.P. (Lond.), Professor of the Principles and Practice of Medicine and Clinical Medicine in the College of Physicians and Surgeons, San Francisco; late A. A. Surgeon U. S. Army. Sixth Edition, Revised and Enlarged by 100 Pages. 8vo. *With Thumb Index in each copy.*
Cloth, $4.50; Leather, $5.50; Half Russia $6.50

Compend of Anatomy, including **Visceral Anatomy.** Fifth Edition. Revised, and greatly Enlarged. With 16 Lithographed Plates and 117 other Illustrations. *Being No. 1 ? Quiz-Compend ? Series.*
Cloth, .80; Interleaved for taking Notes, $1.25

Compend of Materia Medica, Therapeutics and Prescription Writing, with special reference to the Physiological Action of Drugs. Sixth Revised and Improved Edition, with Index, based upon U. S. P. 1890. *Being No. 6 ? Quiz-Compend ? Series.* Cloth, .80. Interleaved for taking Notes, $1.25

Speech and Its Defects. Considered Physiologically, Pathologically and Remedially; being the Lea Prize Thesis of Jefferson Medical College, 1882. Revised and Corrected. 12mo. Cloth, $1.00

POWELL. **Diseases of the Lungs and Pleuræ, Including Consumption.** By R. DOUGLAS POWELL, M.D., F.R.C.P., Physician to the Middlesex Hospital, and Consulting Physician to the Hospital for Consumption and Diseases of the Chest at Brompton. Fourth Edition. With Colored Plates and Wood Engravings. 8vo. Cloth, $4.00

POWER. **Surgical Diseases of Children** and their Treatment by Modern Methods. By D'Arcy Power, M.A., F.R.C.S. (Eng.), Demonstrator of Operative Surgery, St. Bartholomew's Hospital; Surgeon to the Victoria Hospital for Children. Illustrated. 12mo. Cloth, $2.50

PRESTON. Hysteria and Certain Allied Conditions. Their Nature and Treatment. With special reference to the application of the Rest Cure, Massage, Electro-therapy, Hypnotism, etc. By GEORGE J. PRESTON, M.D., Professor of Diseases of the Nervous System, College of Physicians and Surgeons, Baltimore ; Visiting Physician to the City Hospital ; Consulting Neurologist to Bay View Asylum and the Hebrew Hospital ; Member American Neurological Association, etc. With Illustrations. 12mo. Cloth, $2.00

SYNOPSIS OF CONTENTS.—Historical. The Nature of Hysteria ; Etiology and Pathology. Symptomatology. Disturbances of Motion : Tremor, Contracture, Paralysis. Convulsive Attacks : Major and Minor Attacks. Hystero-Epilepsy. The Mental Condition in Hysteria. Visceral and Vasomotor Disturbances. Diagnosis. Treatment : Electro-Therapy, The Rest Cure, Hypnotism, Surgical Interference in the Treatment of Hysteria.

PRITCHARD. Handbook of Diseases of the Ear. By URBAN PRITCHARD, M.D., F.R.C.S., Professor of Aural Surgery, King's College, London, Aural Surgeon to King's College Hospital, Senior Surgeon to the Royal Ear Hospital ; etc. Third Edition, Enlarged. Many Illustrations and Formulæ. 12mo. Cloth, $1.50

PROCTOR'S Practical Pharmacy. Lectures on Practical Pharmacy. With Wood Engravings and 32 Lithographic Fac-simile Prescriptions. By BARNARD S. PROCTOR. Third Edition. Revised and with elaborate Tables of Chemical Solubilities, etc. Cloth, $3.co

REESE'S Medical Jurisprudence and Toxicology. A Text-book for Medical and Legal Practitioners and Students. By JOHN J. REESE, M.D., Editor of Taylor's Jurisprudence, Professor of the Principles and Practice of Medical Jurisprudence, including Toxicology, in the University of Pennsylvania Medical Department. Fourth Edition. Revised by HENRY LEFFMANN, M.D., Pathological Chemist, Jefferson Medical College Hospital ; Chemist, State Board of Health ; Professor of Chemistry, Woman's Medical College of Penna., etc. 12mo. 624 pages. Cloth, $3.00 ; Leather, $3.50

" To the student of medical jurisprudence and toxicology it is invaluable, as it is concise, clear, and thorough in every respect."—*The American Journal of the Medical Sciences.*

REEVES. Medical Microscopy. Illustrated. A Handbook for Physicians and Students, including Chapters on Bacteriology, Neoplasms, Urinary Examination, etc. By JAMES E. REEVES, M.D., Ex-President American Public Health Association, Member Association American Physicians, etc. Numerous Illustrations, some of which are printed in colors. 12mo. Handsome Cloth, $2.50

REEVES. Bodily Deformities and their Treatment. A Handbook of Practical Orthopædics. By H. A. REEVES, M.D., Senior Ass't Surgeon to the London Hospital, Surgeon to the Royal Orthopædic Hospital. 228 Illustrations. Cloth, $1.75

RÉGIS. Mental Medicine. A Practical Manual. By DR. E. RÉGIS, formerly Chief of Clinique of Mental Diseases, Faculty of Medicine of Paris ; Physician of the Maison de Santé de Castel d'Andorte ; Professor of Mental Diseases, Faculty of Medicine, Bordeaux, etc. With a Preface by M. BENJAMIN BALL, Clinical Professor of Mental Diseases, Faculty of Medicine, Paris. Authorized Translation from the Second Edition by H. M. BANNISTER, M.D., late Senior Assistant Physician, Illinois Eastern Hospital for the Insane, etc. With an Introduction by the Author. 12mo. 692 pages. Cloth, $2.00

RICHARDSON. Long Life, and How to Reach It. By J. G. RICHARDSON, Prof. of Hygiene, University of Pennsylvania. Cloth, .40

RICHARDSON'S Mechanical Dentistry. A Practical Treatise on Mechanical Dentistry. By JOSEPH RICHARDSON, D.D.S. Seventh Edition. Thoroughly Revised and in many parts Rewritten by DR. GEO. W. WARREN, Chief of the Clinical Staff, Pennsylvania College of Dental Surgery, Philadelphia. With 691 Illustrations, many of which are from original Wood Engravings. Octavo. 675 pages. Cloth, $5.00 ; Leather, $6.00 ; Half Russia, $7.00

RICHTER'S Inorganic Chemistry. A Text-book for Students. By Prof. VICTOR VON RICHTER, University of Breslau. Fourth American, from Sixth German Edition. Authorized Translation by EDGAR F. SMITH, M.A., PH.D., Prof. of Chemistry, University of Pennsylvania, Member of the Chemical Societies of Berlin and Paris. 89 Illustrations and a Colored Plate. 12mo. Cloth, $1.75

Organic Chemistry. The Chemistry of the Carbon Compounds. Third American Edition, translated from the Last German by EDGAR F. SMITH, M.A., PH.D., Professor of Chemistry, University of Pennsylvania. Illustrated. 12mo. *Preparing.*

ROBERTS. Practice of Medicine. The Theory and Practice of Medicine. By FREDERICK ROBERTS, M.D., Professor of Therapeutics at University College, London. Ninth Edition, with Illustrations. 8vo. Cloth, $4.50; Leather, $5.50

ROBERTS. Fractures of the Radius. A Clinical, Pathological, and Experimental Study. By JOHN B. ROBERTS, M.D., Professor of Anatomy and Surgery in the Philadelphia Polyclinic, etc. 33 Illustrations. 8vo. Cloth, $1.00

ROBINSON. Latin Grammar of Pharmacy and Medicine. By D. H. ROBINSON, PH.D., Professor of Latin Language and Literature, University of Kansas. Introduction by L. E. SAYRE, PH.G., Professor of Pharmacy in, and Dean of the Dept. of Pharmacy, University of Kansas. Third Edition. Revised with the help of Prof. L. E. SAYRE, of University of Kansas, and Dr. CHARLES RICE, of the College of Pharmacy of the city of New York. 12mo. Cloth, $1.75

ST. CLAIR. Medical Latin. Designed expressly for the Elementary Training of Medical Students. By W. T. ST. CLAIR, Instructor in Latin in the Kentucky School of Medicine and in the Louisville Male High School. 12mo. Cloth, $1.00

SANSOM. Diseases of The Heart. The Diagnosis and Pathology of Diseases of the Heart and Thoracic Aorta. By A. ERNEST SANSOM, M.D., F.R.C.P., Physician to the London Hospital, etc. With Illustrations. 8vo. Cloth, $6.00

SAYRE. Organic Materia Medica and Pharmacognosy. An Introduction to the Study of the Vegetable Kingdom and the Vegetable and Animal Drugs. Comprising the Botanical and Physical Characteristics, Source, Constituents, and Pharmacopœial Preparations. With Chapters on Synthetic Organic Remedies, Insects Injurious to Drugs, and Pharmacal Botany. By L. E. SAYRE, PH.G., Professor of Pharmacy and Materia Medica in the University of Kansas, Member of the Committee of Revision of the U. S. Pharmacopœia, 1890. A Glossary and 543 Illustrations. 8vo. Cloth, $4.00; Sheep, $5.00; Half Russia, $6.00

SCHAMBERG. Compend of Diseases of the Skin. By JAY F. SCHAMBERG, Instructor in Skin Diseases, Philadelphia Polyclinic; Quiz-Master at University of Pennsylvania. Illustrated. Cloth, .80. Interleaved, $1.25

SCHULTZE. Obstetrical Diagrams. Being a Series of 20 Colored Lithograph Charts, imperial map size, of Pregnancy and Midwifery, with accompanying explanatory (German) text, illustrated by wood-cuts. By DR. B. S. SCHULTZE, Professor of Obstetrics, University of Jena. Second Revised Edition. Price, in Sheets, $26.00; Mounted on Rollers, Muslin Backs, $36.00

SCOVILLE. The Art of Compounding. A Text-book for Students and a Reference Book for Pharmacists. By WILBUR L. SCOVILLE, PH.G., Professor of Applied Pharmacy and Director of the Pharmaceutical Laboratory in the Massachusetts College of Pharmacy. Cloth, $2.50; Sheep, $3.50; Half Russia, $4.50

SEWELL. Dental Surgery, including Special Anatomy and Surgery. By HENRY SEWELL, M.R.C.S., L.D.S., President Odontological Society of Great Britain. 3d Edition, greatly enlarged, with about 200 Illustrations. Cloth, $2.00

SHAWE. Notes for Visiting Nurses, and all those interested in the working and organization of District, Visiting, or Parochial Nurse Societies. By ROSALIND GILLETTE SHAWE, District Nurse for the Brooklyn Red Cross Society. With an Appendix explaining the organization and working of various Visiting and District Nurse Societies, by HELEN C. JENKS, of Philadelphia. 12mo. Cloth, $1.00

SMITH. Abdominal Surgery. Being a Systematic Description of all the Principal Operations. By J. Greig Smith, M.A., F.R.S.E., Surg. to British Royal Infirmary; Lecturer on Surgery, Bristol Medical School; Late Examiner in Surgery, University of Aberdeen, etc. 224 Illustrations. Sixth Edition. Enlarged and Thoroughly Revised. 2 Volumes. Octavo. Cloth, $10.00

SMITH. Electro-Chemical Analysis. By Edgar F. Smith, Professor of Chemistry, University of Pennsylvania. Second Edition, Revised and Enlarged. 28 Illustrations. 12mo. Cloth, $1.25

SMITH AND KELLER. Experiments. Arranged for Students in General Chemistry. By Edgar F. Smith, Professor of Chemistry, University of Pennsylvania, and Dr. H. F. Keller, Professor of Chemistry, Philadelphia High School. Third Edition. 8vo. Illustrated. Cloth, .60

STAMMER. Chemical Problems, with Explanations and Answers. By Karl Stammer. Translated from the Second German Edition, by Prof. W. S. Hoskinson, A.M., Wittenberg College, Springfield, Ohio. 12mo. Cloth, .50

STARLING. Elements of Human Physiology. By Ernest H. Starling, M.D. Lond., M.R.C.P., Joint Lecturer on Physiology at Guy's Hospital, London, etc. With 100 Illustrations. 12mo. 437 pages. Cloth, $1.00

STARR. The Digestive Organs in Childhood. Second Edition. The Diseases of the Digestive Organs in Infancy and Childhood. With Chapters on the Investigation of Disease and the Management of Children. By Louis Starr, M.D., late Clinical Prof. of Diseases of Children in the Hospital of the University of Penn'a; Physician to the Children's Hospital, Phila. Second Edition. Revised and Enlarged. Illustrated by two Colored Lithograph Plates and numerous Wood Engravings. Crown Octavo. Cloth, $2.00

The Hygiene of the Nursery, including the General Regimen and Feeding of Infants and Children, and the Domestic Management of the Ordinary Emergencies of Early Life, Massage, etc. Sixth Edition. Enlarged. 25 Illustrations. 12mo. 280 pages. Cloth, $1.00

STEARNS. Lectures on Mental Diseases. By Henry Putnam Stearns, M.D., Physician Superintendent at the Hartford Retreat, Lecturer on Mental Diseases in Yale University, Member of the American Medico-Psychological Ass'n, Honorary Member of the British Medico-Pyschological Society. With a Digest of Laws of the Various States Relating to Care of Insane. Illustrated.
Cloth, $2.75; Sheep, $3.25

STEVENSON AND MURPHY. A Treatise on Hygiene. By Various Authors. Edited by Thomas Stevenson, M.D., F.R.C.P., Lecturer on Chemistry and Medical Jurisprudence at Guy's Hospital, London, etc., and Shirley F. Murphy, Medical Officer of Health to the County of London. In Three Octavo Volumes.
Vol. I. With Plates and Wood Engravings. Octavo. Cloth, $6.00
Vol. II. With Plates and Wood Engravings. Octavo. Cloth, $6.00
Vol. III. Sanitary Law. Octavo. Cloth, $5.00
* *Special Circular upon application.*

STEWART'S Compend of Pharmacy. Based upon "Remington's Text-Book of Pharmacy." By F. E. Stewart, M.D., ph.g., Quiz-Master in Chem. and Theoretical Pharmacy, Phila. College of Pharmacy; Lect. in Pharmacology, Jefferson Medical College. Fifth Ed. Revised in accordance with U. S. P., 1890. Complete tables of Metric and English Weights and Measures. *?Quiz-Compend?* *Series.* Cloth, .80; Interleaved for the addition of notes, $1.25

STIRLING. Outlines of Practical Physiology. Including Chemical and Experimental Physiology, with Special Reference to Practical Medicine. By W. Stirling, M.D., Sc.D., Professor of Physiology and Histology, Owens College, Victoria University, Manchester. Examiner in Physiology, Universities of Edinburgh and London. Third Edition. 289 Illustrations. Cloth, $2.00

Outlines of Practical Histology. 368 Illustrations. Second Edition. Revised and Enlarged with new Illustrations. 12mo. Cloth, $2.00

STÖHR. **Text-Book of Histology, Including the Microscopical Technique.** By DR. PHILIPP STÖHR, University of Zurich. Authorized Translation by EMMA L. BILLSTEIN, M.D., Demonstrator of Histology and Embryology, Woman's Medical College of Pennsylvania. Edited, with Additions, by DR. ALFRED SCHAPER, Demonstrator of Histology and Embryology, Harvard Medical School, Boston. 268 Illustrations. Octavo. Cloth, $3.00

STRAHAN. **Extra-Uterine Pregnancy.** The Diagnosis and Treatment of Extra-Uterine Pregnancy. Being the Jenks Prize Essay of the College of Physicians of Philadelphia. By JOHN STRAHAN, M.D. (Univ. of Ireland), late Res. Surgeon Belfast Union Infirmary and Fever Hospital. Octavo. Cloth, .75

SUTTON'S Volumetric Analysis. A Systematic Handbook for the Quantitative Estimation of Chemical Substances by Measure, Applied to Liquids, Solids and Gases. Adapted to the Requirements of Pure Chemical Research, Pathological Chemistry, Pharmacy, Metallurgy, Photography, etc., and for the Valuation of Substances Used in Commerce, Agriculture, and the Arts. By FRANCIS SUTTON, F.C.S. Seventh Edition, Revised and Enlarged, with 112 Illustrations. 8vo.
Cloth, $4.50

SWAIN. **Surgical Emergencies,** together with the Emergencies Attendant on Parturition and the Treatment of Poisoning. A Manual for the Use of Student, Practitioner, and Head Nurse. By WILLIAM PAUL SWAIN, F.R.C.S., Surgeon to the South Devon and East Cornwall Hospital, England. Fifth Edition. 12mo. 149 Illustrations. Cloth, $1.75

SWANZY. **Diseases of the Eye and their Treatment.** A Handbook for Physicians and Students. By HENRY R. SWANZY, A.M., M.B., F.R.C.S.I., Surgeon to the National Eye and Ear Infirmary; Ophthalmic Surgeon to the Adelaide Hospital, Dublin. Sixth Edition, Thoroughly Revised and Enlarged. 158 Illustrations, one Plain Plate, and a Zephyr Test Card. 12mo. Cloth, $3.00

" Is without doubt the most satisfactory manual we have upon diseases of the eye. It occupies the middle ground between the students' manuals, which are too brief and concise, and the encyclopedic treatises, which are too extended and detailed to be of special use to the general practitioner."—*Chicago Medical Recorder.*

SYMONDS. **Manual of Chemistry,** for Medical Students. By BRANDRETH SYMONDS, A.M., M.D., Ass't Physician Roosevelt Hospital, Out-Patient Department; Attending Physician Northwestern Dispensary, New York. Second Edition. 12mo. Cloth, $2.00

TAFT'S Operative Dentistry. A Practical Treatise on Operative Dentistry. By JONATHAN TAFT, D.D.S. Fifth Revised and Enlarged Edition. Over 100 Illustrations. 8vo. *Preparing.*

Index of Dental Periodical Literature. 8vo. Cloth, $2.00

TALBOT. **Irregularities of the Teeth,** and Their Treatment. By EUGENE S. TALBOT, M.D., Professor of Dental Surgery Woman's Medical College, and Lecturer on Dental Pathology in Rush Medical College, Chicago. Second Edition, Revised and Enlarged by about 100 pages. Octavo. 234 Illustrations (169 of which are original). 261 pages. Cloth, $3.00

TANNER'S Memoranda of Poisons and their Antidotes and Tests. By THOS. HAWKES TANNER, M.D., F.R.C.P. 7th American, from the Last London Edition. Revised by JOHN J. REESE, M.D., Professor Medical Jurisprudence and Toxicology in the University of Pennsylvania. 12mo. Cloth, .75

TAYLOR. **Practice of Medicine.** A Manual. By FREDERICK TAYLOR, M.D., Physician to, and Lecturer on Medicine at, Guy's Hospital, London; Physician to Evelina Hospital for Sick Children, and Examiner in Materia Medica and Pharmaceutical Chemistry, University of London. Cloth, $2.00; Sheep, $2.50

TAYLOR AND WELLS. Diseases of Children. A Manual for Students and Physicians. By JOHN MADISON TAYLOR, A.B., M.D., Professor of Diseases of Children, Philadelphia Polyclinic; Assistant Physician to the Children's Hospital and to the Orthopedic Hospital; Consulting Physician to the Elwyn and the Vineland Training Schools for Feeble-Minded Children; Neurologist to the Howard Hospital, etc.; and WILLIAM H. WELLS, M.D., Adjunct-Professor of Obstetrics and Diseases of Infancy in the Philadelphia Polyclinic; late Assistant Demonstrator of Clinical Obstetrics and Diseases of Infancy in Jefferson Medical College. With Illustrations. *In Press.*

PROPOSED CONTENTS AND ARRANGEMENT.—I. Clinical Investigation. II and III. Hygiene and Diet. IV. Care of Children of Feeble Resistance, including Systematic Developmental Methods. V. Diseases Occurring At or Near Birth. VI. Acute Infectious Diseases. VII. General Diseases, Tuberculosis, Syphilis, Malaria, Rachitis, Rheumatism, etc. VIII. Diseases of Digestive Organs, including Parasites. IX. Diseases of the Liver, Cecum, and Appendix. X. Diseases of the Peritoneum, Intestinal Malformations and Obstructions. XI. Diseases of the Respiratory Organs. XII. Diseases of the Heart. XIII. Diseases of the Blood and Blood-making Organs. XIV. Nervous Diseases (including Diabetes). XV. Diseases of the Nose, Pharynx, and Naso-Pharynx. XVI. Genito-Urinary Diseases. XVII. Diseases of Degeneracy, Thyroid Thymus Glands, Dwarfs and Dwarfing, Cretins, Leprosy, Idiocy, Feeblemindedness, and Insanity, etc. XVIII. Diseases of the Skin. XIX. Injuries and Shock. XX. Emergencies—Medical and Surgical. XXI. Diseases of the Bones and Joints. XXII. Curvatures of the Spine. XXIII. Pott's Disease. XXIV. Tumors.

TEMPERATURE Charts for Recording Temperature, Respiration, Pulse, Day of Disease, Date, Age, Sex, Occupation, Name, etc. Put up in pads; each .50

THOMPSON. Urinary Organs. Diseases of the Urinary Organs. Containing 32 Lectures. By Sir HENRY THOMPSON, F.R.C.S., Emeritus Professor of Clinical Surgery in University College. Eighth London Edition. 121 Illustrations. Octavo. 470 pages. Cloth, $3.00

THORINGTON. Retinoscopy (The Shadow Test) in the Determination of Refraction at One Metre Distance with the Plane Mirror. By JAMES THORINGTON, M.D., Adjunct Professor of Diseases of the Eye in the Philadelphia Polyclinic; Ophthalmologist to the Vineland Training School and to the M. E. Orphanage; Lecturer on the Anatomy, Physiology, and Care of the Eyes in the Philadelphia Manual Training Schools, etc. With 24 Illustrations, many of which are Original. Second Edition, Enlarged. 12mo. *In Press.*

TOMES' Dental Anatomy. A Manual of Dental Anatomy, Human and Comparative. By C. S. TOMES, D.D.S. 235 Illustrations. 4th Ed. 12mo. Cloth, $3.50

Dental Surgery. A System of Dental Surgery. By JOHN TOMES, F.R.S. Fourth Edition, Thoroughly Revised. By C. S. TOMES, D.D.S. With 289 Illustrations. 12mo. 717 pages. Cloth, $4.00

TREVES. German-English Medical Dictionary. By FREDERICK TREVES, F.R.C.S., assisted by DR. HUGO LANG, B.A. (Munich). 12mo. ½ Russia, $3.25

Physical Education, Its Effects, Value, Methods, etc. Cloth, .75

TUKE. Dictionary of Psychological Medicine. Giving the Definition, Etymology, and Synonyms of the Terms used in Medical Psychology, with the Symptoms, Pathology, and Treatment of the recognized forms of Mental Disorders, together with the Law of Lunacy in Great Britain and Ireland. Edited by D. HACK TUKE, M.D., LL.D., Examiner in Mental Physiology in the University of London. Two Volumes. Octavo. 1477 pages. Cloth, $10.00

"This is an elaborate and valuable contribution to the literature of medical psychology, and will be found a valuable work of reference. . . . A comprehensive standard book."—*The British Medical Journal.*

TURNBULL'S Artificial Anæsthesia. The Advantages and Accidents of Artificial Anæsthesia; Its Employment in the Treatment of Disease; Modes of Administration; Considering their Relative Risks; Tests of Purity; Treatment of Asphyxia; Spasms of the Glottis; Syncope, etc. By LAURENCE TURNBULL, M.D., PH.G., Aural Surgeon to Jefferson College Hospital, etc. Fourth Edition, Revised and Enlarged. 54 Illustrations. 12mo. Cloth, $2.50

TUSON. **Veterinary Pharmacopœia,** including the outlines of Materia Medica and Therapeutics. By RICHARD V. TUSON, late Professor at the Royal Veterinary College. Fifth Edition. Revised and Edited by JAMES BAYNE, F.C.S., Professor of Chemistry and Toxicology at the Royal Veterinary College. 12mo. Cloth, $2.25

TUSSEY. **High Altitude Treatment for Consumption.** The Principles or Guides for a Better Selection or Classification of Consumptives Amenable to High Altitude Treatment, and to the Selection of Patients who may be More Successfully Treated in the Environment to which They were Accustomed Previous to Their Illness. By A. EDGAR TUSSEY, M.D., Adjunct Professor of Diseases of the Chest in the Philadelphia Polyclinic and School for Graduates in Medicine, etc. 12mo. Cloth, $1.50

TYSON. The Practice of Medicine. A Text-Book for Physicians and Students, with Special Reference to Diagnosis and Treatment. By JAMES TYSON, M.D., Professor of Clinical Medicine in the University of Pennsylvania, Physician to the University and to the Philadelphia Hospitals, etc. Illustrated. 8vo. *Just Ready.* Cloth, $5.50; Leather, $6.50; Half Russia, $7.50

"Few teachers in the country can claim a longer apprenticeship in the laboratory and at the bedside, none a more intimate acquaintance with students, since in one capacity or another he has been associated with the University of Pennsylvania and the Philadelphia Hospital for nearly thirty years. Moreover, he entered medicine through the portal of pathology, a decided advantage in the writer of a text-book. . . . The typography is decidedly above works of this class issued from our publishing houses. There is no American Practice of the same attractive appearance. The print is unusually sharp and clear, and the quality of the paper particularly good. . . . It is a piece of good, honest work, carefully conceived and conscientiously carried out."—*University Medical Magazine.*

*** Sample Pages and Illustrations Sent Free upon Application.

Guide to the Examination of Urine. Ninth Edition. For the Use of Physicians and Students. With Colored Plate and Numerous Illustrations Engraved on Wood. Ninth Edition. Revised. 12mo. 276 pages. Cloth, $1.25
*** *A French translation of this book has just appeared in Paris.*

Handbook of Physical Diagnosis. 3d Edition. Revised and Enlarged. With New Illustrations. 12mo. *In Press.*

Cell Doctrine. Its History and Present State. Second Edition. Cloth, $1.50

UNITED STATES PHARMACOPŒIA. 1890. Seventh Decennial Revision. Cloth, $2.50 (Postpaid, $2.77); Sheep, $3.00 (Postpaid, $3.27); Interleaved, $4.00 (Postpaid, $4.50); printed on one side of page only. Unbound, $3.50 (Postpaid, $3.90).

Select Tables from the U. S. P. (1890). Being Nine of the Most Important and Useful Tables, printed on Separate Sheets. Carefully put up in Patent Envelope. .25

VAN HARLINGEN on Skin Diseases. A Practical Manual of Diagnosis and Treatment with special reference to Differential Diagnosis. By ARTHUR VAN HARLINGEN, M.D., Professor of Diseases of the Skin in the Philadelphia Polyclinic; Clinical Lecturer on Dermatology at Jefferson Medical College. Third Edition. Revised and Enlarged. With Formulæ and Illustrations, several being in Colors. 580 pages. Cloth, $2.75

"As would naturally be expected from the author, his views are sound, his information extensive, and in matters of practical detail the hand of the experienced physician is everywhere visible."—*The Medical News.*

VAN NUYS on The Urine. Chemical Analysis of Healthy and Diseased Urine, Qualitative and Quantitative. By T. C. VAN NÜYS, Professor of Chemistry Indiana University. 39 Illustrations. Octavo. Cloth, $1.00

VIRCHOW'S Post-mortem Examinations. A Description and Explanation of the Method of Performing them in the Dead-House of the Berlin Charité Hospital, with especial reference to Medico-legal Practice. By Prof. VIRCHOW. Translated by Dr. T. P. SMITH. Illustrated. Third Edition, with Additions. Cloth, .75

VOSWINKEL. Surgical Nursing. A Manual for Nurses. By BERTHA M. VOSWINKEL, Graduate Episcopal Hospital, Philadelphia; Nurse in Charge Children's Hospital, Columbus, O. 111 Illustrations. 12mo. 168 pages. Cloth, $1.00

WALKER. Students' Aid in Ophthalmology. By GERTRUDE A. WALKER, A.B., M.D., Clinical Instructor in Diseases of the Eye at Woman's Medical College of Pennsylvania. 40 Illustrations and Colored Plate. 12mo. Cloth, $1.50

WALSHAM. Surgery; its Theory and Practice. For Students and Physicians. By WM. J. WALSHAM, M.D., F.R.C.S., Senior Ass't Surg. to, and Dem. of Practical Surg. in, St. Bartholomew's Hospital, Surg. to Metropolitan Free Hospital, London. Fifth Edition, Revised and Enlarged. With 380 Engravings. 815 pages. Cloth, $2.00 ; Leather, $2.50

WARING. Practical Therapeutics. A Manual for Physicians and Students. By EDWARD J. WARING, M.D. Fourth Edition. Revised, Rewritten, and Rearranged. Crown Octavo. Cloth, $2.00 ; Leather, $3.00

WARREN. Compend Dental Pathology and Dental Medicine. Containing all the most noteworthy points of interest to the Dental Student and a Chapter on Emergencies. By GEO. W. WARREN, D.D.S., Clinical Chief, Penn'a College of Dental Surgery, Phila. Third Edition, Enlarged. Illustrated. *Being No. 13 ? Quiz-Compend ? Series.* 12mo. Cloth, .80
Interleaved for the addition of Notes, $1.25

Dental Prosthesis and Metallurgy. 129 Illustrations. Cloth, $1.25

WATSON on Amputations of the Extremities and Their Complications. By B. A. WATSON, M.D. 250 Illustrations. Cloth, $5.50

Concussions. An Experimental Study of Lesions arising from Severe Concussions. 8vo. Paper cover, $1.00

WATTS' Inorganic Chemistry. (Being the 14th Edition of FOWNE'S INORGANIC CHEMISTRY.) By HENRY WATTS, F.R.S. Illustrated. 12mo. Cloth, $2.00

Organic Chemistry. Second Edition. (Being the 13th Edition of FOWNE'S ORGANIC CHEMISTRY.) Illustrated. 12mo. Cloth, $2.00

WELLS. Compend of Gynecology. By WM. H. WELLS, M.D., Assistant Demonstrator of Obstetrics, Jefferson Medical College, Philadelphia; Fellow of the College of Physicians of Philadelphia. 150 Illustrations. *? Quiz-Compend? Series No. 7.* 12mo. Cloth, .80; Interleaved for Notes, $1.25

WESTLAND. The Wife and Mother. A Handbook for Mothers. By A. WESTLAND, M.D., late Resident Physician, Aberdeen Royal Infirmary. Clo. $1.50

WETHERED. Medical Microscopy. A Guide to the Use of the Microscope in Practical Medicine. By FRANK J. WETHERED, M.D , M.R.C.P., Demonstrator of Practical Medicine, Middlesex Hospital Medical School; Assistant Physician, late Pathologist, City of London Hospital for Diseases of Chest, etc. With a Colored Plate and 101 Illustrations. 406 Pages. 12mo. Cloth, $2.00

WEYL. Sanitary Relations of the Coal-Tar Colors. By THEODORE WEYL. Authorized Translation by HENRY LEFFMANN, M.D., PH.D. 12mo. 154 pages. Cloth, $1.25

WHITACRE. Laboratory Text-Book of Pathology. By HORACE J. WHITACRE, M.D., Demonstrator of Pathology, Medical College of Ohio, Cincinnati. Illustrated with 121 original Illustrations. 8vo. Cloth, $1.50

WHITE. The Mouth and Teeth. By J. W. WHITE, M.D., D.D.S. Cloth, .40

WHITE AND WILCOX. Materia Medica, Pharmacy, Pharmacology, and Therapeutics. A Handbook for Students. By W. HALE WHITE, M.D., F.R.C.P., etc., Physician to and Lecturer on Materia Medica and Therapeutics, Guy's Hospital; Examiner in Materia Medica to the Conjoint Board, etc. Third American Edition. Revised by REYNOLD W. WILCOX, M.A., M.D., LL.D., Professor of Clinical Medicine and Therapeutics at the New York Post-Graduate Medical School and Hospital; Visiting Physician St. Mark's Hospital; Assistant Visiting Physician Bellevue Hospital. Third Edition, thoroughly Revised. 12mo.
Cloth, $2.75; Leather, $3.25

WILSON. Handbook of Hygiene and Sanitary Science. By GEORGE WILSON, M.A., M.D., F.R.S.E., Medical Officer of Health for Mid-Warwickshire, England. With Illustrations. Eighth Edition. 12mo. *Preparing.*

WILSON. The Summer and its Diseases. By JAMES C. WILSON, M.D., Prof. of the Practice of Med. and Clinical Medicine, Jefferson Med. Coll., Phila. Cloth, .40

WILSON. System of Human Anatomy. 11th Revised Edition. Edited by HENRY EDWARD CLARK, M.D., M.R.C.S. 492 Illustrations, 26 Colored Plates, and a Glossary of Terms. Thick 12mo. Cloth, $5.00

WINCKEL. Diseases of Women. Third Edition. Including the Diseases of the Bladder and Urethra. By Dr. F. WINCKEL, Professor of Gynecology and Director of the Royal University Clinic for Women in Munich. Translated by special authority of Author and Publisher, under the Supervision of, and with an Introduction by, THEOPHILUS PARVIN, M.D., Professor of Obstetrics and Diseases of Women and Children in Jefferson Medical College, Philadelphia. With 152 Engravings on Wood, most of which are original. 3d Edition, Revised and Enlarged. *In Preparation.*

Text-Book of Obstetrics; Including the Pathology and Therapeutics of the Puerperal State. Authorized Translation by J. CLIFTON EDGAR, A.M., M.D., Adjunct Professor to the Chair of Obstetrics, Medical Department, University City of New York. With nearly 200 Handsome Illus., the majority of which are original with this work. Octavo. Cloth, $5.co; Leather, $6.00

WINDLE. Surface Anatomy and Landmarks. By B. C. A. WINDLE, D.Sc., M.D., Professor of Anatomy in Mason College, Birmingham, etc. Second Edition, Revised by T. MANNERS SMITH, M.R.C.S., with Colored and other Illustrations. 12mo. Cloth, $1.00

WOAKES. Deafness, Giddiness, and Noises in the Head. By EDWARD WOAKES, M.D., Senior Aural Surgeon, London Hospital; assisted by CLAUD WOAKES, M.R.C.S., Assistant Surgeon to the London Throat Hospital. Fourth Edition. Illustrated. 12mo. Cloth, $2.00

WOAKES. Post-Nasal Catarrh and Diseases of the Nose, causing Deafness. By EDWARD WOAKES, M.D., Senior Aural Surgeon to the London Hospital for Diseases of the Throat and Chest. 26 Illustrations. Cloth, $1.co

WOOD. Brain Work and Overwork. By Prof. H. C. WOOD, Clinical Professor of Nervous Diseases, University of Pennsylvania. 12mo. Cloth, .40

WOODY. Essentials of Chemistry and Urinalysis. By SAM E. WOODY, A.M., M.D., Professor of Chemistry and Public Hygiene, and Clinical Lecturer on Diseases of Children, in the Kentucky School of Medicine. Fourth Edition. Illustrated. 12mo. *In Press.*

WYTHE. Dose and Symptom Book. The Physician's Pocket Dose and Symptom Book. Containing the Doses and Uses of all the Principal Articles of the Materia Medica, and Officinal Preparations. By JOSEPH H. WYTHE, A.M., M.D. 17th Edition, Revised. Cloth, .75; Leather, with Tucks and Pocket, $1.00

YEO. Manual of Physiology. Sixth Edition. A Text-book for Students of Medicine. By GERALD F. YEO, M.D., F.R.C.S., Professor of Physiology in King's College, London. Sixth Edition; revised and enlarged by the author. With 254 Wood Engravings and a Glossary. Crown Octavo.
Cloth, $2.50; Leather, $3.00

BLAKISTON'S ? QUIZ=COMPENDS ?

The Best Series of Manuals for the Use of Students.

Price of each, Cloth, .80.   Interleaved for taking Notes, $1.25.

☞ These Compends are based on the most popular text-books and the lectures of prominent professors, and are kept constantly revised, so that they may thoroughly represent the present state of the subjects upon which they treat. The authors have had large experience as Quiz-Masters and attachés of colleges, and are well acquainted with the wants of students. They are arranged in the most approved form, thorough and concise, containing over 600 fine illustrations, inserted wherever they could be used to advantage. Can be used by students of *any* college, and contain information nowhere else collected in such a condensed, practical shape.

ILLUSTRATED CIRCULAR FREE.

No. 1. **HUMAN ANATOMY.**   Fifth Revised and Enlarged Edition.   Including Visceral Anatomy. Can be used with either Morris's or Gray's Anatomy. 117 Illustrations and 16 Lithographic Plates of Nerves and Arteries, with Explanatory Tables, etc. By SAMUEL O. L. POTTER, M.D., Professor of the Practice of Medicine, College of Physicians and Surgeons, San Francisco; late A. A. Surgeon, U. S. Army.

No. 2. **PRACTICE OF MEDICINE.** Part I. Fifth Edition, Revised, Enlarged, and Improved. By DAN'L E. HUGHES, M.D., Physician-in-Chief, Philadelphia Hospital, late Demonstrator of Clinical Medicine, Jefferson Medical College, Philadelphia.

No. 3. **PRACTICE OF MEDICINE.** Part II. Fifth Edition, Revised, Enlarged, and Improved. Same author as No. 2.

No. 4. **PHYSIOLOGY.**   Eighth Edition, with new Illustrations and a table of Physiological Constants. Enlarged and Revised. By A. P. BRUBAKER, M.D., Professor of Physiology and General Pathology in the Pennsylvania College of Dental Surgery; Demonstrator of Physiology, Jefferson Medical College, Philadelphia.

No. 5. **OBSTETRICS.** Fifth Edition. By HENRY G. LANDIS, M.D. Revised and Edited by WM. H. WELLS, M.D., Assistant Demonstrator of Obstetrics, Jefferson Medical College, Philadelphia. Enlarged. 47 Illustrations.

No. 6.   **MATERIA MEDICA, THERAPEUTICS, AND PRESCRIPTION WRITING.** Sixth Revised Edition (U. S. P. 1890). By SAMUEL O. L. POTTER, M.D., Professor of the Practice of Medicine, College of Physicians and Surgeons, San Francisco.

No. 7. **GYNECOLOGY.** A New Book. By WM. H. WELLS, M.D., Assistant Demonstrator of Obstetrics, Jefferson Medical College, Philadelphia. 150 Illustrations.

No. 8. **DISEASES OF THE EYE AND REFRACTION.** A New Book. Including Treatment and Surgery and a Section on Local Therapeutics. By GEORGE M. GOULD, M.D., and W. L. PYLE, M.D. With Formulæ, Glossary, several useful Tables, and 111 Illustrations, several of which are colored.

No. 9. **SURGERY, Minor Surgery, and Bandaging.** Fifth Edition, Enlarged and Improved. By ORVILLE HORWITZ, B.S., M.D., Clinical Professor of Genito-Urinary Surgery and Venereal Diseases in Jefferson Medical College; Surgeon to Philadelphia Hospital, etc. With 98 Formulæ and 71 Illustrations.

No. 10. **MEDICAL CHEMISTRY.** Fourth Edition. Including Urinalysis, Animal Chemistry, Chemistry of Milk, Blood, Tissues, the Secretions, etc. By HENRY LEFFMANN, M.D., Professor of Chemistry in Pennsylvania College of Dental Surgery and in the Woman's Medical College, Philadelphia.

No. 11. **PHARMACY.** Fifth Edition. Based upon Prof. Remington's Text-Book of Pharmacy. By F. E. STEWART, M.D., PH.G., late Quiz-Master in Pharmacy and Chemistry, Philadelphia College of Pharmacy; Lecturer at Jefferson Medical College.

No. 12. **VETERINARY ANATOMY AND PHYSIOLOGY.** Illustrated. By WM. R. BALLOU, M.D., Professor of Equine Anatomy at New York College of Veterinary Surgeons; Physician to Bellevue Dispensary, etc. With 29 graphic Illustrations.

No. 13. **DENTAL PATHOLOGY AND DENTAL MEDICINE.** Second Edition, Illustrated. Containing all the most noteworthy points of interest to the Dental Student and a Section on Emergencies. By GEO. W. WARREN, D.D.S., Chief of Clinical Staff, Pennsylvania College of Dental Surgery, Philadelphia.

No. 14. **DISEASES OF CHILDREN.** Colored Plate. By MARCUS P. HATFIELD, Professor of Diseases of Children, Chicago Medical College. Second Edition, Enlarged.

No. 15. **GENERAL PATHOLOGY AND MORBID ANATOMY.** 91 Illustrations. By H. NEWBERRY HALL, PH.G., M.D., Professor of Pathology and Medical Chemistry, Chicago Post-Graduate Medical School.

No. 16. **DISEASES OF THE SKIN.** By JAY F. SCHAMBERG, M.D., Instructor at Philadelphia Polyclinic.

Price, each, strongly bound in cloth, .80. Interleaved for taking Notes, $1.25.

THE PHYSICIAN'S VISITING LIST.

(LINDSAY & BLAKISTON'S.)

Special Improved Edition for 1898.

In order to improve and simplify this Visiting List we have done away with the two styles hitherto known as the "25 and 50 Patients plain." We have allowed more space for writing the names, and added to the special memoranda page a column for the "Amount" of the weekly visits and a column for the "Ledger Page." To do this without increasing the bulk or the price, we have condensed the reading matter in the front of the book and rearranged and simplified the memoranda pages, etc., at the back.

The Lists for 75 Patients and 100 Patients will also have special memoranda page as above, and hereafter will come in two volumes only, dated January to June, and July to December. While this makes a book better suited to the pocket, the chief advantage is that it does away with the risk of losing the accounts of a whole year should the book be mislaid.

The changes and improvements made in 1896 met with such general favor that the sale increased more than ten per cent. over the previous year.

CONTENTS.

PRELIMINARY MATTER.—Calendar, 1896-1897—Table of Signs, to be used in keeping records—The Metric or French Decimal System of Weights and Measures—Table for Converting Apothecaries' Weights and Measures into Grams—Dose Table, giving the doses of official and unofficial drugs in both the English and Metric Systems—Asphyxia and Apnea—Complete Table for Calculating the Period of Utero-Gestation—Comparison of Thermometers.

VISITING LIST.—Ruled and dated pages for 25, 50, 75, and 100 patients per day or week, with blank page opposite each on which is an amount column, column for ledger page, and space for special memoranda.

SPECIAL RECORDS for Obstetric Engagements, Deaths, Births, etc., with special pages for Addresses of Patients, Nurses, etc., Accounts Due, Cash Account, and General Memoranda.

SIZES AND PRICES.

REGULAR EDITION, as Described Above.

BOUND IN STRONG LEATHER COVERS, WITH POCKET AND PENCIL.

For 25 Patients weekly, with Special Memoranda Page, ...$1 00
  50   "   "   "   "   " 1 25
  50   "   "   "   "   "   2 vols. { January to June } { July to December } 2 00
  75   "   "   "   "   "   2 vols. { January to June } { July to December } 2 00
 100   "   "   "   "   "   2 vols. { January to June } { July to December } 2 25

PERPETUAL EDITION, without Dates.

No. 1. Containing space for over 1300 names, with blank page opposite each Visiting List page. Bound in Red Leather cover, with Pocket and Pencil, ...$1 25
No. 2. Same as No. 1. Containing space for 2600 names, with blank page opposite, ... 1 50

MONTHLY EDITION, without Dates.

No. 1. Bound, Seal leather, without Flap or Pencil, gilt edges, ... 75
No. 2. Bound, Seal leather, with Tucks, Pencil, etc., gilt edges, ... 1 00

☞ All these prices are net. No discount can be allowed retail purchasers.

Circular and sample pages upon application.

P. BLAKISTON, SON & CO., PUBLISHERS, PHILADELPHIA.

JUST PUBLISHED.

Hemmeter. Diseases of the Stomach. Colored Illustrations.

THEIR SPECIAL PATHOLOGY, DIAGNOSIS, AND TREATMENT. With Sections on Anatomy, Dietetics, Surgery of Stomach, etc. By JOHN C. HEMMETER, M.D., PHILOS.D., Clinical Professor of Medicine at the Baltimore Medical College, Consultant to the Maryland General Hospital, etc. With Colored and other Illustrations, many of which are original and have been specially prepared for this volume. Octavo, 778 pages.

Cloth, $6.00 ; Leather, $7.00 ; Half Russia, $8.00

***This work has been prepared with great care and forms the only complete practical text-book in the English language. The author brings to his own large experience a vast knowledge of the literature of the subject. His chief effort has been to furnish the general practitioner with a work from which he can readily acquaint himself with all that has been done in this important branch of medicine, to fit himself to make examinations, to take advantage of new methods of diagnosis, and to treat this very difficult class of diseases rationally and successfully.

The illustrations have been selected and engraved with great care. A number of them are original; these have been drawn by the author or prepared by an artist under his immediate directions, and will, we believe, prove most satisfactory.

SYNOPSIS OF CONTENTS.—Anatomy and Histology of the Stomach and Intestines—Physiology of Digestion—Pepsinogen and Pepsin—The Bile—Formed or Organized Ferments (Bacteria)—Effects of Digestive Secretions—Qualitative and Quantitative Methods for Testing the Motor, Secretory, and Absorptive Functions—Absorption from the Stomach—Methods for Determining the Location, Size, and Capacity of the Stomach—Gastrodiaphany of Einhorn—The Stomach-Tube and Technics of Its Introduction—Examination of Stomach Contents—Test-Meals—Methods for Qualitative and Quantitative Analysis of Stomach Contents—Tests for Blood in Stomach Contents—Examinations of Portions of Mucosa or Tissue Found in the Washwater and Vomited Matter—The Diagnostic Significance of Fragments of Mucosa and of Gastric Exfoliations and Neoplastic Tissue Occurring in the Washwater and Vomited Matter—Occurrence of Secretions in the Empty Stomach—Stimulations to Secretions of Gastric Juice—Chemical Examination of Gastric Juice—Quantitative Analysis of the Stomach Acids—Dietetics—Mechanical Methods of Treatment—Uses and Abuses of Mineral (Spring) Waters—Alcohol and Alcoholic Beverages, Effect on Digestion, etc.—Surgical Treatment of Gastric Diseases—Influence of Gastric Diseases on Other Organs and on Metabolism—The Influence of Diseases of Other Organs on the Stomach—Condition of the Urine in Gastric Diseases—Acute Gastritis—Chronic Gastritis—Gastric Ulcer—Carcinoma—Sarcoma of the Stomach—Syphilis of the Stomach—Tuberculosis of the Stomach—Ulcus Carcinomatosum, Cancerous Ulcer of the Stomach—Benign Tumors—Atony—Motor Insufficiency—Dilatation—Gastroptosis, Prolapses of the Stomach—Nervous Affections of the Stomach—Neuroses of Secretion—Neuroses of Motility.

***The Sections on Dietetics are exhaustive and particularly valuable to the general practitioner.

www.ingramcontent.com/pod-product-compliance
Lightning Source LLC
Chambersburg PA
CBHW051442170526
45166CB00001B/84